# Interventional Pharmacology

*Editor*

GEORGE D. DANGAS

# INTERVENTIONAL CARDIOLOGY CLINICS

www.interventional.theclinics.com

*Consulting Editors*
SAMIN K. SHARMA
IGOR F. PALACIOS

October 2013 • Volume 2 • Number 4

**ELSEVIER**

1600 John F. Kennedy Boulevard • Suite 1800 • Philadelphia, Pennsylvania, 19103-2899

http://www.theclinics.com

**INTERVENTIONAL CARDIOLOGY CLINICS Volume 2, Number 4**
**October 2013 ISSN 2211-7458, ISBN-13: 978-0-323-22725-4**

Editor: Barbara Cohen-Kligerman
Developmental Editor: Susan Showalter

*Interventional Cardiology Clinics* (ISSN 2211-7458) is published quarterly by Elsevier Inc., 360 Park Avenue South, New York, NY 10010-1710. Months of issue are January, April, July, and October. Subscription prices are USD 188 per year for US individuals, USD 126 per year for US students, USD 281 per year for Canadian individuals, USD 144 per year for Canadian students, USD 281 per year for international individuals, and USD 144 per year for international students. To receive student/resident rate, orders must be accompanied by name of affiliated institution, date of term, and the *signature* of program/residency coordinator on institution letterhead. Orders will be billed at individual rate until proof of status is received. Foreign air speed delivery is included in all *Clinics* subscription prices. All prices are subject to change without notice. **POSTMASTER:** Send address changes to *Interventional Cardiology Clinics*, Elsevier Health Sciences Division, Subscription Customer Service, 3251 Riverport Lane, Maryland Heights, MO 63043. **Customer Service: Telephone: 1-800-654-2452** (U.S. and Canada); **1-314-447-8871** (outside U.S. and Canada). **Fax: 1-314-447-8029. E-mail: journalscustomerservice-usa@elsevier.com** (for print support); **journalsonlinesupport-usa@elsevier.com** (for online support).

*Reprints.* For copies of 100 or more of articles in this publication, please contact the Commercial Reprints Department, Elsevier Inc., 360 Park Avenue South, New York, NY 10010-1710. Tel.: 212-633-3874; Fax: 212-633-3820; E-mail: reprints@elsevier.com.

Printed and bound by CPI Group (UK) Ltd, Croydon, CR0 4YY

Transferred to digital print 2012

# Contributors

## CONSULTING EDITORS

**SAMIN K. SHARMA, MD, FSCAI, FACC**
Director of Clinical Cardiology; Director of
Cardiac Catheterization Laboratory, Mount
Sinai Medical Center, New York, New York

**IGOR F. PALACIOS, MD, FSCAI**
Director of Interventional Cardiology,
Cardiology Division, Heart Center,
Massachusetts General Hospital; Associate
Professor of Medicine, Harvard Medical
School, Boston, Massachusetts

## EDITOR

**GEORGE D. DANGAS, MD, PhD**
Director of Cardiovascular Innovation,
Department of Cardiology, The Zena and
Michael A. Wiener Cardiovascular Institute;
Professor of Medicine and Surgery, Icahn
School of Medicine at Mount Sinai, New York,
New York

## AUTHORS

**OGHENEOCHUKO AJARI, MS, MBBS**
Cardiovascular Division, Department of
Medicine, Beth Israel Deaconess Medical
Center, Harvard Medical School, Boston,
Massachusetts

**DOMINICK J. ANGIOLILLO, MD, PhD**
Division of Cardiology, Department of
Medicine, Shands Jacksonville, University of
Florida College of Medicine—Jacksonville,
Jacksonville, Florida

**JAYANT BAGAI, MD**
Division of Cardiovascular Medicine,
Tennessee Valley VA Healthcare System,
Vanderbilt University Medical Center,
Nashville, Tennessee

**SUBHASH BANERJEE, MD**
Division of Cardiovascular Medicine, VA North
Texas Healthcare System, The University of
Texas Southwestern Medical Center at Dallas,
Dallas, Texas

**PADDY M. BARRETT, MD**
Clinician Scholar, Scripps Translational
Science Institute, La Jolla, California

**EMMANOUIL S. BRILAKIS, MD, PhD**
Division of Cardiovascular Medicine, VA North
Texas Healthcare System, The University of
Texas Southwestern Medical Center at Dallas,
Dallas, Texas

**DAVID A. BURKE, MD**
Division of Cardiovascular Medicine,
Department of Medicine, Beth Israel
Deaconess Medical Center, Harvard Medical
School, Boston, Massachusetts

**DAVIDE CAPODANNO, MD, PhD**
Cardiovascular Department, Ferrarotto
Hospital, University of Catania; Excellence
Through Newest Advances (ETNA) Foundation,
Catania, Italy

**PIERA CAPRANZANO, MD**
Cardiovascular Department, Ferrarotto
Hospital, University of Catania, Catania, Italy

**BIMMER E. CLAESSEN, MD, PhD**
Department of Cardiology, Academic Medical Center, University of Amsterdam, Amsterdam, The Netherlands

**MADELEINE COCHET, BS**
Cardiovascular Division, Department of Medicine, Beth Israel Deaconess Medical Center, Harvard Medical School, Boston, Massachusetts

**GEORGE D. DANGAS, MD, PhD**
Director of Cardiovascular Innovation, Department of Cardiology, The Zena and Michael A. Wiener Cardiovascular Institute; Professor of Medicine and Surgery, Icahn School of Medicine at Mount Sinai, New York, New York

**JOSEPH ROBERT DUNFORD**
Faculty of Medical Sciences, Institute of Cellular Medicine, Newcastle University; Cardiothoracic Centre, Freeman Hospital, Newcastle upon Tyne Hospitals NHS Foundation Trust, Newcastle upon Tyne, United Kingdom

**KRISTIN FEENEY, BS**
Cardiovascular Division, Department of Medicine, Beth Israel Deaconess Medical Center, Harvard Medical School, Boston, Massachusetts

**C. MICHAEL GIBSON, MS, MD**
Cardiovascular Division, Department of Medicine, Beth Israel Deaconess Medical Center, Harvard Medical School, Boston, Massachusetts

**GONZALO ROMERO GONZALEZ, MBBS**
Cardiovascular Division, Department of Medicine, Beth Israel Deaconess Medical Center, Harvard Medical School, Boston, Massachusetts

**ADITYA GOVINDAVARJHULLA, MBBS**
Cardiovascular Division, Department of Medicine, Beth Israel Deaconess Medical Center, Harvard Medical School, Boston, Massachusetts

**RAVITEJA REDDY GUDDETI, MBBS**
Cardiovascular Division, Department of Medicine, Beth Israel Deaconess Medical Center, Harvard Medical School, Boston, Massachusetts

**PAUL A. GURBEL, MD**
Cardiac Catheterization Laboratory, Sinai Center for Thrombosis Research, Baltimore, Maryland

**RIM HALABY, BS**
Cardiovascular Division, Department of Medicine, Beth Israel Deaconess Medical Center, Harvard Medical School, Boston, Massachusetts

**JOSÉ P.S. HENRIQUES, MD, PhD**
Department of Cardiology, Academic Medical Center, University of Amsterdam, Amsterdam, The Netherlands

**BARRY T. KATZEN, MD**
Founder and Medical Director, Baptist Cardiac and Vascular Institute, Miami, Florida

**FARMAN KHAN, MBBS**
Cardiovascular Division, Department of Medicine, Beth Israel Deaconess Medical Center, Harvard Medical School, Boston, Massachusetts

**NISHARAHMED KHERADA, MD**
Hypertension Section, The Icahn School of Medicine at Mount Sinai, New York, New York

**SHANKAR KUMAR, MBBS**
Cardiovascular Division, Department of Medicine, Beth Israel Deaconess Medical Center, Harvard Medical School, Boston, Massachusetts

**VIJAY KUNADIAN, MBBS, MD, FRCP, FACC, FESC**
Faculty of Medical Sciences, Institute of Cellular Medicine, Newcastle University; Cardiothoracic Centre, Freeman Hospital, Newcastle upon Tyne Hospitals NHS Foundation Trust, Newcastle upon Tyne, United Kingdom

**EMILY LARKIN, BS**
Cardiovascular Division, Department of Medicine, Beth Israel Deaconess Medical Center, Harvard Medical School, Boston, Massachusetts

**ROXANA MEHRAN, MD**
Professor of Medicine (Cardiology), The Icahn School of Medicine at Mount Sinai; Cardiovascular Research Foundation, New York, New York

**DANIEL NETHALA, BS**
Cardiovascular Division, Department of
Medicine, Beth Israel Deaconess Medical
Center, Harvard Medical School, Boston,
Massachusetts

**HARDIK PATEL, MBBS**
Cardiovascular Division, Department of
Medicine, Beth Israel Deaconess Medical
Center, Harvard Medical School, Boston,
Massachusetts

**SAPAN PATEL, MBBS**
Cardiovascular Division, Department of
Medicine, Beth Israel Deaconess Medical
Center, Harvard Medical School, Boston,
Massachusetts

**DUANE S. PINTO, MD, MPH, FACC, FSCAI**
Director, Cardiac Intensive Care Unit;
Associate Professor of Medicine, Division of
Cardiovascular Medicine, Department of
Medicine, Beth Israel Deaconess Medical
Center, Harvard Medical School, Boston,
Massachusetts

**MATTHEW J. PRICE, MD**
Assistant Professor, Scripps Translational
Science Institute; Director, Cardiac
Catheterization Laboratory, Scripps
Green Hospital, La Jolla, California

**PRASHANTH SADDALA, MBBS**
Cardiovascular Division, Department of
Medicine, Beth Israel Deaconess Medical
Center, Harvard Medical School, Boston,
Massachusetts

**VISHNU VARDHAN SERLA, MBBS**
Cardiovascular Division, Department of
Medicine, Beth Israel Deaconess Medical
Center, Harvard Medical School, Boston,
Massachusetts

**MEHDI H. SHISHEHBOR, DO, MPH, PhD**
Director, Endovascular Services, Heart and
Vascular Institute, Cleveland Clinic, Cleveland,
Ohio

**HANNAH SINCLAIR, MBBS**
Faculty of Medical Sciences, Institute of
Cellular Medicine, Cardiothoracic Centre,
Freeman Hospital, Newcastle upon Tyne
Hospitals NHS Foundation Trust, Newcastle
University, Newcastle upon Tyne,
United Kingdom

**STEVEN R. STEINHUBL, MD**
Department of Cardiology, Geisinger Medical
Center, Danville, Pennsylvania

**AARON SUTTON**
Faculty of Medical Sciences, Institute of
Cellular Medicine, Cardiothoracic Centre,
Freeman Hospital, Newcastle upon Tyne
Hospitals NHS Foundation Trust, Newcastle
University, Newcastle upon Tyne, United
Kingdom

**DANIEL SWARBRICK, MBBS**
Faculty of Medical Sciences, Institute of
Cellular Medicine, Newcastle University;
Cardiothoracic Centre, Freeman Hospital,
Newcastle upon Tyne Hospitals NHS
Foundation Trust, Newcastle upon Tyne,
United Kingdom

**CORRADO TAMBURINO, MD, PhD**
Cardiovascular Department, Ferrarotto
Hospital, University of Catania; Excellence
Through Newest Advances (ETNA) Foundation,
Catania, Italy

**UDAYA S. TANTRY, PhD**
Cardiac Catheterization Laboratory, Sinai
Center for Thrombosis Research, Baltimore,
Maryland

**DIVYA YADAV, MD**
Cardiovascular Division, Department of
Medicine, Beth Israel Deaconess Medical
Center, Harvard Medical School, Boston,
Massachusetts

**GREGORY W. YOST, DO**
Department of Cardiology, Geisinger Medical
Center, Danville, Pennsylvania

**MARCELO ZACARKIM, MD**
Cardiovascular Division, Department of
Medicine, Beth Israel Deaconess Medical
Center, Harvard Medical School, Boston,
Massachusetts

# Contents

**Preface: Interventional Pharmacology**                                    xiii

George D. Dangas

**Basics of Antithrombotic Therapy for Cardiovascular Disease: Pharmacologic Targets of Platelet Inhibitors and Anticoagulants**                                    499

Piera Capranzano and Dominick J. Angiolillo

Arterial thrombus formation is the common pathophysiologic process of cardio-vascular disease manifestations, requiring interplay between platelets and coagulation factors. Current platelet inhibitors block the formation of thromboxane $A_2$ and interfere with adenosine diphosphate stimulation mediated by the P2Y12 receptor. Novel antiplatelet agents blocking these and other pathways are under clinical development. Thrombin represents a bridge between platelets and coagulation. Indirect and direct thrombin inhibitors are pivotal in clinical settings. Other key coagulation factors include factors IX and X, which are therapeutic targets of current and novel anticoagulants. This article reviews the pathophysiology of arterial thrombosis and current and novel antiplatelet and anticoagulant agents.

**Balance of Ischemia and Bleeding in Selecting an Antithrombotic Regimen**                                    515

Bimmer E. Claessen, George D. Dangas, and Roxana Mehran

Complications after percutaneous coronary intervention (PCI) are of 2 types: ischemic and bleeding. This article provides strategies to individualize pharmacologic regimens after PCI based on periprocedural risk assessment. A practical method to assess whether a patient is at risk for ischemic or bleeding complications is the use of risk scores. Patients at a low risk of bleeding benefit from aggressive antithrombotic therapy. Patients at a high risk of bleeding benefit from selective use of antithrombotic agents. As a large number of antithrombotic agents are currently available, individualization of the antithrombotic drug regimens should be considered in every patient.

**Aspirin, Platelet P2Y12 Receptor Inhibitors, and Other Oral Antiplatelets: Comparative Pharmacology and Role in Elective PCI**                                    527

Vijay Kunadian, Hannah Sinclair, Aaron Sutton, and George D. Dangas

Angina pectoris accounts for a large burden of disease worldwide. Antiplatelet agents play a crucial role in inhibiting the platelet response to vascular injury after percutaneous coronary intervention (PCI) for the management of coronary artery disease. Antiplatelet agents are also essential in the longer term, because the metallic structure of stents is inherently thrombogenic. This article examines the use of aspirin, P2Y12 inhibitors, and other oral antiplatelets in the setting of elective PCI. Dual antiplatelet therapy in elective PCI is now standard therapy. The clinical use of novel antiplatelet therapy in this setting requires further evaluation.

**Role of Parenteral Agents in Percutaneous Coronary Intervention for Stable Patients**    537

David A. Burke and Duane S. Pinto

Numerous agents are available for anticoagulation during percutaneous coronary intervention (PCI), and various antiplatelet agents are also used. With all of the medications available, an assessment must be made regarding the ischemic risk and risk of bleeding for an individual patient during elective PCI when selecting the optimal medical strategy to support PCI. Whether new antiplatelet medications will enhance or reduce complications when paired with various newer anticoagulant agents requires further investigation. This article summarizes existing data examining the benefits and limitations of the various anticoagulant and antiplatelet medications, and summarizes guidelines for their use.

**Combination Antithrombotic Management for Non–ST Segment Elevation Acute Coronary Syndromes**    553

Jayant Bagai, Subhash Banerjee, and Emmanouil S. Brilakis

Patients with non–ST segment elevation acute coronary syndromes (NSTEACS) are at high risk for subsequent thrombotic events. Combination antithrombotic management with anticoagulant and antiplatelet medications can improve outcomes in these high-risk patients. If an early invasive strategy is planned, unfractionated heparin or bivalirudin are the anticoagulants of choice, whereas in those in whom an early conservative strategy is planned enoxaparin or fondaparinux may be preferred. All patients with NSTEACS should receive aspirin and continue it indefinitely unless they cannot tolerate it. A second antiplatelet agent should be administered both for an early invasive or early conservative strategy.

**Combination Antithrombotic Management of STEMI with Pharmacoinvasive Strategy, Primary PCI, or Rescue PCI**    573

Piera Capranzano, Corrado Tamburino, and George D. Dangas

The mainstay of acute ST segment elevation myocardial infarction (STEMI) emergent management consists of reperfusion therapy combined with antithrombotic treatment. Primary percutaneous coronary intervention (PCI) is the preferred reperfusion strategy for STEMI. Rescue PCI consists of urgent transfer for PCI of patients with failed fibrinolysis. The pharmacoinvasive strategy consists of administration of fibrinolysis followed by immediate transfer to a PCI-capable hospital for routine early catheterization. This article provides an overview of data and recommendations on primary PCI, rescue PCI, and pharmacoinvasive strategy as well as of the antithrombotic regimens used to support STEMI reperfusion approaches.

**The Optimal Duration of Dual Combination Antiplatelet Therapy After Stent Implantation and Perioperative Management Issues**    585

Nisharahmed Kherada, Roxana Mehran, and George D. Dangas

Impending risk of stent thrombosis (ST) after percutaneous coronary intervention (PCI) has mandated post-PCI use of dual antiplatelet therapy (DAPT) with aspirin and a P2Y12 inhibitor. As the optimal duration of DAPT remains controversial, premature discontinuation of it potentiates the risk of ST, myocardial infarction or death; while use of DAPT itself increases the risk of bleeding. Similarly, perioperative DAPT management is still ill defined, where there is higher operative risk of bleeding on antiplatelet therapy and higher ST risk during this thrombogenic period if the patient is off antiplatelet therapy. Additional clinical investigation is warranted in these fields.

**Triple Antiplatelet Therapy and Combinations with Oral Anticoagulants After Stent Implantation** 595

Vijay Kunadian, Joseph Robert Dunford, Daniel Swarbrick, Rim Halaby, Ogheneochuko Ajari, Madeleine Cochet, Kristin Feeney, Emily Larkin, Gonzalo Romero Gonzalez, Aditya Govindavarjhulla, Daniel Nethala, Hardik Patel, Raviteja Reddy Guddeti, Farman Khan, Shankar Kumar, Sapan Patel, Prashanth Saddala, Vishnu Vardhan Serla, Marcelo Zacarkim, Divya Yadav, and C. Michael Gibson

Triple oral anticoagulation or triple antiplatelet therapies may be administered for various reasons. They reduce cardiac complications following percutaneous coronary intervention and stroke or other thromboembolic phenomenon in conditions such as atrial fibrillation. There is an elevated risk of severe bleeding, so it is necessary to balance risk and benefits. Newer oral anticoagulants and antiplatelet drugs may be considered; the number of options is increasing. This article examines triple therapies and the efficacy and safety of combinations of traditional anticoagulant and antiplatelet drugs, and reviews clinical trial data on novel agents. Guidelines to inform clinical decision-making are presented.

**The Role of Platelet Function Testing in Risk Stratification and Clinical Decision-Making** 607

Paul A. Gurbel and Udaya S. Tantry

Clopidogrel (a widely used second-generation thienopyridine) therapy is associated with an unpredictable pharmacodynamic response whereby approximately 1 in 3 patients will have a high on-treatment platelet reactivity to adenosine diphosphate. High on-treatment platelet reactivity is an established risk factor for ischemic event occurrence in patients undergoing percutaneous coronary intervention. Platelet function testing may have a role in monitoring therapeutic efficacy when clopidogrel is the chosen agent and in safety when more potent drugs are used, especially in patients with high bleeding risk. At this time, it seems most reasonable to assess platelet function in high-risk clopidogrel-treated patients.

**Pharmacogenomics in Interventional Pharmacology: Present Status and Future Directions** 615

Paddy M. Barrett and Matthew J. Price

Pharmacogenomics offers the possibility of tailoring a drug to a patient's unique genetic signature, improving the likelihood of clinical efficacy while minimizing risks. Clopidogrel, a platelet P2Y12 receptor inhibitor that forms the cornerstone of dual antiplatelet therapy in patients with unstable coronary artery disease and those undergoing percutaneous coronary intervention, is the first broadly used drug in cardiovascular medicine in which genotyping may help optimize outcomes. This article describes techniques to identify the genetic determinants of drug response, their application (ie, clopidogrel), and the challenges to integration of pharmacogenomics into the practice of interventional cardiology.

**Antithrombotic Strategies in Endovascular Interventions: Current Status and Future Directions** 627

Mehdi H. Shishehbor and Barry T. Katzen

Despite increasing numbers of endovascular interventions to treat arterial and venous disease, scant level 1 evidence is available regarding the role of antithrombotic and antiplatelet therapy in patients undergoing these procedures. The current practice in this regard is heterogeneous and has mainly been driven by data from coronary artery disease and percutaneous coronary intervention. This article discusses the role of antithrombotic and antiplatelet agents for endovascular intervention.

**Antithrombotic Strategies in Valvular and Structural Heart Disease Interventions: Current Status and Future Directions**    **635**

Davide Capodanno and Corrado Tamburino

Antithrombotic prophylaxis is the cornerstone of adjunctive pharmacologic therapy in patients undergoing transcatheter intervention for valvular and structural heart disease. However, drugs and doses of antiplatelet and anticoagulant agents are mostly empiric for these indications and typically administered at the operator's discretion. This article describes the rationale for antithrombotic management of patients undergoing transcatheter aortic valve implantation, percutaneous mitral valve repair with the Mitraclip system, patent foramen ovale, and atrial septal defect closure, as well as common strategies for managing antiplatelet and anticoagulant therapy in patients with valvular and structural heart disease undergoing transcatheter procedures.

**Monitoring and Reversal of Anticoagulation and Antiplatelets**    **643**

Gregory W. Yost and Steven R. Steinhubl

Since percutaneous transluminal coronary angioplasty was first described and the breakthrough studies of the role of stents were reported, the evolution in anticoagulation and antiplatelet therapy used during percutaneous coronary intervention (PCI) has reduced periprocedural ischemic events and stent thrombosis. Although greater combinations and doses of anticoagulation with antiplatelets seem to provide the best protection against thrombogenic and embolic events, there is a significant trade-off with a higher risk of major and minor bleeding episodes. This review article expands on each of the commonly used antiplatelet and anticoagulants used at time of PCI, focusing on drug monitoring and reversal.

**Vasoactive and Antiarrhythmic Drugs During Percutaneous Coronary Intervention**    **665**

Bimmer E. Claessen and José P.S. Henriques

The objective in percutaneous coronary intervention (PCI) is to treat flow-limiting atherothrombotic coronary plaques mechanically. Many types of antithrombotic drugs are used to prevent ischemic complications during manipulation of catheters, guidewires, balloons, and stents in coronary arteries while minimizing the risk of bleeding. However, many other types of pharmacologic agents are also used to facilitate PCI. This review focuses on the most commonly used adjunct drugs during PCI. In addition, a recommendation of which drugs should be stopped or interrupted in patients undergoing PCI is provided.

**Index**    **671**

# INTERVENTIONAL CARDIOLOGY CLINICS

**FORTHCOMING ISSUES**

*January 2014*
**Carotid and Cerebrovascular Disease**
Christopher J. White and Kenneth Rosenfield,
*Editors*

*April 2014*
**Approaches to Left Atrial Appendage
Exclusion**
Randall Lee and Moussa Mansour, *Editors*

*July 2014*
**Renal Complications in the Catheterization
Laboratory**
Hitinder S. Gurm and Judith Kooiman, *Editors*

**RECENT ISSUES**

*July 2013*
**Percutaneous Ventricular Support**
Howard A. Cohen and Jose P.S. Henriques,
*Editors*

*April 2013*
**Saphenous Vein Graft Lesions and
Thrombectomy for Acute Myocardial
Infarction**
Amar Krishnaswamy and Samir R. Kapadia,
*Editors*

*January 2013*
**Congenital and Structural Heart Disease**
Damien Kenny and Ziyad M. Hijazi, *Editors*

ISSUES OF RELATED INTEREST

*Cardiology Clinics*, August 2013 (Vol. 31, No. 3)
**Interventions for Structural Heart Disease**
Ray Matthews, *Editor*
Available at: http://www.cardiology.theclinics.com/

*Heart Failure Clinics*, October 2013 (Vol. 9, No. 4)
**Atrial Fibrillation and Heart Failure**
Mark O'Neill, Andrew Grace, and Sanjiv M. Narayan, *Editors*
Available at: http://www.heartfailure.theclinics.com/

**DOWNLOAD
Free App!**

*Review Articles*
THE CLINICS

**NOW AVAILABLE FOR YOUR iPhone and iPad**

# Preface
# Interventional Pharmacology

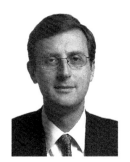

George D. Dangas, MD, PhD
*Editor*

The field of Interventional Pharmacology has advanced tremendously during recent years. This is due not only to the development of new medical therapy options but also to the employment of complex combination strategies with established and emerging interventional devices within different cardiovascular disease states. For example, the field of acute myocardial infarction was one of the first to be intensively explored. Indeed, it has experienced a dramatic improvement in clinical outcomes (both morbidity and mortality) thanks to the often complicated interplay of oral and parenteral antithrombotic, antiplatelet and fibrinolytic agents in several combination strategies that also depend on the interventional devices to be used, the hospital's capabilities, interhospital transferring times, and, of course, many specific patient characteristics. It's easy to understand that the number of possible combinations of all the above treatments is large.

One can further appreciate what the expansion of Interventional Pharmacology options may mean for other cardiovascular diseases, such as stable and unstable angina, chronic (long-term) therapy, endovascular intervention, structural heart disease, and so many other emerging fields. Therefore, rigorous clinical investigation is of paramount importance for our application of the various new therapies as is their incorporation within the already complex clinical treatment pathways. Since every new drug is often approved on a single indication

and as a sole therapy, additional robust clinical data are typically required for its successful incorporation in multidrug and multidevice treatments. The continuous identification of new therapeutic targets and the development of new/novel drugs expand even further the current role of Interventional Pharmacology.

The classic target of this field had been the suppression of complications from endovascular thrombosis in coronary heart disease, and incredible advances have recently made difficult-to-achieve major incremental benefits (we are "victims of our own success" in a way). Targeting improvements in safety outcomes (including lowering of bleeding complications, for example), while ischemic outcomes may remain largely unchanged, has provided additional clinical benefits in recent years.

Endovascular thrombosis is not unique in coronary artery disease. The great fund of knowledge acquired from many decades of research on this subject can be used in principle in other types of cardiovascular disease since the interventional device treatment options have been expanding. Of course, we need to appropriately adapt our research methodology. Another recent quest is that of personalized medicine and the role of genetic predisposition. Interventional cardiology and endovascular therapy have the unique advantage of direct access to the arterial (or venous) treatment site with broad options of local imaging, blood and

interventional.theclinics.com

*Intervent Cardiol Clin 2 (2013) xiii–xiv*
http://dx.doi.org/10.1016/j.iccl.2013.06.006
2211-7458/13/$ – see front matter © 2013 Published by Elsevier Inc.

tissue sampling, as well as various methods of drug delivery. This fact has enabled tremendous clinical developments and will continue to do so in the future.

This concise issue attempts to traverse the basic principles, current status, and future directions of Interventional Pharmacology for cardiovascular disease states. I would like to congratulate the experts who graciously accepted the invitation to contribute to this effort.

George D. Dangas, MD, PhD
Department of Cardiology
The Zena and Michael A. Wiener
Cardiovascular Institute
Icahn School of Medicine at Mount Sinai
One Gustave L. Levy Place, Box 1030
New York, NY 10029, USA

E-mail address:
george.dangas@mountsinai.org

# Basics of Antithrombotic Therapy for Cardiovascular Disease
## Pharmacologic Targets of Platelet Inhibitors and Anticoagulants

Piera Capranzano, MD[a], Dominick J. Angiolillo, MD, PhD[b],*

## KEYWORDS

- Thrombosis • Platelets • Coagulation • Antiplatelets • Anticoagulants

## KEY POINTS

- Arterial thrombus formation is the common pathophysiologic process of different cardiovascular disease manifestations. Platelets and coagulation factors are pivotal in this process.
- Key targets within the platelet and coagulation cascade have been identified for the development of pharmacologic strategies aimed to reduce ischemic events.
- Recently developed antiplatelet agents have yielded a greater reduction in ischemic events but are associated with an increased risk of bleeding, especially in specific subgroups.
- Recently developed anticoagulant agents have more favorable pharmacologic properties and a better safety and efficacy profile.
- New antithrombotic strategies are being development with the aim to find an optimal balance between ischemic and bleeding risk.

Atherosclerotic cardiovascular disease comprises coronary artery disease (CAD), cerebrovascular disease, and peripheral artery disease (PAD). CAD manifestations include stable CAD and acute coronary syndrome (ACS), which embraces a spectrum of clinical presentations, ranging from unstable angina to non-ST elevation (NSTE) myocardial infarction (MI), and ST elevation MI (STEMI). The common pathophysiologic processes of these cardiovascular disease conditions and their clinical manifestations are atherosclerotic plaque progression, thrombosis, or embolization. Mural thrombus formation may be the consequence of either the spontaneous disruption of an atherosclerotic plaque, as in the setting of an ACS, or of iatrogenic endothelial denudation, as in the setting of percutaneous coronary intervention (PCI).[1] Indeed, spontaneous or iatrogenic erosion of the endothelial surface or rupture of atherosclerotic plaque triggers platelet and coagulation

Disclosures: Dominick J. Angiolillo: Received payment as an individual for: a) Consulting fee or honorarium from Bristol Myers Squibb, Sanofi-Aventis, Eli Lilly, Daiichi Sankyo, The Medicines Company, AstraZeneca, Merck, Evolva, Abbott Vascular and PLx Pharma; b) Participation in review activities from Johnson & Johnson, St. Jude, and Sunovion. Institutional payments for grants from Bristol Myers Squibb, Sanofi-Aventis, Glaxo Smith Kline, Otsuka, Eli Lilly, Daiichi Sankyo, The Medicines Company, AstraZeneca, Evolva; and has other financial relationships with Esther and King Biomedical Research Grant. Piera Capranzano has nothing to disclose.
a Cardiovascular Department, Ferrarotto Hospital, University of Catania, Citelli 1, Catania 95124, Italy; b Division of Cardiology, Department of Medicine, Shands Jacksonville, University of Florida College of Medicine–Jacksonville, 655 West 8th Street, Jacksonville, FL 32209, USA
* Corresponding author.
E-mail address: dominick.angiolillo@jax.ufl.edu

Intervent Cardiol Clin 2 (2013) 499–513
http://dx.doi.org/10.1016/j.iccl.2013.06.003
2211-7458/13/$ – see front matter © 2013 Elsevier Inc. All rights reserved.

activation, leading to arterial thrombosis, which blocks blood flow and oxygen supply (ischemia) in the affected arteries.[1,2] The mechanisms of arterial thrombosis require a close interplay between platelets, endothelium, coagulation factors and the extracellular matrix of the vessel wall. In particular, arterial thrombosis comprises three basic pathways: (1) platelet adhesion, activation, and aggregation; (2) blood coagulation with fibrin formation; and (3) fibrinolysis. This article reviews the pathophysiology of the arterial thrombosis cascade and provides a general overview of current and novel antiplatelet and anticoagulant agents.

## ROLE OF PLATELETS AND COAGULATION FACTORS IN THROMBUS FORMATION

Platelet-activated thrombus formation proceeds in three stages: (1) an initiation phase involving platelet adhesion; (2) an extension phase including activation, additional recruitment, and aggregation

of platelets; and (3) a perpetuation phase characterized by continued platelet stimulation and stabilization of clots.[1,3]

Under physiologic conditions, endothelial cells exhibit antithrombotic properties. The endothelial discontinuity of endothelial barrier exposes the subendothelial layer, which contains thrombogenic components, such as collagen, von Willebrand factor (vWF), and other molecules (ie, fibronectin), that bind to platelet receptors, inducing platelet adhesion.[3,4] The latter is mainly mediated by interaction between the glycoprotein (GP) Ib/V/IX receptor complex on the platelet surface to vWF, which is required for initiation of platelets adhesion under high shear rate conditions, and GP VI and GP Ia to collagen at sites of vascular injury.[4] These interactions allow the arrest and activation of adherent platelets (**Fig. 1**).[5]

Platelet activation and aggregation in the extension phase can be induced by multiple pathways (**Fig. 2**).[3,5,6] When activated platelets adhere to sites of vascular injury, the local platelet activating

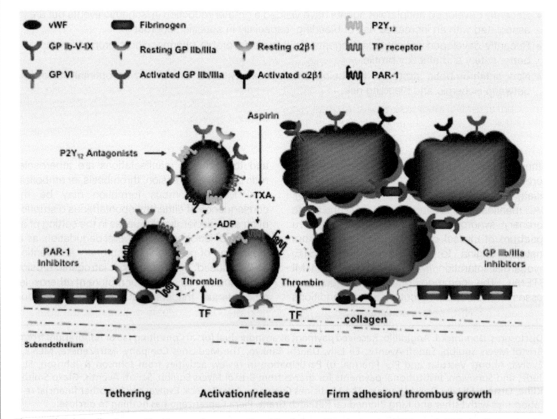

**Fig. 1.** Platelet adhesion, activation, and aggregation. The interaction between GP Ib and vWF mediates platelets tethering, enabling subsequent interaction between GP VI and collagen. This triggers the shift of integrins to a high-affinity state and the release of adenosine diphosphate (ADP) and thromboxane A2 (TXA$_2$), that bind to the purinergic (P2Y$_{12}$) and TP receptors, respectively. Tissue factor (TF) locally triggers thrombin formation, which contributes to platelet activation via binding to the platelet protease activated receptor (PAR-1). (*From* Angiolillo DJ, Ueno M, Goto S. Basic principles of platelet biology and clinical implications. Circ J 2010;74:597–607; with permission.)

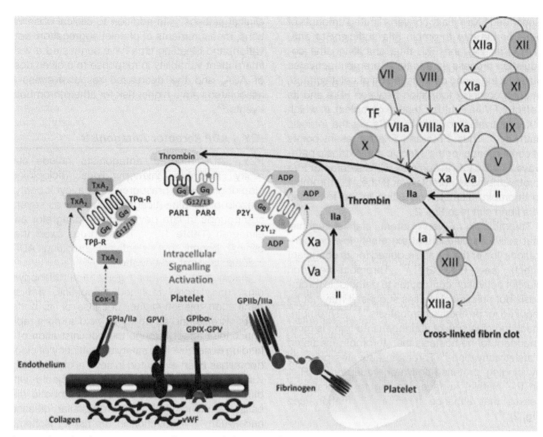

**Fig. 2.** The platelet activation pathways and the coagulation cascade. Major platelet activation pathways are those stimulated by thromboxane A2 (TXA$_2$), adenosine diphosphate (ADP), and thrombin. These agonists bind and activate their respective receptors, which in turn stimulate the activation of associated G-proteins, ultimately activating GP IIb/IIIa and promoting the interaction of adjacent platelets within the clot. In addition to its role in platelet activation, thrombin generated through the activity of the coagulation cascade or by the prothrombinase complex (factor Xa or Va) on the surface of activated platelets converts fibrinogen to fibrin, which adds stability to the growing plug. TP, thromboxane receptor. (*From* Angiolillo DJ, Ferrerio JL. Antiplatelet and anticoagulant therapy for atherothrombotic disease: the role of current and emerging agents. Am J Cardiovasc Drugs 2013. [Epub ahead of print]; with permission.)

factors help recruit additional circulating platelets to extend and stabilize the plug.[4] These platelet-activating factors include adenosine diphosphate (ADP), thromboxane A2 (TXA$_2$), serotonin, collagen, and thrombin.[3] ADP is one of the most important mediators of thrombosis. Platelets express two ADP-specific purinergic receptors: P2Y$_1$ and P2Y$_{12}$.[7] Activation of the P2Y$_1$ receptor leads to signaling events that initiate a weak and transient phase of platelet aggregation.[7] In contrast, activation of the P2Y$_{12}$ receptor results in activation of the GP IIb/IIIa receptor, granule release, amplification of platelet aggregation, and stabilization of the platelet aggregate.[7] TXA$_2$ is another key platelet agonist, which derived from arachidonic acid through conversion by cyclooxygenase-1 (COX-1) and thromboxane synthase.[8] The binding of these agonists to their respective receptors ultimately activates the GP IIb/IIIa receptor, which promotes the interaction of adjacent platelets through fibrinogen (see **Fig. 2**).[6] The perpetuation phase of thrombus formation is mediated by cell-to-cell, contact-dependent mechanisms, mostly intermediated by vWF under high shear stress conditions, that lead to changes in platelet morphology, expression of procoagulant and proinflammatory activities, and platelet aggregation.[3]

The platelet-clot is stabilized by fibrin derived from the coagulation cascade (see **Fig. 2**).[6] Initiation of blood coagulation occurs mainly through tissue factor (TF), a membrane GP that, after vessel wall injury, becomes exposed to circulating blood and forms a complex with the zymogen factor (F) VIIa.[9] The TF-FVIIa complex activates FX into FXa and FIX into FIXa (extrinsic pathway).[9]

Generated FXa initially converts limited amounts of prothrombin into thrombin FIIa sufficient to activate FVIII, FV, and FXI, thus amplifying the coagulation process. In addition, thrombin activates platelets triggering coagulation on platelet surface, through complex formation between FIXa and its cofactor FVIIIa (intrinsic tenase complex), in which FIX is activated to FIXa by FXIa via the intrinsic pathway.[10] Thus, FIXa and FXa represent points of convergence for the intrinsic and extrinsic pathways. Finally, FXa in complex with its cofactor FVa (prothrombinase complex) activates prothrombin to thrombin, ultimately resulting in the formation of a fibrin clot (see **Fig. 2**).

Thrombin is a very potent platelet agonist that activates platelets at extremely low concentrations (lower than those required for its coagulant effect) (see **Fig. 2**).[11,12] Thrombin-mediated platelet activation contributes to pathologic thrombosis but preclinical studies suggest it may not be required for protective hemostasis.[11–15] Thrombin-mediated cleavage of fibrinogen into fibrin is more important for hemostasis than thrombin-mediated platelet activation.[16] Thrombin activates platelets by binding protease-activated receptor (PAR)-1 on the platelet surface, leading to several processes that enhance thrombus formation (see **Fig. 2**).[16,17]

## OVERVIEW OF ANTIPLATELET AGENTS FOR ATHEROSCLEROTIC DISEASES
### Aspirin

Aspirin (acetylsalicylic acid [ASA]), permanently inactivate platelet COX-1, blocking the production of $TXA_2$.[18] Aspirin is rapidly absorbed in the stomach and upper intestine. Peak plasma levels occur 30 to 40 minutes after ASA ingestion, and platelet inhibition is evident by 1 hour. In contrast, it can take up to 3 to 4 hours to reach peak plasma levels after the administration of enteric-coated ASA. Aspirin is the cornerstone of oral antiplatelet therapy for the prevention of atherothrombotic events.[18] Indeed, several large-scale clinical trials and meta-analyses have consistently demonstrated the benefit of ASA in significantly reducing fatal and nonfatal recurrent ischemic events in subjects with a large spectrum of atherosclerotic diseases manifestations.[19] Although ASA is recommended for secondary prevention in all patients who have experienced ischemic cerebrovascular events or ACS and/or undergoing PCI, it is associated with limitations.[20,21] These include a dose-dependent increased risk for bleeding and residual morbidity and mortality higher than those for more recently developed antiplatelet agents when used as monotherapy in different clinical settings.[22] In addition to clinical observations, measurements of platelet aggregation, activation, and bleeding time have suggested a wide interpatient variability in response to a given dose of ASA, and the decreased responsiveness is associated with a higher risk for atherothrombotic events.[23]

### P2Y$_{12}$ ADP Receptor Antagonists

P2Y$_{12}$ ADP receptor antagonists include currently available thienopyridines (ticlopidine, clopidogrel, and prasugrel) and a cyclopentyl-triazolo-pyrimidine (ticagrelor), as well as several compounds in late development (cangrelor and elinogrel) (**Table 1**).[5,24] These drugs exert their clinical benefit by selectively inhibiting ADP-induced platelet aggregation.

Clopidogrel, a second-generation thienopyridine, has largely replaced ticlopidine, a first-generation thienopyridine, because of its better safety profile and its ability to yield a more rapid antiplatelet effect through the administration of a loading dose.[25,26] The safety and efficacy of clopidogrel has been evaluated in several clinical trials, which have been performed in subjects with different manifestations of atherothrombotic disease, including CAD, cerebrovascular disease, and PAD.[27–34] Reduction in the risk of ischemic events observed in trials of clopidogrel plus aspirin in subjects with ACS and/or undergoing PCI have led to the use of dual antiplatelet therapy as standard-of-care therapy in these patient populations.[20,21] However, dual antiplatelet therapy has been associated with increased bleeding risk. Much evidence has demonstrated wide response variability to clopidogrel.[35] Of importance, inadequate inhibition of the ADP platelet activation pathway increases risk for thrombotic events.[35]

Prasugrel is a third-generation thienopyridine that, similarly to clopidogrel, is orally administered as a prodrug, needing conversion to an active metabolite to block the P2Y$_{12}$ receptor irreversibly.[36] However, prasugrel compared with clopidogrel is more efficiently metabolized, more rapidly reaching higher concentrations of its active metabolite, resulting in faster onset of action, enhanced platelet inhibition, and lower interindividual response variability, even when compared with higher loading (600 mg) and maintenance doses (150 mg) of clopidogrel.[36–38] Prasugrel has been compared with clopidogrel in the TRITON-TIMI 38 trial in subjects with ACS undergoing PCI, providing lower ischemic events, driven by a reduction in MI, and higher bleeding complications, but with a more favorable net clinical benefit.[39] Prasugrel was compared with

**Table 1**
**Properties of current and emerging P2Y$_{12}$ ADP receptor antagonists**

| Agent | Class | Mechanism of Action | Mode of Administration | Frequency of Maintenance Dose Administration | Approval or Development Status |
|---|---|---|---|---|---|
| Ticlopidine | Thienopyridine (First generation) | Prodrug, irreversible | Oral | Daily | Approved 1991 |
| Clopidogrel | Thienopyridine (Second generation) | Prodrug, irreversible | Oral | Daily | Approved 1997 |
| Prasugrel | Thienopyridine (Third generation) | Prodrug, irreversible | Oral | Daily | Approved 2009 |
| Ticagrelor | Cyclopentyl-triazolo-pyrimidine | Direct-acting, reversible | Oral | Twice daily | Approved 2011 |
| Cangrelor | ATP analog | Direct-acting, reversible | IV | — | Phase 3 CHAMPION-PLATFORM and CHAMPION-PCI trials terminated 2009; CHAMPION-PHOENIX terminated 2013 |
| Elinogrel | Quinazolinedione | Direct-acting, reversible | IV and oral | Twice daily | Phase 2 trials terminated |

clopidogrel also in the large spectrum of medically managed subjects with ACS (TRILOGY-ACS trial), but failed to show superiority.[40] Prasugrel (60 mg loading dose and 10 mg daily maintenance dose) is currently approved for the prevention of atherothrombotic events in patients with ACS undergoing PCI with no previous cerebrovascular events. Other contraindications include patients at high risk for bleeding and hypersensitivity. Dose modulation (prasugrel 5 mg) is suggested in older and low-weight patients.

Ticagrelor is a direct-acting oral agent that, compared with clopidogrel, provides higher and more consistent degree of platelet inhibition and a more rapid time to maximal platelet inhibition.[41] In the PLATO trial, ticagrelor was compared with clopidogrel in subjects with ACS who were managed invasively or medically. It showed superior efficacy, including lower cardiovascular mortality. Although overall major bleeding events were not increased, ticagrelor was associated with increased spontaneous bleeding and higher rates of fatal intracranial hemorrhages.[42] Ticagrelor (180 mg loading dose and 90 mg bid maintenance dose) is currently approved for the prevention of atherothrombotic events in patients

with ACS who are managed invasively or medically with no previous hemorrhagic stroke. Other contraindications include patients at high risk for bleeding, severe hepatic impairment, and hypersensitivity.

Cangrelor is a direct-acting, intravenously administered, highly selective, P2Y$_{12}$ antagonist, with a short half-life ($\sim$2.6 minutes).[43] It provides, in a dose-dependent manner, a nearly complete inhibition of ADP-induced platelet aggregation, with a rapid onset and offset of action and recovery of platelet function within approximately 30 to 60 minutes after discontinuation.[43] Cangrelor has been compared with clopidogrel in three large-scale randomized trials in subjects undergoing PCI, mostly for ACS. The first two trials (CHAMPION-PCI and PLATFORM), which differed in the timing of study treatment start, failed to show any significant difference between the two treatments in ischemic events, probably in part due to a difficult adjudication of periprocedural MI.[44,45] A recent trial (CHAMPION-PHOENIX), which used a more stringent definition of periprocedural MI, showed that cangrelor compared with clopidogrel significantly reduced ischemic events at 48 hours in about 11,000 subjects undergoing

PCI, including stable CAD and ACS subjects.[46] The pharmacologic profiles of cangrelor make it an attractive strategy for bridging therapy of patients on dual antiplatelet therapy who are scheduled for surgery. The BRIDGE trial compared cangrelor (0.75 μg/kg/min) versus placebo for at least 48 hours, with the study drug discontinued approximately 1 to 6 hours before surgery, in subjects with ACS (N = 210) on a thienopyridine scheduled for cardiac surgery.[47] Cangrelor compared with placebo was shown to consistently achieve and maintain adequate platelet inhibition at levels known to be associated with a low risk of thrombotic events, at the price of an increase in minor bleeding.[47]

Elinogrel is a direct-acting agent associated with more rapid onset and offset effects than clopidogrel.[48] It can be administered both orally and intravenously. A phase 2 trial (INNOVATE-PCI) showed that elinogrel (80–120 mg intravenous loading dose plus 50–150 mg bid) achieved more potent and rapid platelet inhibition than clopidogrel in subjects undergoing elective PCI (N = 652), with no significant increase in major or minor bleeding. However, bleeding requiring medical attention was more frequent with elinogrel.[49,50] In addition, liver enzymes elevation was more common with elinogrel than with clopidogrel. Elinogrel has been evaluated in another small phase 2A dose-escalation investigation in subjects with STEMI, in which it was shown that the incidence of bleeding was infrequent and similar in subjects treated with all doses of elinogrel (10, 20, 40, and 60 mg administered as a single intravenous bolus before the start of primary PCI) versus placebo.[51] In addition, no differences in serious adverse events, laboratory values, corrected thrombolysis in MI frame count, or ST-resolution were demonstrated between elinogrel and placebo. Currently there are no planned phase III investigations with elinogrel.

## GP IIb/IIIa Inhibitors

GP IIb/IIIa antagonists interfere with platelet cross-linking and clot formation by competing with fibrinogen and vWF for GP IIb/IIIa binding.[4] GP IIb/IIIa inhibitors are only intravenously administered within the hospital setting in patients with ACS and/or undergoing PCI and are not used in the long-term care of patients with atherothrombotic disease. Investigations of oral GP IIb/IIIa inhibitors have been halted due to negative results from several large trials. The three parenteral GP IIb/IIIa inhibitors in clinical use are abciximab, eptifibatide, and tirofiban.

Abciximab is a monoclonal antibody with a rapid onset and a short plasma half-life (<10 min).[52] However, because of its high binding affinity for the receptor, it has a biologic half-life of 12 to 24 hours. An estimated 30% of GP IIb/IIIa receptors are still occupied by abciximab 8 days after completion of infusion.[52] The efficacy and safety of abciximab in subjects undergoing PCI, including primary PCI for STEMI, have been evaluated in several trials, predating the use of clopidogrel.[53–56] Overall, these trials have shown that abciximab significantly improved PCI outcomes.[53–56] When abciximab was compared with placebo in subjects undergoing PCI and receiving pretreatment (>2 hours) with clopidogrel 600 mg, additional benefits associated with abciximab were found only in high-risk subjects with NSTE-ACS with elevated levels of troponin, but not in those at low-to-intermediate risk undergoing elective PCI.[57,58] These observations suggest that when adequate inhibition of ADP-induced platelet aggregation is achieved, GP IIb/IIIa inhibitors should be restricted only to patients with high-risk of ACS with positive cardiac markers. The issue of whether abciximab remains beneficial after adequate clopidogrel loading was tested also in subjects with STEMI (n = 800) in the BRAVE 3 trial, which showed no benefits in terms of infarct size before discharge.[59] However, the infarct size 30 days after primary PCI for anterior STEMI was reduced by the use of an intracoronary bolus of abciximab in the INFUSE-MI trial.[60]

Eptifibatide is a small, reversible, and highly selective, synthetic heptapeptide with a rapid onset, a short plasma half-life (mean 1 hour) and a renal clearance accounting for 40% of total body clearance.[52] Recover of platelet aggregation occurs within 2 to 4 hours after infusion discontinuation. Several randomized clinical trials have shown the efficacy and safety of eptifibatide in subjects with NSTE-ACS or undergoing PCI.[61–63] The EARLY-ACS trial demonstrated that upstream administration of eptifibatide versus provisional eptifibatide after angiography resulted in similar 30-day rates of ischemic complications during PCI in subjects with NSTE-ACS.[64] Major and minor bleeding events were significantly higher with early eptifibatide versus delayed eptifibatide.[64] Overall, these findings do not support the use of upstream compared with selective downstream GP IIb/IIIa inhibition in patients with ACS undergoing PCI.

Tirofiban is a nonpeptide, tyrosine-derived, highly selective inhibitor associated with a rapid onset, a short plasma half-life (about 2 hours) and a renal clearance ranging from 25% to 50%.[52] The efficacy and safety of tirofiban in subjects with ACS-PCI have been investigated in several trials.[65,66]

## PHOSPHODIESTERASE INHIBITORS

Cilostazol is indicated for symptomatic relief of intermittent claudication from PAD and does not have an indication for treatment of patients with CAD although it has been studied extensively in adjunct to aspirin and clopidogrel. Cilostazol is an inhibitor of phosphodiesterase type III with both antiplatelet and vasodilatory effects[67] and is associated with more potent platelet inhibitory effects when added to aspirin and clopidogrel.[68] During PCI, cilostazol added to aspirin and clopidogrel (triple therapy) was associated with a significantly reduced risk of stent thrombosis, angiographic restenosis, and clinical ischemic events without increased bleeding risk versus aspirin plus clopidogrel, especially among patients with diabetes.[69] A Food and Drug Administration (FDA) warning indicates that cilostazol should be avoided in patients with congestive heart of any severity because of an increased mortality risk. Cilostazol is also frequently associated with headache, palpitations, and diarrhea.

Dipyridamole selectively inhibits the cyclic guanosine monophosphate (cGMP) phosphodiesterase type V enzyme, thus augmenting the antiplatelet effects of the nitric oxide–cGMP signaling pathway.[70] In a large ESPS II trial, dipyridamole with or without ASA effectively prevented stroke recurrence.[71] The ESPRIT trial demonstrated that dipyridamole plus ASA versus aspirin alone might not only provide protection against stroke recurrence but also against MI or death from vascular causes.[72] Results of the PRoFESS trial showed that there was no significant difference in the risk of fatal or disabling stroke in subjects receiving dipyridamole plus ASA versus clopidogrel.[73]

## PAR-1 ANTAGONISTS

PAR-1 inhibitors block the binding of thrombin to PAR-1, thus inhibiting thrombin-induced platelets activation and aggregation. Preclinical observations showed PAR-1 receptor inhibition does not interfere with thrombin-mediated fibrin generation that is essential for hemostasis.[13] Two PAR-1 inhibitors are under clinical development for the prevention of arterial thrombosis: vorapaxar and atopaxar.[74]

Vorapaxar is a highly selective, orally active, potent, and competitive PAR-1 antagonist. Phase I and II studies have shown that adding vorapaxar to aspirin plus clopidogrel does not significantly increase bleeding, although it may have the potential for reducing ischemic events. These results set the rationale for two large-scale phase III trials: the TRACER and TRA 2P-TIMI 50.[75,76] The TRACER trial randomized 12,944 high-risk subjects with NSTE-ACS, most already on dual antiplatelet therapy, to vorapaxar or placebo, and was halted prematurely due to a lack of reduction in overall ischemic events and a significant increase in the risk of major bleeding, including intracranial hemorrhage, in the investigational arm.[75] In the TRA 2P-TIMI 50 trial, vorapaxar (2.5-mg daily) compared with placebo significantly reduced ischemic events at the cost of increased moderate or severe bleeding, including intracranial hemorrhage, in subjects with a history of MI, ischemic stroke, or PAD (n = 26,449).[76] Notably, after an interim analysis, the data and safety monitoring board recommended discontinuation of vorapaxar in patients with a history of stroke, due to unacceptable risk of intracranial hemorrhage without an improvement in major vascular events, including ischemic stroke, as also shown by a subsequent subanalysis.[77] In contrast, another prespecified subanalysis of the TRA 2P-TIMI 50 showed that, in subjects with a history of MI, vorapaxar reduced ischemic events but increased the risk of moderate or severe bleeding.[78] Also, subjects with PAD experienced less acute limb ischemia and peripheral arterial revascularization with vorapaxar, despite the higher risk of bleeding.[79]

Clinical development of atopaxar is still in the early stage. Two phase II studies, the LANCELOT-ACS and the LANCELOT-CAD, have suggested a good safety profile of the drug in subjects with ACS and CAD, respectively.[80,81] However, the highest doses of atopaxar compared with placebo were more commonly associated to QTc prolongation and transient liver enzymes elevation. Phase III investigations are not currently ongoing for atopaxar.

A meta-analysis of eight phase II and III trials of PAR-1 antagonists in subjects with CAD (N = 41,647) highlighted a higher risk of major bleeding, including intracranial hemorrhage, with the novel agents compared with placebo, paralleled by a significantly lower risk of MI, that was consistently noted in studies of vorapaxar and atopaxar.[82] Interestingly, a significant interaction was found between bleeding with PAR-1 antagonists and the use of $P2Y_{12}$ inhibitors, suggesting that future studies on these novel agents in subjects not receiving a $P2Y_{12}$ inhibitor or studies versus $P2Y_{12}$ inhibitors on a background of aspirin therapy might be considered.

## OTHER NOVEL ANTIPLATELET AGENTS

Other agents are targeted to inhibit $TXA_2$-induced platelet activation mediated by $TXA_2$ receptors

(TPs).[83] The rationale for the development of TP antagonists (eg, terutroban) is that platelets may continue to be exposed to TXA$_2$ despite complete COX-1 blockade using aspirin. Preclinical and clinical studies are currently ongoing for this family of platelet inhibitors as well as for other targets, including those targeted to inhibit serotonin and collagen receptors.

## OVERVIEW OF ANTICOAGULANT AGENTS FOR ATHEROSCLEROTIC DISEASES

Anticoagulants are classified according to the target coagulation enzyme that is being inhibited (eg, antifactor IIa or antithrombins, antifactor Xa, antifactor IXa) (Fig. 3).[84] They are further categorized based on whether inhibitory effects are direct or indirect (ie, warranting a cofactor).

## THROMBIN INHIBITORS
### Indirect Thrombin Inhibitors

Indirect thrombin inhibitors include unfractionated heparin (UFH) and low-molecular weight heparin (LMWH). Thrombin has an active site and two exosites, one of which—exosite 1—binds to its fibrin substrate, orientating it toward the active site. UFH binds to exosite 2 on thrombin and to antithrombin, forming a ternary complex, which is

necessary for the inhibition of thrombin by antithrombin.[85] In contrast to thrombin inhibition, inactivation of factor Xa does not require the formation of the ternary complex. The ratio of anti-Xa to anti-IIa activity for UFH is equal to 1. LMWH derived from the fragmentation or the depolymerization of heparin by chemical or enzymatic process. Because most LMWH chains are not sufficiently long to form the ternary complex necessary for the inactivation of thrombin, their action is mainly directed against factor Xa; therefore, the ratio of anti-IIa to anti-Xa activity varies from 1.9 to 3.8 (enoxaparin).[86]

The pharmacologic properties of UFH and LMWH are compared in Table 2. The UFH has important limitations due to the quite variable pharmacokinetic and pharmacodynamic profiles, the significant nonspecific protease binding, the inability to inhibit fibrin-bound thrombin, the prothrombotic effect on platelets activation and aggregation, and, finally, the life-threatening risk of heparin-induced thrombocytopenia (HIT). Although, to a lesser extent, part of these limitations are also associated with LMWH.

UFH and LMWH are routinely used in interventional practice as the standard anticoagulation for the treatment of patients with ACS and in the PCI setting.[19,20] In these populations, LMWH compared with UFH was associated with an

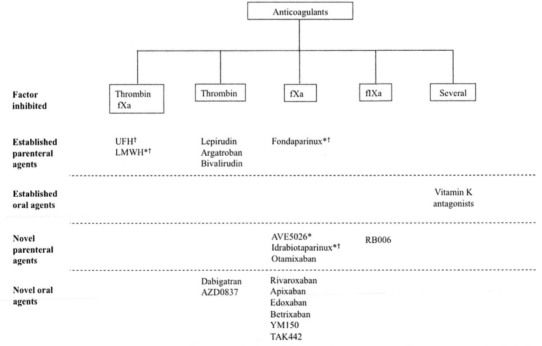

Fig. 3. Established and new anticoagulants classified according to the target coagulation enzyme that is being inhibited. LMWH, low-molecular weight heparin; UFH, unfractionated heparin. *Subcutaneously administered. †Indirect inhibitors.

**Table 2**
**Comparison of pharmacologic properties of current anticoagulants**

| Property | UFH | LMWH | Fondaparinux | Bivalirudin |
|---|---|---|---|---|
| Predictability in pharmacologic profile | − | ++ | +++ | +++ |
| Cofactor required | +++ | +++ | +++ | − |
| Renal clearance | − | ++ | +++ | ++ |
| Nonspecific protein binding | +++ | + | − | − |
| Platelet activation | +++ | + | − | − |
| Rebound of thrombin generation after discontinuation | +++ | + | − | − |
| Inhibition of bound thrombin | − | − | − | +++ |
| Neutralization by platelet factor 4 | +++ | + | + | + |
| Inhibition of thrombin generation | + | ++ | ++ | +++ |

overall better efficacy profile and a similar safety, while being more practical because, unlike UFH, it does not require anticoagulation monitoring and dose adjustment.

### Direct Thrombin Inhibitors

Direct thrombin inhibitors (DTIs) inhibit soluble and clot-bound thrombin without depending on antithrombin for anticoagulant activity. Indeed, they are physically small molecules that do not interact with exosite 2 and that bind directly to the active site of thrombin and inhibit all its proteolytic activity without the need for antithrombin as an intermediary molecule. They have high specificity and potency for thrombin inhibition and do not promote platelet aggregation. Given their potential benefits compared with heparins, parenteral DTIs have undergone extensive appraisal in subjects with ACS or HIT, or those undergoing PCI. Three parenteral agents are currently available for clinical use in these populations: recombined hirudin (lepirudin), argatroban, and bivalirudin.[87] The oral agent dabigatran, although approved for clinical use as a replacement for warfarin in patients with atrial fibrillation (AF), its clinical investigation has been halted in the setting of ACS after the very high bleeding rates observed in adjunct to dual antiplatelet therapy in the phase II RE-DEEM trial.[88]

Lepirudin is a peptide that binds to the catalytic site and exosite 1 of thrombin with very high affinity. It has a half-life of 80 minutes and is primarily cleared by the kidneys. It is approved for treatment of patients with HIT. No studies have evaluated the role of lepirudin in contemporary PCI.

Argatroban is a synthetic peptide competitive inhibitor of thrombin, binding to a site near the catalytic site.[87] It has a short half-life (45 minutes) and it is mainly metabolized by the liver, requiring dose adjustment in patients with hepatic dysfunction. It

is approved for treatment of patients with HIT. Few small studies have evaluated the effects of argatroban during PCI; it is approved in this setting as an alternative anticoagulant only in patients with HIT.[20]

Bivalirudin (hirulog-1) is a 20-amino acid polypeptide and is a synthetic version of hirudin that binds to the catalytic site and exosite 1 of thrombin. This binding is reversible and is associated with the cleavage near the amino-terminal of bivalirudin by thrombin itself.[89] When bivalirudin is cleaved, the bond between exosite 1 and the amino-terminal of the bivalirudin segment is weakened, leading to their dissociation and to restoration of normal thrombin activity.[89] Bivalirudin has a half-life of 25 minutes, which is prolonged by renal insufficiency, and is primarily cleared via proteolysis, with renal excretion accounting for less than 20% of its degradation. The pharmacologic properties of bivalirudin compared with those of heparins are listed in **Table 2**.

Currently, it is the only DTI extensively evaluated in several powered clinical trials with respect to its use in coronary intervention in patients with stable CAD and in those with ACS, including NSTEMI and STEMI.[90–93] Trials on bivalirudin are consistent in showing that bivalirudin compared with heparin plus GPIIb/IIIa is associated with comparable ischemic outcomes and reduced major bleeding with a favorable impact on survival. Bivalirudin is currently approved for use during PCI as an alternative to UFH and in patients with HIT.

### FACTOR-XA INHIBITORS
### Indirect Factor-Xa Inhibitors

Fondaparinux is the prototype of the indirect factor Xa inhibitors. Other agents are variants of fondaparinux and include idraparinux, idrabiotaparinux, and SR123781 A. All these agents are subcutaneously administrated. Only fondaparinux has been investigated in the setting of ACS-PCI.

Fondaparinux, a synthetic analogous of the antithrombin-binding pentasaccharide sequence found in heparin, binds to antithrombin with very high specificity, enhancing the ability of antithrombin to neutralize factor Xa and, hence, the formation of thrombin. Fondaparinux has almost complete bioavailability after subcutaneous injection with rapid absorption, achieving a steady state after 3 to 4 daily doses. Its plasma half-life of approximately 17 hours allows once-daily administration at fixed dosages. It has a highly predictable anticoagulant effect and, thus, there is no need for laboratory monitoring. The pharmacologic properties of fondaparinux compared with those of heparins are listed in **Table 2**.

The efficacy and safety of fondaparinux (2.5 mg subcutaneous daily) compared with heparin were tested in subjects with ACS.[94–96] In the NSTE-ACS population, fondaparinux was associated with superior net clinical benefit compared with enoxaparin.[94–96] In subjects with STEMI, fondaparinux compared with UFH reduced the combined endpoint of death or MI in subjects treated with thrombolysis, whereas those who underwent primary PCI had no significant benefit with fondaparinux.[96] Of concern, subjects who underwent primary PCI with fondaparinux had more catheter-related thrombi, more coronary complications, and a trend toward higher death or MI compared with UFH. Fondaparinux is recommended for patients with NSTE-ACS in whom an early conservative or a delayed invasive strategy of management is considered and for patients with STEMI who are receiving fibrinolytic therapy. Fondaparinux should not be used in patients with acute STEMI who are undergoing primary PCI. Despite guideline recommendations for the use of fondaparinux in ACS, fondaparinux is not approved for such use by the FDA in the United States.

### Direct Factor-Xa Inhibitors

Direct factor Xa inhibitors include parenteral agents, such as DX9065a and otamixaban, and several orally active drugs, including rivaroxaban, apixaban, edoxaban, darexaban, LY517717, and betrixaban. Only otamixaban, rivaroxaban, and apixaban have advanced to phase III clinical investigation in the setting of ACS-PCI.

Otamixaban is an intravenous direct, reversible, selective inhibitor of factor Xa. It has an initial half-life of 30 minutes and a rapid on-off anticoagulant activity. It is mainly cleared unchanged via the biliary system with a no significant renal excretion (<25%), suggesting no need for dose modification in case of renal insufficiency. Due to its predictable pharmacodynamic there is no need for anticoagulation monitoring. The SEPIA-ACS1 TIMI 42 trial showed a marked reduction in death or MI, and similar bleeding rates with otamixaban at midrange doses, compared with UFH plus eptifibatide.[97] These positive findings set the rationale for investigation of otamixaban in the ongoing phase III TAO trial, which is a randomized, double-blind, triple-dummy controlled trial testing the efficacy of otamixaban compared with UFH plus eptifibatide in subjects with NSTE-ACS who are treated with dual oral antiplatelet therapy and an invasive strategy.

Rivaroxaban is an orally active oxazolidone derivative that acts by directly and selectively inhibiting both free factor Xa and factor Xa bound in the prothrombinase complex. Rivaroxaban has a rapid and predictable anticoagulant effect with no need for dose adjustment and routine laboratory monitoring. The half-life is 9 to 13 hours and renal elimination accounts for 33%. It is approved for stroke prevention in AF. A recent phase III trial (ATLAS ACS 2-TIMI 51) has evaluated rivaroxaban (2.5 or 5.0 mg bid) versus placebo plus low-dose aspirin (75–100 mg/day), with or without a thienopyridine, in 15,526 subjects with ACS.[98] Rivaroxaban reduced the incidence of ischemic outcomes at the cost of increased bleeding. The 2.5 mg bid dose had the better benefit-risk balance, due to a lower bleeding risk than the 5 mg bid dose, with a significant mortality reduction.[98]

Apixaban is a potent direct inhibitor of both free and prothrombin-bound factor Xa, has a minimal affinity for factor IIa, has a half-life of 8 to 15 hours, and is eliminated mainly via the fecal route (~75%). It is approved for stroke prevention in AF. A recent phase III APPRAISE-2 trial evaluated apixaban 5 mg bid versus placebo on top of standard antiplatelet therapy, in subjects with high-risk for ACS.[99] The trial was stopped prematurely, after recruiting 7392 of the preplanned 10,800 subjects, because an interim analysis showed that the increase of major bleeding with apixaban, including increases in fatal and intracranial bleeding, was not counterbalanced by the expected decrease in recurrent ischemic events compared with placebo. Importantly, the decrease in ischemic events was offset by an increase in bleeding both in subjects taking only aspirin and in those on dual antiplatelet therapy.

## OTHER ANTICOAGULANTS UNDER CLINICAL DEVELOPMENT

Investigations are ongoing on novel anticoagulants using recombinant proteins that are directed at the initiation of coagulation targeting TF or factor VII. Another novel anticoagulant approach involves using RNA aptamer technology to target coagulation factors (eg, factor IXa). The advantage of this approach is the ability to initiate rapid anticoagulation that can be reversed immediately with a complementary RNA strand. The clinical safety and pharmacodynamic profiles of REG1, consisting of RB006 (drug), an injectable synthetic RNA aptamer that specifically binds and inhibits factor IXa, and RB007 (antidote), a complementary oligonucleotide that neutralizes the effect of RB006, has been evaluated in phase Ib and IIb studies, in subjects with stable CAD or ACS undergoing PCI and receiving standard antiplatelet therapy. In the phase IIb RADAR trial, the REG1 system, with reversal from 50% to 100% compared with UFH or LMWH, reduced major bleeding and ischemic events in 640 subjects with ACS undergoing cardiac catheterization.[100] A large-scale phase III clinical investigations is planned with the REG1.

## SUMMARY

Arterial thrombus formation is the common pathophysiologic process of different cardiovascular disease manifestations. Platelets and coagulation factors are key components in this process. Identification of key targets within the platelet and coagulation cascade has been pivotal for the development of strategies aimed to reduce ischemic recurrences. Although recent advances have yielded a greater reduction in ischemic events through their ability to achieve more potent blockade thrombotic processes, this has come at an increased risk of bleeding complications. Indeed, the future of antithrombotic therapies will rely on identifying treatment strategies that are able to find the fine balance between ischemic and bleeding risk. Emerging treatment regimens will represent a step forward toward reaching these goals.

## REFERENCES

1. Davi G, Patrono C. Platelet activation and atherothrombosis. N Engl J Med 2007;357:2482–94.
2. Libby P, Theroux P. Pathophysiology of coronary artery disease. Circulation 2005;111:3481–8.
3. Brass LF. Thrombin and platelet activation. Chest 2003;124:18S–25S.
4. Varga-Szabo D, Pleines I, Nieswandt B. Cell adhesion mechanisms in platelets. Arterioscler Thromb Vasc Biol 2008;28:403–12.
5. Angiolillo DJ, Ueno M, Goto S. Basic principles of platelet biology and clinical implications. Circ J 2010;74:597–607.
6. Angiolillo DJ, Ferrerio JL. Antiplatelet and anticoagulant therapy for atherothrombotic disease: the role of current and emerging agents. Am J Cardiovasc Drugs 2013. [Epub ahead of print].
7. Dorsam RT, Kunapuli SP. Central role of the P2Y12 receptor in platelet activation. J Clin Invest 2004;113:340–5.
8. Offermanns S. Activation of platelet function through G protein-coupled receptors. Circ Res 2006;99:1293–304.
9. Mackman N, Tilley RE, Key NS. Role of the extrinsic pathway of blood coagulation in hemostasis and thrombosis. Arterioscler Thromb Vasc Biol 2007;27:1687–93.
10. Monroe DM, Hoffman M, Roberts HF. Platelet and thrombin generation. Arterioscler Thromb Vasc Biol 2002;22:1381–9.
11. Brummel KE, Paradis SG, Butenas S, et al. Thrombin functions during tissue factor-induced blood coagulation. Blood 2002;100:148–52.
12. Mann KG. Thrombin formation. Chest 2003;124:4S–10S.
13. Derian CK, Damiano BP, Addo MF, et al. Blockade of the thrombin receptor protease-activated receptor-1 with a small-molecule antagonist prevents thrombus formation and vascular occlusion in nonhuman primates. J Pharmacol Exp Ther 2003;304:855–61.
14. Kato Y, Kita Y, Hirasawa-Taniyama Y, et al. Inhibition of arterial thrombosis by a protease-activated receptor 1 antagonist, FR171113, in the guinea pig. Eur J Pharmacol 2003;473:163–9.
15. Vandendries ER, Hamilton JR, Coughlin SR, et al. Par4 is required for platelet thrombus propagation but not fibrin generation in a mouse model of thrombosis. Proc Natl Acad Sci U S A 2007;104:288–92.
16. Coughlin SR. Protease-activated receptors in hemostasis, thrombosis and vascular biology. J Thromb Haemost 2005;3:1800–14.
17. Leger AJ, Covic L, Kuliopulos A. Protease-activated receptors in cardiovascular diseases. Circulation 2006;114:1070–7.
18. Patrono C. Aspirin as an antiplatelet drug. N Engl J Med 1994;330:1287–94.
19. Baigent C, Blackwell L, Collins R, et al. Aspirin in the primary and secondary prevention of vascular disease: collaborative meta-analysis of individual participant data from randomised trials. Lancet 2009;373:1849–60.
20. Wijns W, Kolh P, Danchin N, et al. Guidelines on myocardial revascularization. Task Force on Myocardial Revascularization of the European Society of Cardiology (ESC) and the European Association for Cardio-Thoracic Surgery (EACTS); European Association for Percutaneous Cardiovascular Interventions (EAPCI). Eur Heart J 2010;31:2501–55.

21. Levine GN, Bates ER, Blankenship JC, et al, American College of Cardiology Foundation, American Heart Association Task Force on Practice Guidelines, Society for Cardiovascular Angiography and Interventions. 2011 ACCF/AHA/SCAI Guideline for Percutaneous Coronary Intervention. A report of the American College of Cardiology Foundation/American Heart Association Task Force on Practice Guidelines and the Society for Cardiovascular Angiography and Interventions. J Am Coll Cardiol 2011;58:e44–122.

22. Angiolillo DJ. The evolution of antiplatelet therapy in the treatment of acute coronary syndromes: from aspirin to the present day. Drugs 2012;72: 2087–116.

23. Mason PJ, Jacobs AK, Freedman JE. Aspirin resistance and atherothrombotic disease. J Am Coll Cardiol 2005;46:986–93.

24. Ferreiro JL, Angiolillo DJ. New directions in antiplatelet therapy. Circ Cardiovasc Interv 2012;5: 433–45.

25. Bertrand ME, Rupprecht HJ, Urban P, et al, CLASSICS Investigators. Double-blind study of the safety of clopidogrel with and without a loading dose in combination with aspirin compared with ticlopidine in combination with aspirin after coronary stenting: the Clopidogrel Aspirin Stent International Cooperative Study (CLASSICS). Circulation 2000; 102:624–9.

26. Cadroy Y, Bossavy JP, Thalamas C, et al. Early potent antithrombotic effect with combined aspirin and a loading dose of clopidogrel on experimental arterial thrombogenesis in humans. Circulation 2000;101:2823–8.

27. Yusuf S, Zhao F, Mehta SR, et al. Effects of clopidogrel in addition to aspirin in patients with acute coronary syndromes without ST-segment elevation. N Engl J Med 2001;345:494–502.

28. Chen ZM, Jiang LX, Chen YP, et al. Addition of clopidogrel to aspirin in 45,852 patients with acute myocardial infarction: randomised placebo-controlled trial. Lancet 2005;366:1607–21.

29. Sabatine MS, Cannon CP, Gibson CM, et al. Addition of clopidogrel to aspirin and fibrinolytic therapy for myocardial infarction with ST-segment elevation. N Engl J Med 2005;352:1179–89.

30. Mehta SR, Yusuf S, Peters RJ, et al. Effects of pretreatment with clopidogrel and aspirin followed by long-term therapy in patients undergoing percutaneous coronary intervention: the PCI-CURE study. Lancet 2001;358:527–33.

31. Steinhubl SR, Berger PB, Mann JT 3rd, et al. Early and sustained dual oral antiplatelet therapy following percutaneous coronary intervention: a randomized controlled trial. JAMA 2002;288:2411–20.

32. CAPRIE Steering Committee. A randomised, blinded, trial of clopidogrel versus aspirin in patients at risk of ischaemic events (CAPRIE). CAPRIE Steering Committee. Lancet 1996;348: 1329–39.

33. Bhatt DL, Fox KA, Hacke W, et al. Clopidogrel and aspirin versus aspirin alone for the prevention of atherothrombotic events. N Engl J Med 2006;354: 1706–17.

34. Bhatt DL, Flather MD, Hacke W, et al. Patients with prior myocardial infarction, stroke, or symptomatic peripheral arterial disease in the CHARISMA trial. J Am Coll Cardiol 2007;49:1982–8.

35. Ferreiro JL, Angiolillo DJ. Clopidogrel response variability: current status and future directions. Thromb Haemost 2009;102:7–14.

36. Capranzano P, Ferreiro JL, Angiolillo DJ. Prasugrel in acute coronary syndrome patients undergoing percutaneous coronary intervention. Expert Rev Cardiovasc Ther 2009;7:361–9.

37. Brandt JT, Payne CD, Wiviott SD, et al. A comparison of prasugrel and clopidogrel loading doses on platelet function: magnitude of platelet inhibition is related to active metabolite formation. Am Heart J 2007;153:66.e9–16.

38. Wiviott SD, Trenk D, Frelinger AL, et al. Prasugrel compared with high loading- and maintenance-dose clopidogrel in patients with planned percutaneous coronary intervention: the Prasugrel in Comparison to Clopidogrel for Inhibition of Platelet Activation and Aggregation-Thrombolysis in Myocardial Infarction 44 trial. Circulation 2007; 116:2923–32.

39. Wiviott SD, Braunwald E, McCabe CH, et al. Prasugrel versus clopidogrel in patients with acute coronary syndromes. N Engl J Med 2007;357:2001–15.

40. Roe MT, Armstrong PW, Fox KA, et al, TRILOGY ACS Investigators. Prasugrel versus clopidogrel for acute coronary syndromes without revascularization. N Engl J Med 2012;367:1297–309.

41. Capodanno D, Dharmashankar K, Angiolillo DJ. Mechanism of action and clinical development of ticagrelor, a novel platelet ADP P2Y12 receptor antagonist. Expert Rev Cardiovasc Ther 2010;8: 151–8.

42. Wallentin L, Becker RC, Budaj A, et al. Ticagrelor versus clopidogrel in patients with acute coronary syndromes. N Engl J Med 2009;361:1045–57.

43. Ferreiro JL, Ueno M, Angiolillo DJ. Cangrelor: a review on its mechanism of action and clinical development. Expert Rev Cardiovasc Ther 2009;7: 1195–201.

44. Harrington RA, Stone GW, McNulty S, et al. Platelet Inhibition with Cangrelor in Patients Undergoing PCI. N Engl J Med 2009;361:2318–29.

45. Bhatt DL, Lincoff AM, Gibson CM, et al, CHAMPION PLATFORM Investigators. Intravenous Platelet Blockade with Cangrelor during PCI. N Engl J Med 2009;361:2330–41.

46. Bhatt DL, Stone GW, Mahaffey KW, et al, the CHAM-PION PHOENIX Investigators. Effect of Platelet Inhibition with Cangrelor during PCI on Ischemic Events. N Engl J Med 2013;368(14):1303–13.

47. Angiolillo DJ, Firstenberg MS, Price MJ, et al. Bridging antiplatelet therapy with cangrelor in patients undergoing cardiac surgery: a randomized controlled trial. JAMA 2012;307:265–74.

48. Ueno M, Rao SV, Angiolillo DJ. Elinogrel: pharmacological principles, preclinical and early phase clinical testing. Future Cardiol 2010;6:445–53.

49. Welsh RC, Rao SV, Zeymer U, et al, On behalf of the INNOVATE PCI investigators. A Randomized, Double-Blind, Active Controlled Phase 2 Trial to Evaluate a Novel Selective and Reversible Intravenous and Oral P2Y12 Inhibitor Elinogrel versus Clopidogrel in Patients Undergoing Non-urgent Percutaneous Coronary Intervention; the INNOVATE-PCI Trial. Circ Cardiovasc Interv 2012;5:336–46.

50. Angiolillo DJ, Welsh RC, Trenk D, et al. Pharmacokinetic and pharmacodynamic effects of elinogrel: results of the platelet function substudy from the intravenous and oral administration of elinogrel to evaluate tolerability and efficacy in nonurgent percutaneous coronary intervention patients (INNOVATE-PCI) trial. Circ Cardiovasc Interv 2012;5:347–56.

51. Berger JS, Roe MT, Gibson CM, et al. Safety and feasibility of adjunctive antiplatelet therapy with intravenous elinogrel, a direct-acting and reversible P2Y12 ADP-receptor antagonist, before primary percutaneous intervention in patients with ST-elevation myocardial infarction: the Early Rapid ReversAl of platelet thromboSis with intravenous Elinogrel before PCI to optimize reperfusion in acute Myocardial Infarction (ERASE MI) pilot trial. Am Heart J 2009;158:998–1004.

52. Kleiman NS. Pharmacokinetics and pharmacodynamics of glycoprotein IIb-IIIa inhibitors. Am Heart J 1999;138:263–75.

53. The EPISTENT Investigators. Randomised placebo-controlled and balloon-angioplasty-controlled trial to assess safety of coronary stenting with use of platelet glycoprotein-IIb/IIIa blockade. Lancet 1998;352:87–92.

54. Use of a monoclonal antibody directed against the platelet glycoprotein IIb/IIIa receptor in high-risk coronary angioplasty. The EPIC Investigation. N Engl J Med 1994;330:956–61.

55. Platelet glycoprotein IIb/IIIa receptor blockade and low-dose heparin during percutaneous coronary revascularization. The EPILOG Investigators. N Engl J Med 1997;336:1689–96.

56. Stone GW, Grines CL, Cox DA, et al. Comparison of angioplasty with stenting, with or without abciximab, in acute myocardial infarction. N Engl J Med 2002;346:957–66.

57. Kastrati A, Mehilli J, Schuhlen H, et al. A clinical trial of abciximab in elective percutaneous coronary intervention after pretreatment with clopidogrel. N Engl J Med 2004;350:232–8.

58. Kastrati A, Mehilli J, Neumann FJ, et al. Abciximab in patients with acute coronary syndromes undergoing percutaneous coronary intervention after clopidogrel pretreatment: the ISAR-REACT 2 randomized trial. JAMA 2006;295:1531–8.

59. Mehilli J, Kastrati A, Schulz S, et al, Bavarian Reperfusion Alternatives Evaluation-3 (BRAVE-3) Study Investigators. Abciximab in patients with acute ST-segment-elevation myocardial infarction undergoing primary percutaneous coronary intervention after clopidogrel loading: a randomized double-blind trial. Circulation 2009;119:1933–40.

60. Stone, Maehara A, Witzenbichler B, et al, INFUSE-AMI Investigators. Intracoronary abciximab and aspiration thrombectomy in patients with large anterior myocardial infarction: the INFUSE-AMI randomized trial. JAMA 2012;307:1817–26.

61. Randomised placebo-controlled trial of effect of eptifibatide on complications of percutaneous coronary intervention: IMPACT-II. Integrilin to Minimise Platelet Aggregation and Coronary Thrombosis-II. Lancet 1997;349:1422–8.

62. Inhibition of platelet glycoprotein IIb/IIIa with eptifibatide in patients with acute coronary syndromes. The PURSUIT Trial Investigators. Platelet Glycoprotein IIb/IIIa in Unstable Angina: Receptor Suppression Using Integrilin Therapy. N Engl J Med 1998; 339:436–43.

63. ESPRIT Investigators. Enhanced Suppression of the Platelet IIb/IIIa Receptor with Integrilin Therapy. Novel dosing regimen of eptifibatide in planned coronary stent implantation (ESPRIT): a randomised, placebo-controlled trial. Lancet 2000;356: 2037–44.

64. Giugliano RP, White JA, Bode C, et al. Early versus delayed, provisional eptifibatide in acute coronary syndromes. N Engl J Med 2009;360:2176–90.

65. Inhibition of the platelet glycoprotein IIb/IIIa receptor with tirofiban in unstable angina and non-Q-wave myocardial infarction. Platelet Receptor Inhibition in Ischemic Syndrome Management in Patients Limited by Unstable Signs and Symptoms (PRISM-PLUS) Study Investigators. N Engl J Med 1998;338:1488–97.

66. Topol EJ, Moliterno DJ, Herrmann HC, et al. Comparison of two platelet glycoprotein IIb/IIIa inhibitors, tirofiban and abciximab, for the prevention of ischemic events with percutaneous coronary revascularization. N Engl J Med 2001; 344:1888–94.

67. Meadows TA, Bhatt DL. Clinical aspects of platelet inhibitors and thrombus formation. Circ Res 2007; 100:1261–75.

68. Angiolillo DJ, Capranzano P, Goto S, et al. A randomized study assessing the impact of cilostazol on platelet function profiles in patients with diabetes mellitus and coronary artery disease on dual antiplatelet therapy: results of the OPTIMUS-2 study. Eur Heart J 2008;29:2202–11.

69. Lee S, Park S, Kim Y, et al. Drug-eluting stenting followed by cilostazol treatment reduces late restenosis in patients with diabetes mellitus the DECLARE-DIABETES Trial (A Randomized Comparison of Triple Antiplatelet Therapy with Dual Antiplatelet Therapy After Drug-Eluting Stent Implantation in Diabetic Patients). J Am Coll Cardiol 2008;51:1181–7.

70. Aktas B, Utz A, Hoenig-Liedl P, et al. Dipyridamole enhances NO/cGMP-mediated vasodilator-stimulated phosphoprotein phosphorylation and signaling in human platelets: in vitro and in vivo/ex vivo studies. Stroke 2003;34:764–9.

71. Diener HC, Cunha L, Forbes C, et al. European Stroke Prevention Study. 2. Dipyridamole and acetylsalicylic acid in the secondary prevention of stroke. J Neurol Sci 1996;143:1–13.

72. Halkes PH, van Gijn J, Kappelle LJ, et al. Aspirin plus dipyridamole versus aspirin alone after cerebral ischaemia of arterial origin (ESPRIT): randomised controlled trial. Lancet 2006;367:1665–73.

73. Sacco RL, Diener HC, Yusuf S, et al. Aspirin and extended-release dipyridamole versus clopidogrel for recurrent stroke. N Engl J Med 2008;359: 1238–51.

74. Angiolillo DJ, Capodanno D, Goto S. Platelet thrombin receptor antagonism and atherothrombosis. Eur Heart J 2010;31:17–28.

75. Tricoci P, Huang Z, Held C, et al, The TRACER Investigators. Thrombin-Receptor Antagonist Vorapaxar in Acute Coronary Syndromes. N Engl J Med 2012;366:20–33.

76. Morrow DA, Braunwald E, Bonaca MP, et al, TRA 2P–TIMI 50 Steering Committee and Investigators. Vorapaxar in the secondary prevention of atherothrombotic events. N Engl J Med 2012;366: 1404–13.

77. Morrow DA, Alberts MJ, Mohr JP, et al, For the Thrombin Receptor Antagonist in Secondary Prevention of Atherothrombotic Ischemic Events—TIMI 50 Steering Committee and Investigators. Efficacy and Safety of Vorapaxar in Patients With Prior Ischemic Stroke. Stroke 2013;44(3): 691–8.

78. Scirica BM, Bonaca MP, Braunwald E, et al, TRA 2P-TIMI 50 Steering Committee Investigators. Vorapaxar for secondary prevention of thrombotic events for patients with previous myocardial infarction: a prespecified subgroup analysis of the TRA 2P-TIMI 50 trial. Lancet 2012;380: 1317–24.

79. Bonaca MP, Morrow DA, Braunwald E. Vorapaxar for secondary prevention in patients with peripheral artery disease: Results from the peripheral artery disease cohort of the TRA 2P-TIMI 50 trial. American Heart Association Emerging Science Series Report. Available at: http://my.americanheart.org/professional/Sessions/AdditionalMeetings/EmergingScienceSeries/2012-Emerging-Science-Series%C2%97-June-20-2012_UCM_441183_Article.jsp. Accessed June, 2012.

80. O'Donoghue ML, Bhatt DL, Wiviott SD, et al, LANCELOT-ACS Investigators. Safety and tolerability of atopaxar in the treatment of patients with acute coronary syndromes: the lessons from antagonizing the cellular effects of Thrombin—Acute Coronary Syndromes Trial. Circulation 2011;123:1843–53.

81. Wiviott SD, Flather MD, O'Donoghue ML, et al, LANCELOT-CAD Investigators. Randomized trial of atopaxar in the treatment of patients with coronary artery disease: the lessons from antagonizing the cellular effect of Thrombin–Coronary Artery Disease Trial. Circulation 2011;123:1854–63.

82. Capodanno D, Bhatt DL, Goto S, et al. Safety and efficacy of protease-activated receptor-1 antagonists in patients with coronary artery disease: a meta-analysis of randomized clinical trials. J Thromb Haemost 2012;10:2006–15.

83. Chamorro A. TP receptor antagonism: a new concept in atherothrombosis and stroke prevention. Cerebrovasc Dis 2009;27(Suppl 3):20–7.

84. Eikelboom JW, Weitz JI. New anticoagulants. Circulation 2010;121:1523–32.

85. Bjork I, Lindahl U. Mechanism of the anticoagulant action of heparin. Mol Cell Biochem 1982; 48:161–82.

86. Choay J, Petitou M, Lormeau JC, et al. Structure-activity relationship in heparin: a synthetic pentasaccharide with high affinity for antithrombin III and eliciting high anti-factor Xa activity. Biochem Biophys Res Commun 1983;116:492–9.

87. Di Nisio M, Middeldorp S, Buller HR. Direct thrombin inhibitors. N Engl J Med 2005;353:1028–40.

88. Oldgren J, Budaj A, Granger CB, et al, RE-DEEM Investigators. Dabigatran vs. placebo in patients with acute coronary syndromes on dual antiplatelet therapy: a randomized, double-blind, phase II trial. Eur Heart J 2011;32:2781–9.

89. Witting JI, Bourdon P, Brezniak DV, et al. Thrombin-specific inhibition by and slow cleavage of hirulog-1. Biochem J 1992;283:737–43.

90. Lincoff AM, Bittl JA, Harrington RA, et al. Bivalirudin and provisional glycoprotein IIb/IIIa blockade compared with heparin and planned glycoprotein IIb/IIIa blockade during percutaneous coronary intervention: REPLACE-2 randomized trial. JAMA 2003;289:853–63.

91. Stone GW, McLaurin BT, Cox DA, et al, ACUITY Investigators. Bivalirudin for patients with acute coronary syndromes. N Engl J Med 2006;355:2203–16.

92. Stone GW, Witzenbichler B, Guagliumi G, et al. Bivalirudin during primary PCI in acute myocardial infarction. N Engl J Med 2008;358:2218–30.

93. Kastrati A, Neumann FJ, Schulz S, et al, ISAR-REACT 4 Trial Investigators. Abciximab and heparin versus bivalirudin for non-ST-elevation myocardial infarction. N Engl J Med 2011;365:1980–9.

94. Yusuf S, Mehta SR, Chrolavicius S, et al. Comparison of fondaparinux and enoxaparin in acute coronary syndromes. N Engl J Med 2006;354:1464–76.

95. Steg PG, Jolly SS, Mehta SR, et al. Low-dose vs standard-dose unfractionated heparin for percutaneous coronary intervention in acute coronary syndromes treated with fondaparinux: the FUTURA/OASIS-8 randomized trial. JAMA 2010;304:1339–49.

96. Yusuf S, Mehta SR, Chrolavicius S, et al. Effects of fondaparinux on mortality and reinfarction in patients with acute ST-segment elevation myocardial infarction: the OASIS-6 randomized trial. JAMA 2006;295:1519–30.

97. Sabatine MS, Antman EM, Widimsky P, et al. Otamixaban for the treatment of patients with non-ST-elevation acute coronary syndromes (SEPIA-ACS1 TIMI 42): a randomised, double-blind, active-controlled, phase 2 trial. Lancet 2009;374:787–95.

98. Mega JL, Braunwald E, Wiviott SD, et al, ATLAS ACS 2–TIMI 51 Investigators. Rivaroxaban in patients with a recent acute coronary syndrome. N Engl J Med 2012;366:9–19.

99. Alexander JH, Lopes RD, James S, et al, APPRAISE-2 Investigators. Apixaban with antiplatelet therapy after acute coronary syndrome. N Engl J Med 2011;365:699–708.

100. Povsic TJ, Vavalle JP, Aberle LH, et al, On behalf of the RADAR Investigators. A Phase 2, randomized, partially blinded, active-controlled study assessing the efficacy and safety of variable anticoagulation reversal using the REG1 system in patients with acute coronary syndromes: results of the RADAR trial. Eur Heart J 2012. [Epub ahead of print].

# Balance of Ischemia and Bleeding in Selecting an Antithrombotic Regimen

Bimmer E. Claessen, MD, PhD[a],*,
George D. Dangas, MD, PhD[b], Roxana Mehran, MD[c,d]

## KEYWORDS

- Bleeding - Ischemia - Antithrombotic drugs - Percutaneous coronary intervention
- Risk assessment - Individualized medicine

## KEY POINTS

- The risk of developing ischemic and bleeding complications should be evaluated in every patient undergoing percutaneous coronary intervention.
- In general, aggressive antithrombotic therapy is associated with a reduction in ischemic events but an increase in bleeding risk.
- The large number of currently available antithrombotic drugs allows extensive pharmacologic personalization.
- Novel antithrombotic agents are currently being evaluated in randomized clinical trials and may be a welcome addition to clinical practice in the near future.

## INTRODUCTION

In the United States, coronary revascularization by means of percutaneous coronary intervention (PCI) is performed more than 1 million times each year.[1] However, PCI has only been associated with improved clinical outcomes when performed for acute coronary syndromes (ACSs).[2,3] In patients with stable coronary artery disease, there is an ongoing debate concerning the clinical usefulness of PCI. Although PCI is strongly associated with relief of anginal complaints and a reduction in the need for medication,[4] no study to date has shown an improvement in terms of hard clinical end points (ie, cardiac or all-cause mortality). Therefore, minimizing the number of ischemic and bleeding complications after PCI is an important priority for interventional cardiologists.

Rates of adverse outcomes after PCI vary widely. In general, adverse outcomes are more common after PCI for ACSs compared with elective PCI. Moreover, rates of ischemic and bleeding complications tend to be lower in the selected patient populations of randomized clinical trials compared with unselected cohorts in observational studies.

Disclosures: Dr Roxana Mehran: Institutional Research Grant Support: The Medicines Company, Bristol-Myers Squibb/Sanofi and Lilly/Daichii Sankyo; Consulting: Abbott Vascular, Astra Zeneca, Boston Scientific, Covidien, Janssen (J+J), Regado Biosciences, Maya Medical, and Merck.
Dr George D. Dangas: Institutional Research Grant Support: The Medicines Company, BMS/Sanofi and Lilly/DSI; Consulting: Abbott Vascular, Astra Zeneca, Janssen (J+J), Regado Biosciences, The Medicines Company, BMS/Sanofi, and Merck.
[a] Department of Cardiology, Academic Medical Center, University of Amsterdam, Meibergdreef 9, Amsterdam 1105AZ, The Netherlands; [b] Department of Cardiology, The Zena and Michael A. Wiener Cardiovascular Institute, The Icahn School of Medicine at Mount Sinai, One Gustave L. Levy Place, Box 1030, New York, NY 10029, USA; [c] Department of Cardiology, The Icahn School of Medicine at Mount Sinai, One Gustave L. Levy Place, Box 1030, New York, NY 10029, USA; [d] Cardiovascular Research Foundation, 111 East 59th Street, New York, NY 10022-1202, USA
* Corresponding author.
E-mail address: b.e.claessen@amc.uva.nl

This article provides pharmacologic treatment strategies to optimize the safety and efficacy of PCI by minimizing the risk of ischemic and bleeding outcomes.

## DEFINITIONS OF MYOCARDIAL INFARCTION, RESTENOSIS, STROKE, STENT THROMBOSIS, AND BLEEDING

Uniform definitions of ischemic and bleeding complications of PCI are needed to adequately evaluate its safety and efficacy. However, until recently there was a large variability in these definitions. In 2007, an academic research consortium (ARC) proposed definitions for several ischemic events, and these definitions have subsequently been widely used in clinical research and practice.[5] Definitions of myocardial infarction (MI), restenosis, and stent thrombosis as proposed by the ARC are shown in Tables 1–3. No definition for stroke was provided by the ARC; however, a useful definition was used in the HORIZONS-AMI (Harmonizing outcomes with revascularization and Stents in Acute Myocardial Infarction) trial: an acute neurologic deficit resulting in death or lasting for more than 24 hours, as classified by a physician, with supporting information, including brain images and neurologic/neurosurgical evaluation.[6]

Before 2011, when standardized bleeding definitions were proposed by the Bleeding Academic Research Consortium (BARC), a wide variety of different definitions for bleeding were used such as those of Thrombolysis in Myocardial Infarction (TIMI),[7] Global Use of Streptokinase and Tpa for Occluded Arteries (GUSTO),[8] Global Registry of Acute Coronary Events (GRACE),[9] and many others. The BARC proposed an objective, hierarchically graded classification for bleeding, which is shown in Table 4. When used in ongoing and future clinical trials and registries, this definition will allow consistent reporting for bleeding events.

## OUTCOMES AFTER ISCHEMIC OR BLEEDING COMPLICATIONS

Both ischemic and bleeding complications are associated with an increased risk of mortality after PCI. A patient-pooled meta analysis of 3 randomized trials comparing bivalirudin and heparin in PCI (n = 17,034) reported a hazard ratio for mortality of 4.2 and 2.9 after TIMI major bleeding and MI, respectively.[10] This study also showed that not all types of bleeding have similar effects on mortality, because there was no increased risk of mortality after bleeding defined as a hematoma greater than or equal to 5 cm at the arterial access site. This finding has also been reported by 2 other studies.[11,12] Mortality is increased not only within the first 30 days after a bleeding event but also thereafter. In contrast, some studies have suggested that MI is only associated with increased mortality within the first 30 days after the event.[12] The novel BARC bleeding definition has been validated in a patient-pooled analysis of 6 randomized trials of patients undergoing PCI.[13] BARC class greater than or equal to 2 bleeding occurred in 9.9% of patients, and was associated with an increased 1-year mortality with an adjusted hazard ratio of 2.72.

It remains unclear how a bleeding event contributes to an increased risk of mortality even beyond the first month after the event. Several studies

**Table 1**
**Definition of MI**

| Classification | Biomarker Criteria | Additional Criteria |
|---|---|---|
| Periprocedural MI PCI | Troponin>3 times URL or CKMB>3 times URL | Baseline value <URL |
| Periprocedural MI CABG | Troponin>5 times URL or CKMB>5 times URL | Baseline value <URL and any of the following: new pathologic Q waves or LBBB, new native or graft vessel occlusion, imaging evidence of loss of viable myocardium |
| Spontaneous | Troponin>URL or CKMB>URL | — |
| Sudden death | Death before biomarkers obtained or before expected to be increased | Symptoms suggesting ischemia and any of the following: new ST elevation or LBBB, documented thrombus by angiography or autopsy |
| Reinfarction | Stable or decreasing values on 2 samples and 20% increase 3–6 h after second sample | If biomarkers increasing or peak not reached then insufficient data to diagnose recurrent MI |

*Abbreviations:* CABG, coronary artery bypass graft surgery; CKMB, creatine kinase MB; LBBB, left bundle branch block; URL, upper range limit.

**Table 2**
**Definition of restenosis**

| Angiographic Restenosis | Clinical Restenosis |
|---|---|
| Diameter stenosis of ≥50% | Diameter stenosis of ≥50% and 1 of the following:<br>1. A positive history of recurrent angina pectoris, presumably related to the target vessel<br>2. Objective signs of ischemia at rest (ECG changes) or during exercise test (or equivalent), presumably related to the target vessel<br>3. Abnormal results of any invasive functional diagnostic test (eg, coronary flow velocity reserve, fractional flow reserve <0.80; IVUS minimum cross-sectional area less than 4 mm$^2$ (and <6.0 mm$^2$ for left main stem)<br>4. A TLR with a diameter stenosis ≥70% even in the absence of the ischemic signs or symptoms mentioned earlier |

*Abbreviations:* ECG, electrocardiogram; IVUS, intravascular ultrasound; TLR, target lesion revascularization.

have reported suboptimal medical therapy in patients with bleeding events such as β-blocker and statin therapy or a reduction in the use of antiplatelet agents, as has been reported in the Prospective Registry Evaluating Myocardial Infarction: Events and Recovery (PREMIER) registry.[14,15] However, patient frailty and comorbidity have also been implicated as causal factors relating bleeding with an increased risk of mortality.

Stent thrombosis (ST) is a serious complication of intracoronary stenting and is associated with high rates of morbidity and mortality.[16–18] Recent studies have suggested that the timing of the ST event (eg, in hospital vs out of hospital, or early vs late/very late) is correlated with the risk of mortality. Early ST or ST occurring in hospital has been associated with worse clinical outcome compared with late/very late ST.[16,19,20]

## RISK ASSESSMENT OF PATIENTS FOR ISCHEMIC AND BLEEDING COMPLICATIONS

Risk factor for ischemic and bleeding events seem to overlap. Because ischemic events such as MI and bleeding are both associated with increased mortality after PCI, identifying patients at higher

**Table 3**
**Definition of stent thrombosis**

| Definite Stent Thrombosis | Probable Stent Thrombosis | Possible Stent Thrombosis |
|---|---|---|
| Angiographic confirmation of stent thrombosis<br>• The presence of a thrombus that originates in the stent or in the segment 5 mm proximal or distal to the stent, and at least 1 of the following within a 48-h time window<br>• Acute onset of ischemic symptoms at rest<br>• New ischemic ECG changes that suggest acute ischemia<br>• Typical increase and decrease in cardiac biomarkers<br>Pathologic confirmation of stent thrombosis<br>• Evidence of recent thrombus within the stent determined at autopsy or via examination of tissue retrieved following thrombectomy | Any unexplained death within the first 30 d<br>Irrespective of the time after the index procedure, any MI that is related to documented acute ischemia in the territory of stent thrombosis and in the absence of any other obvious cause | Any unexplained death from 30 d after intracoronary stenting |

**Table 4**
**Bleeding definition according to the BARC**

| | |
|---|---|
| Type 0 | No bleeding |
| Type 1 | Bleeding that is not actionable and does not cause the patient to seek unscheduled performance of studies, hospitalization, or treatment by a health care professional; may include episodes leading to self-discontinuation of medical therapy by the patient without consulting a health care professional |
| Type 2 | Any overt, actionable sign of hemorrhage (eg, more bleeding than is expected for a clinical circumstance, including bleeding found by imaging alone) that does not fit the criteria for type 3, 4, or 5 but does meet at least 1 of the following criteria: (1) requiring nonsurgical, medical intervention by a health care professional; (2) leading to hospitalization or increased level of care; (3) prompting evaluation |
| Type 3a | Overt bleeding plus hemoglobin reduction of 3 to <5 g/dL (provided hemoglobin reduction is related to bleed)<br>Any transfusion with overt bleeding |
| Type 3b | Overt bleeding plus hemoglobin reduction ≥5 g/dL (provided hemoglobin reduction is related to bleed)<br>Cardiac tamponade<br>Bleeding requiring surgical intervention for control (excluding dental/nasal/skin/hemorrhoid). Bleeding requiring intravenous vasoactive agents |
| Type 3c | Intracranial hemorrhage (does not include microbleeds or hemorrhagic transformation; does include intraspinal)<br>Subcategories confirmed by autopsy or imaging or lumbar puncture<br>Intraocular bleed compromising vision |
| Type 4 | CABG-related bleeding<br>Perioperative intracranial bleeding within 48 h<br>Reoperation after closure of sternotomy for the purpose of controlling bleeding<br>Transfusion of ≥5 U whole blood or packed red blood cells within a 48-h period<br>Chest tube output ≥2L within a 24-h period |
| Type 5 | Fatal bleeding |
| Type 5a | Probable fatal bleeding; no autopsy or imaging confirmation but clinically suspicious |
| Type 5b | Definite fatal bleeding; overt bleeding or autopsy or imaging confirmation |

risk of these two types of complications may allow an individualized pharmacologic approach. Pocock and colleagues[21] investigated predictors of bleeding and MI in 13,819 patients with ACS undergoing an early invasive strategy randomized to heparin plus a glycoprotein IIb/IIIa inhibitor (GPI), bivalirudin plus a GPI, or bivalirudin monotherapy. Predictors of both MI and bleeding included older age and ST-segment deviation greater than or equal to 1 mm at baseline. Moreover, 3 predictors for MI were identified: increased baseline cardiac biomarkers, family history of coronary artery disease, and a history of a prior MI. In addition, there were 8 predictors of bleeding: female sex, baseline anemia, use of heparin plus a GPI compared with bivalirudin monotherapy, increased baseline serum creatinine, increased baseline white blood cell count, no history of a prior PCI, prior stroke and treatment with heparin plus routine upstream GPI compared with deferred selective GPI use. Therefore, estimating an individual patient's risk to develop ischemic complications and bleeding

complications may permit personalized clinical decision making. At present, a large number of risk scores exist for MI, mortality, ST, and bleeding that can be used to assess the risk profile of an individual patient. The GRACE[22] and TIMI risk scores for non–ST-segment elevation ACSs[23] and for ST-segment MI (STEMI)[24] can be easily accessed on the Internet and are widely used in clinical practice to assess the risk of ischemic events. In addition, **Table 5** shows a risk score that can be used to predict the risk of stent thrombosis in patients with STEMI undergoing primary PCI with stent placement.[25]

Two bleeding risk scores that may be particularly useful in clinical practice are the Randomized Evaluation of PCI Linking Angiomax to Reduced Clinical Events (REPLACE) 2/Acute Catheterization and Urgent Intervention Triage Strategy (ACUITY)/ Harmonizing Outcomes with Revascularization and Stents in Acute Myocardial Infarction (HORI-ZONS-AMI) PCI bleeding risk score,[10] and the HAS-BLED risk score, which can be useful in

**Table 5**
**Integer-based risk score for 1-year definite/probable ST in patients with acute coronary syndromes**

| Variable | Integer Assignment for ST Risk Score Calculation | | |
|---|---|---|---|
| Type of acute coronary syndrome | NSTE-ACS without ST changes: +1 | NSTE-ACS with ST deviation: +2 | STEMI: +4 |
| Current smoking | Yes: +1 | | No: +0 |
| Insulin-treated diabetes mellitus | Yes: +2 | | No: +0 |
| History of PCI | Yes: +1 | | No: +0 |
| Baseline platelet count | <250 K/μL: +0 | 250 K/μL–400 K/μL: +1 | >400 K/μL: +2 |
| Absence of early (pre-PCI) heparin[a] | Yes: +1 | | No: 0 |
| Aneurysm or ulceration | Yes: +2 | | No: 0 |
| Baseline TIMI flow grade 0/1 | Yes: +1 | | No: 0 |
| Final TIMI flow grade less than 3 | Yes: +1 | | No: 0 |
| Number of vessels treated | 1 vessel: +0 | 2 vessels: +1 | 3 vessels: +2 |

*Abbreviation:* NSTE-ACS, non–ST-segment elevation ACS.
[a] Includes parenteral heparin or low-molecular-weight heparin.

patients already treated with warfarin for atrial fibrillation.[26] **Table 6** shows the variables of which the aforementioned risk scores consist.

## PHARMACOLOGIC STRATEGIES TO REDUCE ISCHEMIC AND BLEEDING COMPLICATIONS
### Antithrombotic Therapies

Antithrombotic therapy in PCI is focused on minimizing thrombotic complications while limiting the number of bleeding events. **Box 1** shows an overview of currently available antithrombotic drugs. At present, unfractionated heparin and bivalirudin (a direct thrombin inhibitor) are the most widely used antithrombotic drugs during PCI. Several studies have shown a reduction in bleeding compared with unfractionated heparin (with or without a GPI).[10,27–29] Moreover, some studies have reported increased survival with bivalirudin monotherapy compared with heparin with or without a GPI.[30–32] However, several recent meta-analyses suggest that the benefit of bivalirudin is limited to a decrease in bleeding.[27–29] Moreover, in HORIZONS-AMI, bivalirudin monotherapy was associated with an increase rate of acute ST despite the administration of a 600 mg clopidogrel loading dose in most patients.[32] At present, both bivalirudin (level of evidence [LOE] B) and unfractionated heparin (LOE C) hold a class I recommendation in the American College of Cardiology Foundation (ACCF)/American Heart Association (AHA)/Society for Cardiovascular Angiography and Interventions (SCAI) guidelines.[33] Bivalirudin is also an alternative for unfractionated heparin in patients with a history of heparin-induced thrombocytopenia.[34]

Fondaparinux, a pentasaccharide factor Xa inhibitor was compared with unfractionated heparin in patients with STEMI in the 12,092-patient Organization to Assess Strategies in Acute Ischemic Syndromes 6 (OASIS-6) randomized trial.[35] In this trial, fondaparinux was associated with a reduction in death or reinfarction at 3-month to 6-month follow-up. However, this benefit was limited to patients not undergoing primary PCI. In patients undergoing PCI there was a higher rate of guiding catheter thrombosis and more coronary complications such as abrupt coronary artery closure, no reflow, dissection, or perforation. Therefore, current guidelines state that fondaparinux should not be used as the sole anticoagulant to support PCI. The addition of an anticoagulant with anti-IIa activity is advised.[33]

In addition, enoxaparin (a low-molecular-weight heparin) can be used during PCI. Enoxaparin may be particularly useful in patients who have already received 2 or more therapeutic subcutaneous doses. An additional dose of 0.3 mg/kg of intravenous enoxaparin should be administered in patients who have received the last subcutaneous dose of enoxaparin more than 8 hours before PCI or who have received fewer than 2 doses before PCI.

### Antiplatelet Therapy: Aspirin and P2Y12 Inhibitors

An aspirin loading dose of 325 mg orally or 500 mg intravenously is administered before PCI. There is no consensus on the optimal dose of aspirin after PCI. However, several studies have shown a reduction in major bleeding when using a

**Table 6**
**Variables contributing to bleeding in risk scores**

**(A) REPLACE-2/ACUITY/HORIZONS-AMI PCI Bleeding Risk Score**

| | | | | | | | |
|---|---|---|---|---|---|---|---|
| Serum creatinine (mg/dL) | <1.0 (0) | 1.0–<1.2 (+2) | 1.2–<1.4 (+4) | 1.4–<1.6 (+6) | 1.6–<1.8 (+8) | 1.8–<2.0 (+10) | ≥2.0 (+12) |
| Age (y) | <50 (0) | 50–59 (+3) | | 60–69 (+6) | 70–79 (+9) | | ≥80 (+13) |
| Gender | | | Female (+5) | | | | |
| White blood cell count (×10⁹) | <10 (0) | 10–<12 (+1) | 12–<14 (+2) | 14–16 (+4) | 16–<18 (+5) | 18–<20 (+6) | ≥20 (+8) |
| Presentation | Normal biomarkers (elective and NSTEMI) (0) | | NSTEMI-raised biomarkers (+3) | | STEMI (+6) | | |
| Current cigarette smoker | | | Yes (+4) | | | | |
| Antithrombotic medications | Heparin + GPI (0) | | | Bivalirudin monotherapy (−6) | | | |

**(B) HAS-BLED Risk Score**

| | |
|---|---|
| Hypertension | +1 |
| Abnormal renal and liver function | +1 (for each) |
| Stroke | +1 |
| Bleeding | +1 |
| Labile INR | +1 |
| Elderly | +1 |
| Drugs or alcohol | +1 (for each) |

*Abbreviations:* ACUITY, Acute Catheterization and Urgent Intervention Triage Strategy trial; HORIZONS-AMI, Harmonizing Outcomes with Revascularization and Stents in Acute Myocardial Infarction; INR, International Normalized Ratio; NSTEMI, non–ST-segment elevation MI; REPLACE-2, Randomized Evaluation of PCI Linking Angiomax to Reduced Clinical Events 2; STEMI, ST-segment elevation MI.

**Box 1**
**Overview of currently available antithrombotic drugs**

*Parenteral anticoagulants*

Xa/IIa inhibitors:

  Unfractionated heparin

  Enoxaparin

Xa inhibitors:

  Fondaparinux

Direct thrombin inhibitors:

  Argatroban

  Bivalirudin

  Hirudin

*Enteral anticoagulants*

Direct thrombin inhibitors:

  Dabigatran

Xa inhibitors:

  Rivaroxaban

  Apixaban

  Edoxaban

  Otamixaban

  Rivaroxaban

*Parenteral antiplatelet agents*

Cyclooxygenase 1 inhibitor:

  Intravenous aspirin (Aspegic)

Glycoprotein IIb/IIA inhibitors:

  Eptifibatide

  Tirofiban

  Abciximab

P2Y12 antagonists:

  Cangrelor

*Enteral antiplatelet agents*

Cyclooxygenase 1 inhibitor:

  Aspirin

P2Y12 antagonists:

  Clopidogrel

  Prasugrel

  Ticagrelor

Proteinase-activated receptor 1 antagonists:

  Vorapaxar

low maintenance dose of aspirin (ie, <100 mg daily).[36–38] This finding may be explained by doses of as little as 50 mg of aspirin being able to block the enzyme cyclooxygenase 1 (COX-1) in platelets sufficiently to prevent platelet aggregation.[39] Higher doses of aspirin may increase the risk of developing gastro-intestinal bleeding by inhibiting COX-1 in gastric mucosal cells, which inhibits the production of protective prostaglandins.[40]

Clopidogrel, prasugrel, and ticagrelor inhibit platelet activation by antagonizing the adenosine diphosphate receptor P2Y12. Clopidogrel and prasugrel irreversibly inhibit P2Y12, whereas its inhibition by ticagrelor is reversible. Current guidelines recommend a loading dose of either 600 mg of clopidogrel, 60 mg of prasugrel, or 180 mg of ticagrelor before PCI.[33] After balloon angioplasty alone or bare-metal stent (BMS) implantation, P2Y12 inhibitors should be continued for 1 month. After drug-eluting stent implantation, P2Y12 inhibitors should be continued for at least 12 months. Therefore, BMS implantation may be preferred in patients at high risk of bleeding or likely not to be compliant.

Both prasugrel and ticagrelor have been associated with improved clinical outcomes compared with clopidogrel.[41,42] Clopidogrel is a prodrug that requires transformation by cytochrome P-450 (CYP) enzymes to establish its antiplatelet effect. Variability in CYP activity by common polymorphisms resulting in a reduced function has been associated with reduced circulating levels of the active metabolite of clopidogrel, diminished platelet inhibition, and a higher rate of ST.[43] Prasugrel also requires conversion to an active metabolite to act as an antiplatelet agent. However, prasugrel inhibits platelet aggregation faster, more consistently, and to a greater extent than clopidogrel in patients undergoing PCI.[44] Prasugrel was compared with clopidogrel in the large randomized Trial to Assess Improvement in Therapeutic Outcomes by Optimizing Platelet Inhibition with Prasugrel – Thrombolysis in Myocardial Infarction (TRITON-TIMI) 38 trial.[44] In this moderate-risk to high-risk ACS population, prasugrel was associated with a reduction in MI, urgent revascularization, and ST. However, prasugrel was associated with an excess in (fatal) bleeding. Subgroup analyses of TRITON-TIMI 38 have suggested an increased benefit of prasugrel in diabetic patients and patients with STEMI undergoing PCI.[45,46] Prasugrel is contraindicated in patients with a history of prior stroke or transient ischemic attack, and is only recommended in patients more than 75 years old if they have diabetes mellitus or a history of a prior MI.

Ticagrelor is not a prodrug but a direct-acting reversible P2Y12 inhibitor. It is dosed twice daily, whereas clopidogrel and prasugrel are dosed once daily. The 18,624-patient Platelet Inhibition and Patient Outcomes (PLATO) trial comparing ticagrelor with clopidogrel in patients with ACS showed a reduction in death from vascular causes (ticagrelor group 4.0% vs clopidogrel group 5.1%, P<.001) and death from any cause (ticagrelor group 4.5% vs clopidogrel group 5.9%, P<.001). Moreover, definite/probable ST (2.2% vs 2.9%) and MI (5.8% vs 6.9%, P = .005) were lower in patients randomized to treatment with ticagrelor.[41] There were no differences in the rate of overall major bleeding. However, there was a higher rate of major bleeding not related to coronary artery bypass graft surgery with ticagrelor (4.5% vs 3.8%). In patients undergoing PCI, the beneficial effects of ticagrelor were consistent with the overall results in the PLATO trial.[47,48] A post-hoc analysis of the PLATO trial investigating patients with chronic kidney disease has suggested that ticagrelor compared with clopidogrel significantly reduces ischemic end points and mortality with similar rates of major bleeding.[49]

### Antiplatelet Therapy: GPIs

In the current era of dual antiplatelet therapy, the role of GPIs is unclear, because most trials of GPIs in PCI were performed before the introduction of dual antiplatelet therapy. GPIs such as eptifibatide, tirofiban, and abciximab are intravenous antiplatelet agents that antagonize platelet aggregation by inhibiting the glycoprotein IIb/IIIa receptor. GPIs have been associated with an increased risk of bleeding and their use may therefore best be limited to patients not at high risk of developing bleeding complications.[28,50] Clinical trials in patients undergoing elective PCI pretreated with P2Y12 inhibitors have not shown any benefit of GPIs.[51,52] In patients with unstable angina or non–ST-elevation ACS, GPIs may be associated with a reduction in ischemic outcomes.[53] In addition, in patients with STEMI, the use of GPIs is generally limited to patients with large anterior MI or a large thrombus burden who have a high risk of ischemic events and a low risk of bleeding events. Moreover, bolus administration of GPIs can be considered as a bailout strategy in patients with a high risk of ischemic events but also a high risk of bleeding.

### New Oral Anticoagulants After PCI

Novel oral anticoagulant drugs are also being investigated after PCI. The Anti-Xa Therapy to Lower Cardiovascular Events in Addition to

---

**Box 2**
**Algorithm suggesting antithrombotic strategies according to bleeding and ischemic risk**

*Low bleeding risk, low ischemic risk*

Preloading with:

   Aspirin and clopidogrel

Anticoagulant therapy:

   Bivalirudin or unfractionated heparin

Antithrombotic therapy at discharge:

   Aspirin, clopidogrel

*Low bleeding risk, high ischemic risk*

Preloading with:

   Aspirin and prasugrel or ticagrelor[a]

Anticoagulant therapy:

   Heparin plus a glycoprotein IIb/IIIa inhibitor

   Bivalirudin

Antithrombotic therapy at discharge:

   Aspirin, prasugrel, or ticagrelor; consider low-dose rivaroxaban

*High bleeding risk, low ischemic risk*

Preloading with:

   Aspirin and clopidogrel

Anticoagulant therapy:

   Bivalirudin

Antithrombotic therapy at discharge:

   Aspirin, prasugrel, or ticagrelor[a]

*High bleeding risk, high ischemic risk*

Preloading with:

   Aspirin and clopidogrel, ticagrelor, or prasugrel[a]

Anticoagulant therapy:

   Bivalirudin

Antithrombotic therapy at discharge:

   Aspirin, prasugrel, or ticagrelor[a]

Consider:

   Low dose prasugrel (5 mg) and hybrid regiments with prasugrel or ticagrelor for 30 days before switching to clopidogrel

STEMI: prasugrel.
Non–ST-elevation ACSs: ticagrelor.
Prior stroke, <60 kg, ≥75 years, creatinine clearance <60 mL/min: ticagrelor instead of prasugrel.
   [a] General considerations to choose between prasugrel or ticagrelor.

Standard Therapy in Subjects with Acute Coronary Syndrome – Thrombolysis in Myocardial Infarction (ATLAS ACS-TIMI) 51 trial showed a reduction in death from cardiovascular causes, MI, or stroke in patients with a recent ACS with the addition of twice-daily 2.5 mg of the novel oral Xa inhibitor rivaroxaban.[54] The results of additional randomized clinical trials evaluating the use of oral anticoagulant drugs after PCI are eagerly awaited.

## SUMMARY AND RECOMMENDATIONS FOR CLINICAL PRACTICE

In general, a more aggressive anticoagulant regime is associated with a reduction in ischemic events at the cost of an increased risk of bleeding. It is therefore paramount that all patients undergoing PCI should be evaluated for risk of bleeding. Patients at a low risk of bleeding derive benefit from more aggressive antithrombotic therapy. However, patients at a high risk of bleeding benefit from selective use of antithrombotic agents. In contrast, the risk of developing ischemic complications should also be assessed, because patients undergoing PCI for ACSs may benefit from more effective antithrombotic therapy (especially in STEMI).[33]

**Box 2** shows a treatment algorithm suggesting antithrombotic therapeutic options in patients undergoing PCI according to their bleeding and ischemic risks. Many new antithrombotic drugs are still being investigated and there is a large variety of antithrombotic drugs currently available, allowing extensive pharmacologic personalization (see **Box 1**).

## REFERENCES

1. DeFrances CJ, Lucas CA, Vuie VC, et al. 2006 National hospital discharge survey. Hyattsville (MD): National Center for Health Statistics; 2008.
2. Keeley EC, Boura JA, Grines CL. Primary angioplasty versus intravenous thrombolytic therapy for acute myocardial infarction: a quantitative review of 23 randomised trials. Lancet 2003;361(9351): 13–20.
3. Mehta SR, Cannon CP, Fox KA, et al. Routine vs selective invasive strategies in patients with acute coronary syndromes: a collaborative meta-analysis of randomized trials. JAMA 2005;293(23):2908–17.
4. Bucher HC, Hengstler P, Schindler C, et al. Percutaneous transluminal coronary angioplasty versus medical treatment for non-acute coronary heart disease: meta-analysis of randomised controlled trials. BMJ 2000;321(7253):73–7.
5. Cutlip DE, Windecker S, Mehran R, et al. Clinical end points in coronary stent trials: a case for

6. standardized definitions. Circulation 2007;115(17): 2344–51.
6. Mehran R, Brodie B, Cox DA, et al. The Harmonizing Outcomes with RevasculariZatiON and Stents in Acute Myocardial Infarction (HORIZONS-AMI) Trial: study design and rationale. Am Heart J 2008; 156(1):44–56.
7. Chesebro JH, Knatterud G, Roberts R, et al. Thrombolysis in Myocardial Infarction (TIMI) trial, phase I: a comparison between intravenous tissue plasminogen activator and intravenous streptokinase. Clinical findings through hospital discharge. Circulation 1987;76(1):142–54.
8. An international randomized trial comparing four thrombolytic strategies for acute myocardial infarction. The GUSTO investigators. N Engl J Med 1993; 329(10):673–82.
9. Moscucci M, Fox KA, Cannon CP, et al. Predictors of major bleeding in acute coronary syndromes: the Global Registry of Acute Coronary Events (GRACE). Eur Heart J 2003;24(20):1815–23.
10. Mehran R, Pocock S, Nikolsky E, et al. Impact of bleeding on mortality after percutaneous coronary intervention results from a patient-level pooled analysis of the REPLACE-2 (Randomized Evaluation of PCI Linking Angiomax to Reduced Clinical Events), ACUITY (Acute Catheterization and Urgent Intervention Triage Strategy), and HORIZONS-AMI (Harmonizing Outcomes with Revascularization and Stents in Acute Myocardial Infarction) trials. JACC Cardiovasc Interv 2011; 4(6):654–64.
11. White HD, Aylward PE, Gallo R, et al. Hematomas of at least 5 cm and outcomes in patients undergoing elective percutaneous coronary intervention: insights from the SafeTy and Efficacy of Enoxaparin in PCI patients, an internationaL randomized Evaluation (STEEPLE) trial. Am Heart J 2010;159(1): 110–6.
12. Mehran R, Pocock SJ, Nikolsky E, et al. A risk score to predict bleeding in patients with acute coronary syndromes. J Am Coll Cardiol 2010; 55(23):2556–66.
13. Ndrepepa G, Schuster T, Hadamitzky M, et al. Validation of the Bleeding Academic Research Consortium definition of bleeding in patients with coronary artery disease undergoing percutaneous coronary intervention. Circulation 2012;125(11): 1424–31.
14. Suh JW, Mehran R, Claessen BE, et al. Impact of in-hospital major bleeding on late clinical outcomes after primary percutaneous coronary intervention in acute myocardial infarction the HORIZONS-AMI (Harmonizing Outcomes With Revascularization and Stents in Acute Myocardial Infarction) trial. J Am Coll Cardiol 2011;58(17): 1750–6.

15. Wang TY, Xiao L, Alexander KP, et al. Antiplatelet therapy use after discharge among acute myocardial infarction patients with in-hospital bleeding. Circulation 2008;118(21):2139–45.

16. Dangas GD, Claessen BE, Mehran R, et al. Clinical outcomes following stent thrombosis occurring in-hospital versus out-of-hospital: results from the HORIZONS-AMI (Harmonizing Outcomes with Revascularization and Stents in Acute Myocardial Infarction) trial. J Am Coll Cardiol 2012;59(20): 1752–9.

17. de la Torre-Hernandez JM, Alfonso F, Hernandez F, et al. Drug-eluting stent thrombosis: results from the multicenter Spanish registry ESTROFA (Estudio ESpanol sobre TROmbosis de stents FArmacoactivos). J Am Coll Cardiol 2008;51(10):986–90.

18. Iakovou I, Schmidt T, Bonizzoni E, et al. Incidence, predictors, and outcome of thrombosis after successful implantation of drug-eluting stents. JAMA 2005;293(17):2126–30.

19. Kimura T, Morimoto T, Kozuma K, et al. Comparisons of baseline demographics, clinical presentation, and long-term outcome among patients with early, late, and very late stent thrombosis of sirolimus-eluting stents: Observations from the Registry of Stent Thrombosis for Review and Reevaluation (RESTART). Circulation 2010;122(1): 52–61.

20. Lasala JM, Cox DA, Dobies D, et al. Drug-eluting stent thrombosis in routine clinical practice: two-year outcomes and predictors from the TAXUS ARRIVE registries. Circ Cardiovasc Interv 2009; 2(4):285–93.

21. Pocock SJ, Mehran R, Clayton TC, et al. Prognostic modeling of individual patient risk and mortality impact of ischemic and hemorrhagic complications: assessment from the Acute Catheterization and Urgent Intervention Triage Strategy trial. Circulation 2010;121(1):43–51.

22. Granger CB, Goldberg RJ, Dabbous O, et al. Predictors of hospital mortality in the global registry of acute coronary events. Arch Intern Med 2003; 163(19):2345–53.

23. Antman EM, Cohen M, Bernink PJ, et al. The TIMI risk score for unstable angina/non-ST elevation MI: A method for prognostication and therapeutic decision making. JAMA 2000;284(7):835–42.

24. Morrow DA, Antman EM, Charlesworth A, et al. TIMI risk score for ST-elevation myocardial infarction: a convenient, bedside, clinical score for risk assessment at presentation: an intravenous nPA for treatment of infarcting myocardium early II trial substudy. Circulation 2000;102(17):2031–7.

25. Dangas GD, Claessen BE, Mehran R, et al. Development and validation of a stent thrombosis risk score in patients with acute coronary syndromes. JACC Cardiovasc Interv 2012;5(11):1097–105.

26. Lip GY, Frison L, Halperin JL, et al. Comparative validation of a novel risk score for predicting bleeding risk in anticoagulated patients with atrial fibrillation: the HAS-BLED (Hypertension, Abnormal Renal/Liver Function, Stroke, Bleeding History or Predisposition, Labile INR, Elderly, Drugs/Alcohol Concomitantly) score. J Am Coll Cardiol 2011;57(2):173–80.

27. Lee MS, Liao H, Yang T, et al. Comparison of bivalirudin versus heparin plus glycoprotein IIb/IIIa inhibitors in patients undergoing an invasive strategy: a meta-analysis of randomized clinical trials. Int J Cardiol 2011;152(3):369–74.

28. De Luca G, Cassetti E, Verdoia M, et al. Bivalirudin as compared to unfractionated heparin among patients undergoing coronary angioplasty: a meta-analysis of randomised trials. Thromb Haemost 2009;102(3):428–36.

29. Bertrand OF, Jolly SS, Rao SV, et al. Meta-analysis comparing bivalirudin versus heparin monotherapy on ischemic and bleeding outcomes after percutaneous coronary intervention. Am J Cardiol 2012; 110(4):599–606.

30. Lemesle G, De Labriolle A, Bonello L, et al. Impact of bivalirudin on in-hospital bleeding and six-month outcomes in octogenarians undergoing percutaneous coronary intervention. Catheter Cardiovasc Interv 2009;74(3):428–35.

31. Bangalore S, Cohen DJ, Kleiman NS, et al. Bleeding risk comparing targeted low-dose heparin with bivalirudin in patients undergoing percutaneous coronary intervention: results from a propensity score-matched analysis of the Evaluation of Drug-Eluting Stents and Ischemic Events (EVENT) registry. Circ Cardiovasc Interv 2011; 4(5):463–73.

32. Stone GW, Witzenbichler B, Guagliumi G, et al. Bivalirudin during primary PCI in acute myocardial infarction. N Engl J Med 2008;358(21): 2218–30.

33. Levine GN, Bates ER, Blankenship JC, et al. 2011 ACCF/AHA/SCAI guideline for percutaneous coronary intervention. A report of the American College of Cardiology Foundation/American Heart Association Task Force on Practice Guidelines and the Society for Cardiovascular Angiography and Interventions. J Am Coll Cardiol 2011;58(24): e44–122.

34. Mahaffey KW, Lewis BE, Wildermann NM, et al. The anticoagulant therapy with bivalirudin to assist in the performance of percutaneous coronary intervention in patients with heparin-induced thrombocytopenia (ATBAT) study: main results. J Invasive Cardiol 2003;15(11):611–6.

35. Yusuf S, Mehta SR, Chrolavicius S, et al. Effects of fondaparinux on mortality and reinfarction in patients with acute ST-segment elevation myocardial

infarction: the OASIS-6 randomized trial. JAMA 2006;295(13):1519–30.

36. Mahaffey KW, Wojdyla DM, Carroll K, et al. Ticagrelor compared with clopidogrel by geographic region in the Platelet Inhibition and Patient Outcomes (PLATO) trial. Circulation 2011;124(5): 544–54.

37. Jolly SS, Pogue J, Haladyn K, et al. Effects of aspirin dose on ischaemic events and bleeding after percutaneous coronary intervention: insights from the PCI-CURE study. Eur Heart J 2009;30(8): 900–7.

38. Yu J, Mehran R, Dangas GD, et al. Safety and efficacy of high- versus low-dose aspirin after primary percutaneous coronary intervention in ST-segment elevation myocardial infarction: the HORIZONS-AMI (Harmonizing Outcomes With Revascularization and Stents in Acute Myocardial Infarction) trial. JACC Cardiovasc Interv 2012;5(12):1231–8.

39. Montalescot G, Maclouf J, Drobinski G, et al. Eicosanoid biosynthesis in patients with stable angina: beneficial effects of very low dose aspirin. J Am Coll Cardiol 1994;24(1):33–8.

40. Campbell CL, Smyth S, Montalescot G, et al. Aspirin dose for the prevention of cardiovascular disease: a systematic review. JAMA 2007; 297(18):2018–24.

41. Wallentin L, Becker RC, Budaj A, et al. Ticagrelor versus clopidogrel in patients with acute coronary syndromes. N Engl J Med 2009;361(11):1045–57.

42. Wiviott SD, Braunwald E, McCabe CH, et al. Prasugrel versus clopidogrel in patients with acute coronary syndromes. N Engl J Med 2007;357(20): 2001–15.

43. Mega JL, Close SL, Wiviott SD, et al. Cytochrome p-450 polymorphisms and response to clopidogrel. N Engl J Med 2009;360(4):354–62.

44. Wiviott SD, Trenk D, Frelinger AL, et al. Prasugrel compared with high loading- and maintenance-dose clopidogrel in patients with planned percutaneous coronary intervention: the Prasugrel in Comparison to Clopidogrel for Inhibition of Platelet Activation and Aggregation-Thrombolysis in Myocardial Infarction 44 trial. Circulation 2007; 116(25):2923–32.

45. Wiviott SD, Braunwald E, Angiolillo DJ, et al. Greater clinical benefit of more intensive oral antiplatelet therapy with prasugrel in patients with diabetes mellitus in the trial to assess improvement in therapeutic outcomes by optimizing platelet inhibition with prasugrel-Thrombolysis in Myocardial Infarction 38. Circulation 2008;118(16):1626–36.

46. Montalescot G, Wiviott SD, Braunwald E, et al. Prasugrel compared with clopidogrel in patients undergoing percutaneous coronary intervention for ST-elevation myocardial infarction (TRITON-TIMI 38): double-blind, randomised controlled trial. Lancet 2009;373(9665):723–31.

47. Cannon CP, Harrington RA, James S, et al. Comparison of ticagrelor with clopidogrel in patients with a planned invasive strategy for acute coronary syndromes (PLATO): a randomised double-blind study. Lancet 2010;375(9711):283–93.

48. Steg PG, James S, Harrington RA, et al. Ticagrelor versus clopidogrel in patients with ST-elevation acute coronary syndromes intended for reperfusion with primary percutaneous coronary intervention: a Platelet Inhibition and Patient Outcomes (PLATO) trial subgroup analysis. Circulation 2010; 122(21):2131–41.

49. James S, Budaj A, Aylward P, et al. Ticagrelor versus clopidogrel in acute coronary syndromes in relation to renal function: results from the Platelet Inhibition and Patient Outcomes (PLATO) trial. Circulation 2010;122(11):1056–67.

50. Stone GW, Moliterno DJ, Bertrand M, et al. Impact of clinical syndrome acuity on the differential response to 2 glycoprotein IIb/IIIa inhibitors in patients undergoing coronary stenting: the TARGET Trial. Circulation 2002;105(20):2347–54.

51. Valgimigli M, Percoco G, Barbieri D, et al. The additive value of tirofiban administered with the high-dose bolus in the prevention of ischemic complications during high-risk coronary angioplasty: the ADVANCE Trial. J Am Coll Cardiol 2004;44(1):14–9.

52. Kastrati A, Mehilli J, Schuhlen H, et al. A clinical trial of abciximab in elective percutaneous coronary intervention after pretreatment with clopidogrel. N Engl J Med 2004;350(3):232–8.

53. Kastrati A, Mehilli J, Neumann FJ, et al. Abciximab in patients with acute coronary syndromes undergoing percutaneous coronary intervention after clopidogrel pretreatment: the ISAR-REACT 2 randomized trial. JAMA 2006;295(13):1531–8.

54. Mega JL, Braunwald E, Wiviott SD, et al. Rivaroxaban in patients with a recent acute coronary syndrome. N Engl J Med 2012;366(1):9–19.

# Aspirin, Platelet P2Y12 Receptor Inhibitors, and Other Oral Antiplatelets

## Comparative Pharmacology and Role in Elective PCI

Vijay Kunadian, MBBS, MD, FRCP, FESC[a],*,
Hannah Sinclair, MBBS[a], Aaron Sutton[a],
George D. Dangas, MD, PhD[b]

KEYWORDS

• Antiplatelet agents • Percutaneous coronary intervention • Elective angioplasty

KEY POINTS

• Elective angioplasty is commonly performed for stable angina, and stent placement necessitates antiplatelet therapy to prevent stent thrombosis.
• Clopidogrel significantly improves outcomes after PCI, but platelet aggregation may be affected by genetic variability in response to clopidogrel.
• Few studies have evaluated the use of novel antiplatelet therapy after elective PCI.

## INTRODUCTION

Angina pectoris accounts for a large burden of disease worldwide, with an incidence of 3.9% in the United States in 2008.[1] In 2009, it accounted for 34,000 hospital discharges, with an average lifetime cost estimated at $770,000 (2006).[1] In 2009, 1,133,000 in-patient percutaneous coronary interventions (PCI) were performed in the United States.[1] Antiplatelet agents play a crucial role in inhibiting the platelet response to vascular injury after PCI. Antiplatelet agents are also essential in the longer term, because the metallic structure of stents is inherently thrombogenic. The earliest stent trials showed significant in-stent restenosis rate in up to a third of patients in the first 6 months without antiplatelet therapy.[2] This article examines the use of aspirin, P2Y12 inhibitors, and other oral antiplatelets in the setting of elective PCI.

## ANTIPLATELET AGENTS
### Aspirin

Aspirin (acetylsalicylic acid) is an analgesic, antipyretic, anti-inflammatory, and inhibitor of platelet aggregation (**Fig. 1**). It is manufactured by acetylating salicylic acid with acetic anhydride. It irreversibly acetylates the active enzyme site of fatty acid cyclooxygenase (mainly cyclooxygenase-1), thus inhibiting the formation of prostaglandins, prostacyclin, and thromboxanes.[3] Low-dose aspirin (75 mg/day) has been demonstrated

Disclosures: The authors have nothing to disclose.
[a] Faculty of Medical Sciences, Institute of Cellular Medicine, Cardiothoracic Centre, Freeman Hospital, Newcastle upon Tyne Hospitals NHS Foundation Trust, Newcastle University, Newcastle upon Tyne NE2 4HH, UK; [b] Icahn School of Medicine at Mount Sinai, One Gustave L. Levy Place, Box 1030, New York, NY 10029, USA
* Corresponding author. Faculty of Medical Sciences, Institute of Cellular Medicine, Newcastle University, 3rd Floor William Leech Building, Newcastle upon Tyne NE2 4HH, UK.
E-mail address: vijay.kunadian@ncl.ac.uk

Intervent Cardiol Clin 2 (2013) 527–535
http://dx.doi.org/10.1016/j.iccl.2013.05.010
2211-7458/13/$ – see front matter © 2013 Elsevier Inc. All rights reserved.

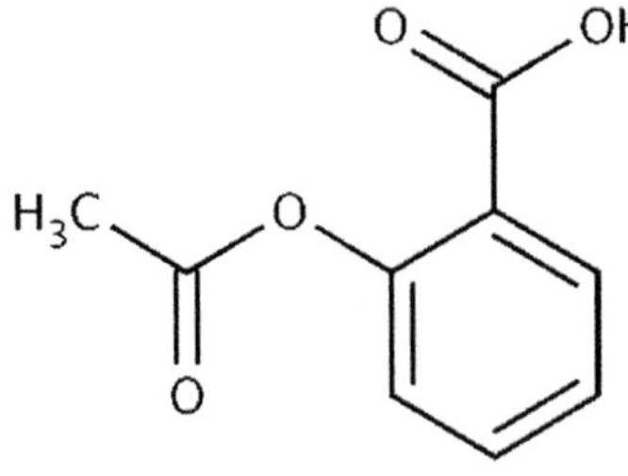

**Fig. 1.** Chemical structure of aspirin.

to completely inhibit platelet thromboxane production.[4]

The first studies evaluating aspirin therapy were performed in the balloon angioplasty era. Thornton and colleagues[5] compared warfarin with aspirin after percutaneous transluminal coronary angioplasty (PTCA) in the first randomized controlled trial to compare the two agents in patients undergoing elective PTCA. This study demonstrated a significant advantage with aspirin in preventing the need for repeat intervention, and also decreased anginal symptoms at 6 months. A meta-analysis by the Antithrombotic Trialists' Collaboration evaluated nine trials involving 3212 patients and demonstrated an unequivocal benefit from aspirin therapy in PCI.[6]

Weil and colleagues[7] demonstrated that low-dose aspirin doubles the risk of hospitalization for peptic ulcer bleeding compared with placebo. A total of 1121 patients with peptic ulcer bleeding were matched with hospital and community control subjects, and 12.8% had been regular users of aspirin.[7] Increasing dose of aspirin increased the risk of gastrointestinal (GI) bleeding, with an odds ratio (OR) of 2.3 for aspirin, 75 mg/day (95% confidence interval [CI], 1.2–4.4); 3.2 for 150 mg/day (95% CI, 1.7–6.5); and 3.9 for 300 mg/day (95% CI, 2.5–6.3).[7] In the Antithrombotic Trialists' Collaboration meta-analysis, there were no significant differences in rates of extracranial bleeding between aspirin less than 75 mg/day (OR, 1.7; 95% CI, 0.8–3.3); 75 to 150 mg/day (OR, 1.5; 95% CI, 1.0–2.3); and 160 to 325 mg/day (OR, 1.4; 95% CI, 1.0–2.0).

## Thienopyridines

The risk of stent thrombosis is highest when circulating blood is exposed to the bare metal of the stent before endothelialization of the stented segment. This led to the development of dual antiplatelet therapy (DAPT) regimens for a defined period of time after PCI. Thienopyridines irreversibly inactivate the platelet adenosine diphospate (ADP) receptor PY2Y12, preventing platelet aggregation and preventing amplification of the platelet

response to thrombin and thromboxane.[3,4] Ticlopidine and clopidogrel are prodrugs, metabolized to their active metabolites in the liver by cytochrome P-4501A.[4,8] They both exhibit time- and dose-dependent inhibition of platelet function, reaching a maximum of 40% to 60% inhibition of ADP-induced aggregation after 3 to 5 days.[8]

## Ticlopidine

Ticlopidine was the first thienopyridine to be evaluated in elective PCI (**Fig. 2**). The Stent Anticoagulation Restenosis Study trial[9] randomized 1965 patients undergoing elective PCI to aspirin alone, aspirin and warfarin, or aspirin and ticlopidine. The primary end point (death, revascularization, angiographic evidence of thrombosis, or myocardial infarction [MI] within 30 days) was seen in 3.6% of those receiving aspirin alone, 2.7% of those on aspirin and warfarin, and 0.5% of those receiving aspirin and ticlopidine (P = .001 for the comparison among all three groups). The group receiving aspirin and ticlopidine had a higher hemorrhagic complication rate (any procedure-related bleeding event requiring transfusion) than the group receiving aspirin alone (5.5% vs 1.8%; P<.001) but a similar hemorrhagic rate to the aspirin and warfarin group (6.2%).

The Stent Anticoagulation Restenosis Study was followed-up by the Full Anticoagulation vs Aspirin and Ticlopidine after Stent Implantation[10] and Intracoronary Stenting and Antithrombotic Regimen[11] trials, evaluating mixed-risk patients (both elective PCI and unplanned procedures after failed PTCA). The Multicenter Aspirin and Ticlopidine Trial after Intracoronary Stenting evaluated high-risk patients (those who required stenting for thrombolysis in myocardial infarction [TIMI] grade 0 or 1 flow post-PTCA, coronary artery dissection post-PTCA, suboptimal result after stenting with residual stenosis >20%, and multiple stent implantations within the same vessel).[12] These studies confirmed superiority of DAPT over aspirin alone or aspirin plus anticoagulation (lower risk of death, MI, or repeat revascularization in the territory of the stented vessel), with a lower risk of bleeding. These benefits persisted for up to 12 months and were independent of stent design.[10–12]

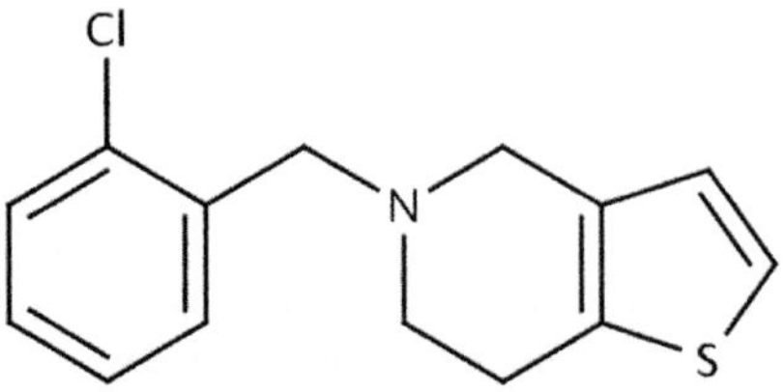

**Fig. 2.** Chemical structure of ticlopidine.

Despite the benefits, ticlopidine has an unfavorable side effect profile. GI side effects occurred in up to half of patients receiving ticlopidine, and skin rashes were also commonly reported.[8] More seriously, neutropenia occurred in 2.3% of patients, and there were several fatalities caused by this side effect.[13] Aplastic anemia and thrombotic thrombocytopenia were also reported. Use of ticlopidine has virtually disappeared since the Clopidogrel Aspirin Stent International Cooperative Study[14] demonstrated equivalent efficacy of clopidogrel and ticlopidine, with the former having a less unfavorable side effect profile.

## Clopidogrel

After the success of ticlopidine in reducing adverse events following PCI, clopidogrel (**Fig. 3**) was developed as a safer and more effective alternative. The Clopidogrel Aspirin Stent International Cooperative Study[14] evaluated the safety and efficacy of aspirin plus clopidogrel, 75 mg/day (with or without a loading dose of 300 mg) to aspirin plus ticlopidine among patients undergoing elective PCI. Forty-eight centers in eight different countries took part in randomizing 1020 patients undergoing elective PCI in this placebo-controlled, double-blind study. The primary end point (major bleeding, neutropenia, or thrombocytopenia) was reached in 9.1% in the ticlopidine group, 6.3% in the clopidogrel 75 mg/day group, and 2.9% in the clopidogrel loading dose group. This is a relative risk reduction of 50% (95% CI, 31%–81%; $P = .005$) between the ticlopidine and combined clopidogrel groups. There was a high rate of discontinuation of the drug in the ticlopidine group (8.2%), mainly caused by an increase in skin disorders, GI disturbances, and allergic adverse events. There were no significant differences in the rate of major adverse cardiac events (MACE) among the groups defined as death from a cardiac cause, MI, or repeat revascularization.

Several other trials corroborated these results, and these were collated in a meta-analysis by Bhatt and colleagues[15] in 2002. This showed a significant reduction in 30-day MACE (death, MI, target vessel revascularization, or subacute stent thrombosis) with clopidogrel compared with ticlopidine and a lower rate of discontinuation because of side effects.

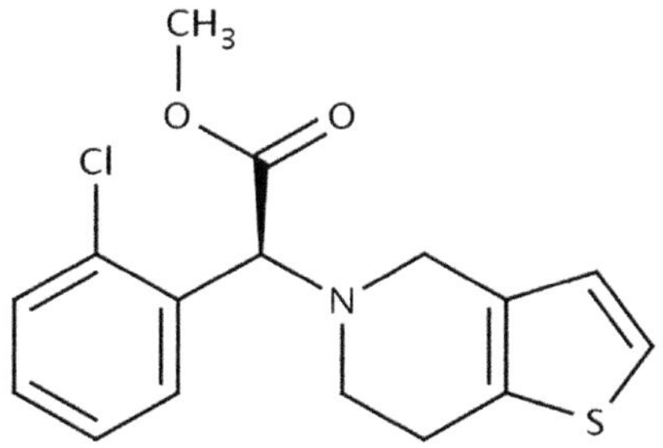

**Loading dose of clopidogrel in elective PCI** The Clopidogrel for the Reduction of Events During Observation[16] trial evaluated the long-term benefit of clopidogrel after stenting, and evaluated the benefits of a loading dose of clopidogrel before elective stenting for stable angina. A total of 2116 patients were randomized to receive a loading dose of 300 mg of clopidogrel or placebo 3 to 24 hours before PCI, and both groups continued 75 mg/day clopidogrel until Day 28. Patients then received either 75 mg/day clopidogrel or placebo until 12 months. There was a nonsignificant reduction in MACE in the loading dose group (6.8% vs 8.3%; 95% CI, −14.2% to 41.8%; $P = .23$), but this became borderline significant when clopidogrel had been given more than 6 hours before PCI (relative risk reduction of 38.6%; 95% CI, −1.6% to 62.9%; $P = .051$). Only just over 60% of patients completed a full 12 months of either clopidogrel or placebo (mainly because of either patient choice or an adverse event), but analysis of the remaining patients showed a 26.9% relative risk reduction in death, MI, and stroke in the long-term clopidogrel group ($P = .02$). There was no significant difference in nonprocedure-related major bleeding between the two groups ($P = .28$).

**A 300- versus 600-mg loading dose of clopidogrel in elective PCI** Trials in acute coronary syndromes (ACS) have demonstrated benefit of a higher loading dose of clopidogrel. However, this does not seem to be the case in elective PCI. In a study of 400 patients who were randomized to receive either 300- or 600-mg loading dose of clopidogrel before elective PCI, there was no significant difference in MACE (combined death, MI, acute neurologic event, stent thrombosis, or repeat revascularization) with 300 mg (6% at 30 days) versus 600 mg clopidogrel (5%; $P = .826$).[17] There was also no difference in major bleeding with the higher loading dose (9% vs 8.5%; $P = 1.00$).[17]

**Interpatient variability in response to clopidogrel** As clopidogrel has become widely used in elective and nonelective PCI, several pitfalls have become apparent with its use. Particular attention has been paid to interpatient variability in response. The first large-scale study was published in 2005[18] and analyzed platelet aggregation in response to clopidogrel in 544 patients with documented vascular disease or recent cerebrovascular event, and those undergoing PCI. This

**Fig. 3.** Chemical structure of clopidogrel.

demonstrated a bell-shaped curve of patient-responsiveness to clopidogrel, and those with a low clopidogrel response have a higher risk of stent thrombosis.[19]

**Genetic polymorphisms** It has been hypothesized that genetic polymorphisms in the hepatic enzymes responsible for metabolism of clopidogrel are implicated in the variation in response to clopidogrel. It requires oxidation by cytochrome P-450 followed by conversion by paraoxonase enzymes to the active metabolite before it can inhibit platelet aggregation.[20] In the Impact of Extent of Clopidogrel-Induced Platelet Inhibition During Elective Stent Implantation on Clinical Event Rate study,[21] patients carrying the loss of function CYP2C19*2 polymorphism in the cytochrome P-450 enzyme had higher residual platelet aggregation after clopidogrel administration, and three times the risk of death and MI at a year after elective PCI. Patients with the QQ192 polymorphism in the paraoxonase enzyme PON1 had lower platelet inhibition and higher rates of stent thrombosis,[20] and there are also polymorphisms that increase the effect of clopidogrel and predispose to a greater risk of bleeding.[21]

**Drug interactions with clopidogrel** Drugs may also affect the metabolism of clopidogrel. Many statins are metabolized by the same P-450 enzyme (CYP3A4) as clopidogrel, but a post hoc analysis of the Clopidogrel for High Atherothrombotic Risk and Ischemic Stabilization, Management, and Avoidance trial[22] did not show a significant difference between patients receiving a CYP3A4-metabolized statin (mainly atorvastatin) and clopidogrel versus those who received a different statin (mainly pravastatin) in MI, stroke, or cardiovascular death (5.9% vs 5.7%, respectively; $P = .69$). Proton pump inhibitors were also implicated in clopidogrel-response variability in several observational trials, especially because they are often prescribed in conjunction with clopidogrel to reduce the risk of GI bleeding. The Clopidogrel and the Optimization of Gastrointestinal Events Trial[23] was a multicenter, double-blind, randomized controlled trial where patients received clopidogrel and either omeprazole or placebo. Those in the omeprazole arm had a significantly reduced rate of upper GI bleeding with no increased risk of cardiovascular events.[23]

**Platelet function tests** The clinical relevance of variability in clopidogrel responsiveness remains unclear. Patients with a low responsiveness to clopidogrel were studied in the Gauging Responsiveness with a VerifyNow Assay—Impact on Thrombosis and Safety trial.[24] A total of 2214 patients were randomized to high-dose (600 mg loading then 150 mg/day thereafter) or standard-dose (no additional loading and 75 mg/day) clopidogrel before PCI with drug eluting stents (for stable angina or non-ST elevation ACS). Platelet function was measured 12 to 24 hours post-PCI with the VerifyNow P2Y12 test, which measures ADP-induced platelet aggregation, and low responders to clopidogrel (defined as a P2Y12 reaction unit [PRU] >230) were enrolled in the trial. There were no significant differences between the two groups in terms of adverse cardiovascular events (death from cardiovascular causes, nonfatal MI, stent thrombosis; 2.3% in both groups; $P = .97$) or major bleeding (1.4% in the standard-dose group, 2.3% in the high-dose group; $P = .10$).

*Prasugrel*
Concerns regarding the variability in clopidogrel responsiveness led to development of third-generation thienopyridines, such as prasugrel (**Fig. 4**). Prasugrel is also a prodrug that requires metabolizing by cytochrome P-450 but has a more rapid onset of action than clopidogrel because of single-step rather than multistep activation.[25]

The Joint Utilization of Medications to Block Platelets Optimally trial[26] randomized 904 patients to either standard clopidogrel therapy (300-mg loading dose followed by 75 mg/day) or low-dose (40-mg loading dose followed by 7.5 mg/day), intermediate-dose (60-mg loading dose followed by 10 mg/day), or high-dose (60-mg loading dose followed by 15 mg/day) prasugrel. Patients then underwent elective or urgent PCI and the clinical end points at 30 days were MACEs (all-cause mortality, MI, stroke, recurrent ischemia requiring hospitalization, target vessel thrombosis) and non-coronary artery bypass grafting–related major bleeding. Bleeding rates in all groups were low but there were no significant differences between

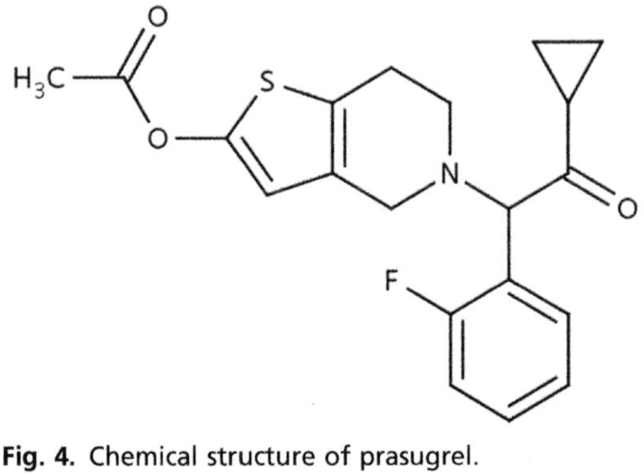

**Fig. 4.** Chemical structure of prasugrel.

groups (1.7% for combined prasugrel group vs 1.2% for clopidogrel). There was a nonsignificant trend toward a lower rate of MACE (7.4% vs 9.4%; $P = .26$) in the combined prasugrel group, but the study was not powered to detect a difference in clinical efficacy.

The Testing Platelet Reactivity in Patients Undergoing Elective Stent Placement on Clopidogrel to Guide Alternative Therapy with Prasugrel trial[27] compared prasugrel with clopidogrel in patients with low platelet responsiveness to clopidogrel. A total of 423 patients were randomized to either clopidogrel, 75 mg/day, or prasugrel, 10 mg/day, after elective PCI, and platelet reactivity was measured at 3 and 6 months by the VerifyNow assay. The prasugrel group demonstrated a consistent decrease in platelet reactivity at 3 months (median PRU was 80 in the prasugrel group at 3 months, vs 241 in the clopidogrel group; $P<.001$). However, there was a very low event rate so the study was unable to conclude whether the change in platelet responsiveness leads to a concomitant reduction in cardiovascular events.

Prasugrel in Comparison to Clopidogrel for Inhibition of Platelet Activation and Aggregation—Thrombolysis in Myocardial Infarction 44[28] was a multicenter, randomized, double-blind controlled trial comparing higher loading (600 mg and 60 mg, respectively) and maintenance (150 mg/day and 10 mg/day, respectively) doses of clopidogrel and prasugrel in 201 subjects undergoing elective PCI. Platelet aggregation measures (light-transmission aggregometry, VerifyNow assay, vasodilator-stimulated phosphoprotein), MACE (cardiovascular death, MI, stroke), and major bleeding rates were the primary end points. Measures of platelet function were significantly more favorable in the prasugrel arm (eg, inhibition of platelet aggregation with 20 μmol/L ADP at 6 hours after loading dose was 74.8% with prasugrel and 31.8% with clopidogrel, $P<.001$; and at 14 days was 61.3% vs 46.1%, $P<.0001$). There were low rates of MACE (3.6% vs 1.7%) and bleeding (2% vs 0%) in both arms, neither of which were statistically significant.[28]

Prasugrel is currently approved for clinical use in Europe and the United States for patients undergoing PCI for ACS only, at a 60-mg loading dose and 10 mg/day maintenance dose.

## NOVEL ANTIPLATELET AGENTS

Ticagrelor, cangrelor, and elinogrel directly and reversibly inhibit the P2Y12 receptor and are classed as cyclopentyltriazolopyrimidines. This reversibility and more rapid onset/offset of action are desirable, especially in patients who may have to undergo major cardiac surgery after angiography or PCI.

### Ticagrelor

Ticagrelor reversibly inhibits the P2Y12 receptor (**Fig. 5**) and does not require hepatic metabolism for its activity.[29] It has a shorter half-life and therefore requires twice-daily dosing.[29] There are currently no trials of ticagrelor in the setting of elective PCI; the main evidence for its use comes from the Platelet Inhibition and Patient Outcomes study consisting of patients with ACS.[30]

The Platelet Inhibition and Patient Outcomes study enrolled 18,624 patients with ACS and randomized them to ticagrelor (180-mg loading dose followed by 90 mg twice daily) or clopidogrel (300- to 600-mg loading dose followed by 75 mg/day). There was a lower rate of death, MI, and stent thrombosis in the ticagrelor group (9.8% vs 11.7%; 95% CI, 0.77–0.92; $P<.001$) and no significant difference in major bleeding between the groups (11.6 vs 11.2%; $P = .43$).[28] However, dyspnea and ventricular pauses were more common in the ticagrelor group.[30] It remains to be seen whether the benefits of ticagrelor are seen in a more stable PCI population.

### Cangrelor

Cangrelor is only available as a parenteral preparation but is a rapid-acting, reversible, direct P2Y12 receptor antagonist. The Cangrelor vs Standard Therapy to Achieve Optimal Management of

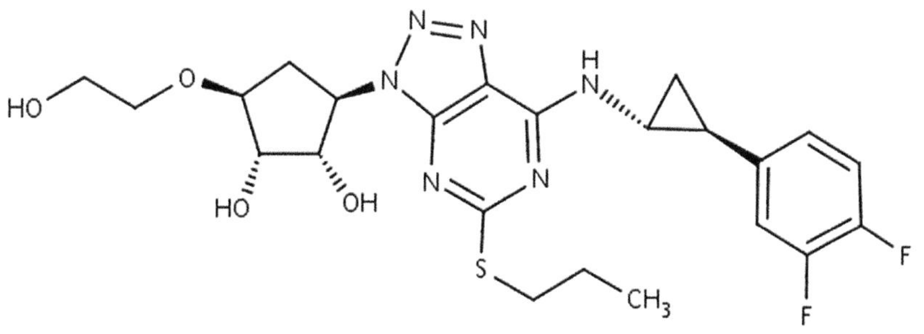

**Fig. 5.** Chemical structure of ticagrelor.

Platelet Inhibition PCI trial[31] recruited mainly patients with ACS, but 15% of subjects were those with stable angina undergoing PCI. It demonstrated that loading with cangrelor rather than oral clopidogrel before PCI was not superior in preventing all-cause mortality, MI, or revascularization at 48 hours (7.5% of patients receiving cangrelor vs 7.1% receiving clopidogrel; $P = .59$). Minor bleeding was more common with cangrelor (3.6% vs 2.9%; $P = .06$).[31] The trial was discontinued early because of futility.

In a previous randomized study among patients who discontinue thienopyridine therapy before cardiac surgery, the use of cangrelor compared with placebo resulted in a higher rate of maintenance of platelet inhibition (primary end point PRU <240; 98.8% vs 19%; relative risk, 5.2 [95% CI, 3.3–8.1]; $P<.001$). Excessive coronary artery bypass grafting surgery–related bleeding occurred in 11.8% versus 10.4% in the cangrelor and placebo groups, respectively (relative risk, 1.1 [95% CI, 0.5–2.5]; $P = .763$).[32]

More recently, in a double-blind, placebo-controlled trial, 11,145 patients who were undergoing either urgent or elective PCI and were receiving guideline-recommended therapy were randomized to receive a bolus and infusion of cangrelor or to receive a loading dose of 600 or 300 mg of clopidogrel. The rate of the primary efficacy end point (a composite of death, MI, ischemia-driven revascularization, or stent thrombosis at 48 hours after randomization) was significantly lower in the cangrelor group versus the clopidogrel group (4.7% vs 5.9%; adjusted OR, 0.78; 95% CI, 0.66–0.93; $P = .005$). The rate of the primary safety end point (severe bleeding at 48 hours) was not different between the two groups (OR, 1.50; 95% CI, 0.53–4.22; $P = .44$). Stent thrombosis was significantly lower in the cangrelor group versus the clopidogrel group (OR, 0.62; 95% CI, 0.43–0.90; $P = .01$). In this study, cangrelor significantly reduced the rate of ischemic events, including stent thrombosis, during PCI, with no significant increase in severe bleeding.[33]

### Elinogrel

Elinogrel is the only available reversible thienopyridine with both oral and intravenous formulations. Like ticagrelor, it does not require hepatic activation and has a half-life of around 9 to 12 hours.[34] The Intravenous and Oral administration of Elinogrel to Evaluate Tolerability and Efficacy in Non-urgent PCI trial[35] is a phase 2b study characterizing the safety, efficacy, and tolerability of elinogrel. In total, 652 patients undergoing elective PCI were randomized to receiving a loading dose of clopidogrel (either 300 or 600 mg at the discretion of the PCI operator) followed by standard 75 mg/day therapy, or elinogrel (randomized to loading doses of 80 mg or 160 mg intravenously) followed by 50, 100, or 150 mg/day oral therapy for 120 days. The 50 mg/day arm was discontinued early because it was deemed that there was an acceptable safety profile for the higher doses. Primary end points were major bleeding or MACE (death, MI, stroke, urgent revascularization, bailout glycoprotein IIb/IIIa use).

There was an increase in bleeding post-procedurally (3.8% vs 8.8%; OR, 2.42; 95% CI, 1.16–5.69) and longer term (6.7% vs 13%; HR, 1.98; 95% CI, 1.10–3.57) in the elinogrel arms. Elinogrel had similar discontinuation rates to clopidogrel, but had a higher frequency of dyspnea and deranged liver transaminases. Analysis of the MACE data showed a trend toward higher event rates in the elinogrel arm (HR, 1.82; 95% CI, 0.96–3.45), although this did not reach statistical significance ($P = .058$). However, the study results should be viewed with caution because it was not powered for efficacy.

## TESTING AND PERSONALIZED ANTIPLATELET THERAPY

Patients with a poor response to antiplatelet therapy carry a higher risk of MI, death, and stent thrombosis post-PCI.[21,36] The mechanisms leading to poor response are multifactorial.[37] However, patients with the reduced function CYP2C19 allele are significantly associated with high on-clopidogrel platelet activity,[38] indicating a poor response to the antiplatelet drug. Therefore, identification of this genotype may play an important role in implementing different therapeutic regimes to reduce nonresponders' risk.

### The VerifyNow Assay

Genetic testing is the gold standard to identify patients with the loss of function CYP2C19*2 polymorphism. However, the cost and time implication of this test are not suitable in the clinical setting and are more appropriate to research. The VerifyNow assay was found to be a suitable platelet function test to monitor response to clopidogrel.[39] Ono and colleagues[40] were able to determine cut off levels using the VerifyNow P2Y12 system for on-clopidogrel patients to predict carriers of CYP2C19 reduced-function allele in patients undergoing PCI. A total of 202 patients with stable coronary artery disease undergoing elective PCI were enrolled. All patients underwent CYP2C19 genotyping and measurement of residual platelet aggregation using the VerifyNow system. All patients were on DAPT; aspirin (100 mg/day); and clopidogrel (loading dose of 300 mg followed by 75 mg/day). A total of 65% of enrolled patients were carriers of CYP2C19 reduced-function allele. Platelet inhibition (measured by PRU) and percent inhibition were reduced in carriers compared with noncarriers (PRU, 290 ± 81.2 vs 217.6 ± 82.4, $P<.001$; percent inhibition, 17.9 ± 17.8 vs 35.5 ± 22.8, $P<.001$). Furthermore, multiple logistic regression analysis identified PRU and percent inhibition as significant predictors of carrier state (OR, 4.95; 95% CI, 2.49–9.85; $P<.001$; and OR, 5.55; 95% CI, 2.80–10.99; $P<.001$, respectively). This was based on cut off values for PRU and percent inhibition of 256% and 26.5% to identify carriers. These findings suggest that cut off levels of PRU and percent inhibition can be used to identify carriers of the CYP2C19 reduced-function allele, providing a more practical alternative to genotype testing.

### The ARMYDA-PROVE Study

The VerifyNow assay has identified other useful therapeutic parameters. Mangiacapra and colleagues[41] were able to identify a therapeutic window based on platelet activity in the Antiplatelet Therapy for Reduction of Myocardial Damage during Angioplasty–Platelet Reactivity for Outcome Validation Effort study. A total of 732 patients on DAPT undergoing elective PCI were recruited. All patients received clopidogrel (600-mg loading dose ≥6 h or a maintenance dose of 75 mg/day for at least 5 days before intervention). All patients were on aspirin (80–100 mg/day) before intervention and continued on it indefinitely postprocedure. Platelet reactivity was measured using the VerifyNow assay before PCI. The primary end point was the 30-day incidence of net adverse clinical events, defined as the occurrence of ischemic (death, MI, or target vessel revascularization) or bleeding events (major bleeding according to the TIMI criteria, or large entry-site hematoma), in relation to PRU distribution. PRU values could significantly discriminate between patients with and without bleeding events (area under the curve, 0.72; 95% CI, 0.65–0.80; $P<.0001$) and those with and without ischemic events (area under the curve, 0.68; 95% CI, 0.61–0.76; $P<.0001$).

The optimal cut offs for bleeding (PRU ≤178) and ischemic events (PRU ≥239) were used to define three groups: (1) low platelet reactivity (LPR) (LPR = PRU ≤178); (2) normal platelet reactivity (NPR) (NPR = PRU 179–238); and (3) high platelet reactivity (HPR) (HPR = PRU ≥239). The incidence of net adverse clinical events was 14.1% in the LPR group; 7.8% in the NPR group

($P = .025$ vs LPR group); and 15.4% in the HPR group ($P = .005$ vs NPR group). According to these results preoperative platelet function provides useful diagnostic information and may influence therapeutic approach.

The previously mentioned studies demonstrate the value of the VerifyNow assay on therapeutics in the PCI setting. Not only has it demonstrated that it can actively predict which patients have the reduced-function CYP2C19 allele and therefore correlate with clopidogrel nonresponders, but it has also provided an optimal platelet function level to reduce adverse events. Use of the VerifyNow assay could help tailor clopidogrel therapy reducing patients' risk of MI and death postelective PCI. By identifying nonresponders to clopidogrel it may justify use of novel P2Y12 receptor blockers, such as prasugrel and ticagrelor.[42] Testing can be used to ensure patients are in therapeutic window to reduce the risk of further ischemic or bleeding events. This may influence the way antiplatelets are prescribed post-PCI with titration of dose or change of antiplatelet to achieve optimal platelet reactivity.

### Mean Platelet Volume

An increase in mean platelet volume (MPV) has been demonstrated to be a significant predictor of cardiovascular adverse events including death in elective and urgent PCI.[43] Furthermore, an increase in MPV, particularly an increase in large reticulated platelets, has been associated with a decreased response to antiplatelet drugs.[36,37,44] Therefore, MPV may well be a predictor of clopidogrel responsiveness.[45] Currently, no large-scale studies have compared MPV as a predictor of poor clopidogrel response with either genetic testing or VerifyNow assay. This may be an important step in adapting antiplatelet therapy against antiplatelet response to patients in the community where MPV is readily available on all full blood counts. Furthermore, a recent study by Ang and colleagues[46] demonstrated that elevated plasma fibrinogen was independently associated with myocardial injury in on-clopidogrel patients undergoing elective PCI. This was significant regardless of platelet reactivity, measured using the VerifyNow assay score.

### SUMMARY

DAPT in elective PCI is now standard therapy and there is a wealth of evidence to support the use of aspirin and clopidogrel in this setting. Fears about the variability in response to clopidogrel have prompted the search for novel antiplatelets, although it remains to be seen whether this variability in platelet function corresponds to a difference in clinical outcome after PCI. The clinical use of novel antiplatelet therapy in the setting requires further evaluation.

## REFERENCES

1. Roger V, Go A, Lloyd-Jones D, et al. Heart disease and stroke statistics: 2012 update. Circulation 2012;125:e2–220.
2. Serruys PW, Strauss BH, Beatt KJ, et al. Angiographic follow-up after placement of a self-expanding coronary-artery stent. N Engl J Med 1991;324:13–7.
3. Meadows TA, Bhatt DL. Clinical aspects of platelet inhibitors and thrombus formation. Circ Res 2007; 100:1261–75.
4. Cattaneo M. Aspirin and clopidogrel: efficacy, safety, and the issue of drug resistance. Arterioscler Thromb Vasc Biol 2004;24:1980–7.
5. Thornton MA, Gruentzig AR, Hollman J, et al. Coumadin and aspirin in prevention of recurrence after transluminal coronary angioplasty: a randomized study. Circulation 1984;69:721–7.
6. Antithrombotic Trialists' Collaboration. Collaborative meta-analysis of randomised trials of antiplatelet therapy for prevention of death, myocardial infarction, and stroke in high risk patients. BMJ 2002; 324:71–86.
7. Weil J, Colin-Jones D, Langman M, et al. Prophylactic aspirin and risk of peptic ulcer bleeding. BMJ 1995;310:827–30.
8. Quinn MJ, Fitzgerald DJ. Ticlopidine and clopidogrel. Circulation 1999;100:1667–72.
9. Leon MB, Baim DS, Popma JJ, et al. A clinical trial comparing three antithrombotic-drug regimens after coronary-artery stenting. Stent anticoagulation restenosis study investigators. N Engl J Med 1998; 339:1665–71.
10. Bertrand M, Legrand V, Boland J, et al. Randomized multicenter comparison of conventional anticoagulation versus antiplatelet therapy in unplanned and elective coronary stenting. The full anticoagulation versus aspirin and ticlopidine (fantastic) study. Circulation 1998;98:1597–603.
11. Kastrati A, Schuhlen H, Hausleiter J, et al. Restenosis after coronary stent placement and randomization to a 4-week combined antiplatelet or anticoagulant therapy: six-month angiographic follow-up of the intracoronary stenting and antithrombotic regimen (ISAR) trial. Circulation 1997;96: 462–7.
12. Urban P, Macaya C, Rupprecht H, et al. Randomized evaluation of anticoagulation versus antiplatelet therapy after coronary stent implantation in high-risk patients: the multicenter aspirin and ticlopidine trial after intracoronary stenting (mattis). Circulation 1998;98:2126–32.
13. Gur H, Wartenfield R, Tanne D, et al. Ticlopidine-induced severe neutropaenia. Postgrad Med J 1998;74:126–7.
14. Bertrand ME, Rupprecht HJ, Urban P, et al. Double-blind study of the safety of clopidogrel with and without a loading dose in combination with aspirin compared with ticlopidine in combination with aspirin after coronary stenting: the clopidogrel aspirin stent international cooperative study (classics). Circulation 2000;102:624–9.
15. Bhatt DL, Bertrand ME, Berger PB, et al. Meta-analysis of randomized and registry comparisons of ticlopidine with clopidogrel after stenting. J Am Coll Cardiol 2002;39:9–14.
16. Steinhubl SR, Berger PB, Mann JT III, et al. Early and sustained dual oral antiplatelet therapy following percutaneous coronary intervention: a randomized controlled trial. J Am Med Assoc 2002;288: 2411–20.
17. Fernandez A, Aboodi M, Milewski K, et al. Comparison of adverse cardiovascular events and bleeding complications of loading dose of clopidogrel 300 mg versus 600 mg in stable patients undergoing elective percutaneous intervention (from the CADICE study). Am J Cardiol 2011;107:6–9.
18. Serebruany V, Steinhubl S, Berger P, et al. Variability in platelet responsiveness to clopidogrel among 544 individuals. J Am Coll Cardiol 2005;45:246–51.
19. Gurbel P, Bliden K, Samara W, et al. Clopidogrel effect on platelet reactivity in patients with stent thrombosis: results of the CREST study. J Am Coll Cardiol 2005;46:1827–32.
20. Bouman H, Schömig E, van Werkum J, et al. Paraoxonase-1 is a major determinant of clopidogrel efficacy. Nat Med 2011;17:110–6.
21. Trenk D, Hochholzer W, Fromm MF, et al. Cytochrome p450 2c19 681g>a polymorphism and high on-clopidogrel platelet reactivity associated with adverse 1-year clinical outcome of elective percutaneous coronary intervention with drug-eluting or bare-metal stents. J Am Coll Cardiol 2008;51:1925–34.
22. Saw J, Brennan D, Steinhubl S, et al. Lack of evidence of a clopidogrel-statin interaction in the charisma trial. J Am Coll Cardiol 2007;50:291–5.
23. Bhatt D, Cryer B, Contant C, et al. Clopidogrel with or without omeprazole in coronary artery disease. N Engl J Med 2010;363:1909–17.
24. Price M, Berger P, Teirstein P, et al. Standard- vs high-dose clopidogrel based on platelet function testing after percutaneous coronary intervention: the gravitas randomized trial. J Am Med Assoc 2011;305:1097–105.
25. Sugidachi A, Asai F, Ogawa T, et al. The in vivo pharmacological profile of cs-747, a novel antiplatelet agent with platelet ADP receptor antagonist properties. Br J Pharmacol 2000;129:1439–46.

26. Wiviott S, Antman E, Winters K, et al. Randomized comparison of prasugrel (cs-747, ly640315), a novel thienopyridine p2y12 antagonist, with clopidogrel in percutaneous coronary intervention: results of the joint utilization of medications to block platelets optimally (jumbo)-TIMI 26 trial. Circulation 2005;111:3366–673.

27. Trenk D, Stone G, Gawaz M, et al. A randomized trial of prasugrel versus clopidogrel in patients with high platelet reactivity on clopidogrel after elective percutaneous coronary intervention with implantation of drug-eluting stents: results of the trigger-PCI (testing platelet reactivity in patients undergoing elective stent placement on clopidogrel to guide alternative therapy with prasugrel) study. J Am Coll Cardiol 2012;59:2159–64.

28. Wiviott S, Trenk D, Frelinger A, et al. Prasugrel compared with high loading- and maintenance-dose clopidogrel in patients with planned percutaneous coronary intervention: the prasugrel in comparison to clopidogrel for inhibition of platelet activation and aggregation-thrombolysis in myocardial infarction 44 trial. Circulation 2007;116:2923–32.

29. Husted S, Emanuelsson H, Heptinstall S, et al. Pharmacodynamics, pharmacokinetics, and safety of the oral reversible p2y12 antagonist azd6140 with aspirin in patients with atherosclerosis: a double-blind comparison to clopidogrel with aspirin. Eur Heart J 2006;27:1038–47.

30. Wallentin L, Becker R, Budaj A, et al. Ticagrelor versus clopidogrel in patients with acute coronary syndromes. N Engl J Med 2009;361:1045–57.

31. Harrington R, Stone G, McNulty S, et al. Platelet inhibition with cangrelor in patients undergoing PCI. N Engl J Med 2009;361:2318–29.

32. Angiolillo DJ, Firstenberg MS, Price MJ, et al. Bridging antiplatelet therapy with cangrelor in patients undergoing cardiac surgery: a randomized controlled trial. J Am Med Assoc 2012;307:265–74.

33. Bhatt DL, Stone GW, Mahaffey KW, et al. Effect of platelet inhibition with cangrelor during PCI on ischemic events. N Engl J Med 2013;368:1303–13.

34. Ueno M, Rao S, Angiolillo D. Elinogrel: pharmacological principles, preclinical and early phase clinical testing. Futures 2010;6:445–53.

35. Welsh R, Rao S, Zeymer U, et al. A randomized, double-blind, active-controlled phase 2 trial to evaluate a novel selective and reversible intravenous and oral p2y12 inhibitor elinogrel versus clopidogrel in patients undergoing nonurgent percutaneous coronary intervention: the innovate-PCI trial. Circ Cardiovasc Interv 2012;5:336–46.

36. Buonamici P, Marcucci R, Migliorini A, et al. Impact of platelet reactivity after clopidogrel administration on drug-eluting stent thrombosis. J Am Coll Cardiol 2007;49:2312–7.

37. Angiolillo DJ, Fernandez-Ortiz A, Bernardo E, et al. Variability in individual responsiveness to clopidogrel: clinical implications, management, and future perspectives. J Am Coll Cardiol 2007;49:1505–16.

38. Price MJ, Murray SS, Angiolillo DJ, et al. Influence of genetic polymorphisms on the effect of high- and standard-dose clopidogrel after percutaneous coronary intervention: the GIFT (genotype information and functional testing) study. J Am Coll Cardiol 2012;59:1928–37.

39. Bouman HJ, Parlak E, van Werkum JW, et al. Which platelet function test is suitable to monitor clopidogrel responsiveness? A pharmacokinetic analysis on the active metabolite of clopidogrel. J Thromb Haemost 2010;8:482–8.

40. Ono T, Kaikita K, Hokimoto S, et al. Determination of cut-off levels for on-clopidogrel platelet aggregation based on functional cyp2c19 gene variants in patients undergoing elective percutaneous coronary intervention. Thromb Res 2011;128:e130–6.

41. Mangiacapra F, Patti G, Barbato E, et al. A therapeutic window for platelet reactivity for patients undergoing elective percutaneous coronary intervention: results of the ARMYDA-PROVE (antiplatelet therapy for reduction of myocardial damage during angioplasty-platelet reactivity for outcome validation effort) study. JACC Cardiovasc Interv 2012;5:281–9.

42. Nijjer SS, Davies JE, Francis DP. Quantitative comparison of clopidogrel 600 mg, prasugrel and ticagrelor, against clopidogrel 300 mg on major adverse cardiovascular events and bleeding in coronary stenting: synthesis of current-oasis-7, triton-timi-38 and plato. Int J Cardiol 2012;158:181–5.

43. Eisen A, Bental T, Assali A, et al. Mean platelet volume as a predictor for long-term outcome after percutaneous coronary intervention. J Thromb Thrombolysis 2013. [Epub ahead of print].

44. Guthikonda S, Alviar CL, Vaduganathan M, et al. Role of reticulated platelets and platelet size heterogeneity on platelet activity after dual antiplatelet therapy with aspirin and clopidogrel in patients with stable coronary artery disease. J Am Coll Cardiol 2008;52:743–9.

45. De Luca G, Secco GG, Iorio S, et al. Short-term effects of aspirin and clopidogrel on mean platelet volume among patients with acute coronary syndromes. A single-center prospective study. Blood Coagul Fibrinolysis 2012;23:756–9.

46. Ang L, Thani KB, Ilapakurti M, et al. Elevated plasma fibrinogen rather than residual platelet reactivity after clopidogrel pre-treatment is associated with an increased ischemic risk during elective percutaneous coronary intervention. J Am Coll Cardiol 2013;61:23–34.

# Role of Parenteral Agents in Percutaneous Coronary Intervention for Stable Patients

David A. Burke, MD, Duane S. Pinto, MD, MPH, FSCAI*

## KEYWORDS

- Anticoagulation • Heparin • Glycoprotein IIb/IIIa receptor inhibition • Abciximab • Eptifibatide
- Antithrombin • Bivalirudin

## KEY POINTS

- Despite significant improvements, it remains important to carefully select anticoagulant agents in the percutaneous treatment of coronary disease with the dual goal of decreasing ischemic events and minimizing bleeding complications.
- In the "elective" population, glycoprotein IIb/IIIa receptor inhibitors tend to be reserved for higher-risk patients, for those not adequately pretreated with thienopyridines, or for those with a suboptimal procedural outcome.
- Unfractionated heparin continues to be a mainstay in the elective PCI population because of its ease of use, simple monitoring, and reversibility.
- Enoxaparin has been shown to have reduced bleeding outcomes, with ischemic events comparable with those in unfractionated heparin in patients undergoing PCI.
- Bivalirudin has become a popular agent across the spectrum of coronary disease, having demonstrated consistent reductions in bleeding and comparable ischemic events when compared with a heparin plus glycoprotein IIb/IIIa receptor inhibitor strategy.

## INTRODUCTION

Optimal anticoagulation has proved to be a key component in the management of patients undergoing percutaneous coronary intervention (PCI). There has been a considerable evolution in pharmacotherapy for PCI since the early days of balloon angioplasty. Medications with variable modes of action are used to reduce complications by inhibiting thrombin formation, platelet activation, and platelet aggregation. These medications have targeted different portions of the coagulation cascade, and newer synthetic agents have been developed to specifically target factor Xa or thrombin in an attempt to minimize ischemic and bleeding complications, goals that are often at odds with one another.

The principal aims of pharmacotherapy during PCI are to avoid the adverse consequences related to iatrogenic plaque rupture from balloon inflation or stent deployment after PCI, and to reduce the risk of thrombus formation on intravascular PCI equipment during the procedure. Growing evidence supports use of a variety of agents in the setting of stable ischemic heart disease, unstable angina, non–ST-elevation myocardial infarction (NSTEMI), and ST-elevation myocardial infarction (STEMI).

Disclosures: The authors have no relevant conflicts of interest to disclose.
Division of Cardiovascular Medicine, Department of Medicine, Beth Israel Deaconess Medical Center, Harvard Medical School, Deaconess Road, Palmer 415, Boston, MA 02215, USA
* Corresponding author. Interventional Cardiology Section, 1 Deaconess Road, Palmer 415, Boston, MA 02215.
E-mail address: dpinto@bidmc.harvard.edu

Intervent Cardiol Clin 2 (2013) 537–551
http://dx.doi.org/10.1016/j.iccl.2013.06.004
2211-7458/13/$ – see front matter © 2013 Elsevier Inc. All rights reserved.

Most data involving newer antithrombotic drugs focus on their use in acute coronary syndromes (ACS). However, the main aims of this article are to summarize the agents available for anticoagulation during elective PCI, to outline their mode of action, and to review the evidence supporting their use.

## ANTIPLATELET THERAPY USING GLYCOPROTEIN IIB/IIIA INHIBITION

Platelet ability to adhere to abnormal surfaces and aggregate is mediated by surface membrane glycoprotein receptors that are expressed in increasing numbers with platelet activation and are potential targets for antiplatelet therapies. The platelet glycoprotein IIb/IIIa receptor plays a central role in platelet aggregation and thus forms an attractive target for therapy.

Abciximab, tirofiban, and eptifibatide are currently available for clinical use. Abciximab is a monoclonal antibody directed against the glycoprotein receptor, whereas tirofiban and eptifibatide are high-affinity non–antibody receptor inhibitors. The use of intravenous glycoprotein IIb/IIIa receptor inhibition (GPI) has been studied in patients with ACS and those undergoing intracoronary stent implantation, and has been associated with improved outcomes (**Fig. 1**).

The use of GPI in patients who are undergoing PCI depends on the clinical setting of PCI and the patient's risk for ischemic complications. Among patients undergoing elective PCI, considered low to intermediate risk for ischemic complications, the ISAR-REACT trial found no benefit for GPI at 30 days or in subsequent follow-up at 1 year in patients who had received clopidogrel (600 mg) at least 2 hours before the procedure.[1,2] The same lack of benefit was apparent for GPI in a subgroup analysis of lower-risk patients from the ESPRIT (Enhanced Suppression of the Platelet IIb/IIIa Receptor with Integrilin Therapy) trial.[3]

These trials were completed before the routine use of stents in patients undergoing PCI, before the use of clopidogrel prior to and/or at high dose before PCI, and before development of more potent oral antiplatelet agents. However, there is evidence that GPI did provide benefit among patients with ACS and some patients undergoing elective procedures (**Table 1**).

Based on available data, many operators limit the use of GPI in elective PCI to those patients considered higher risk, those who have not already received appropriate pretreatment with

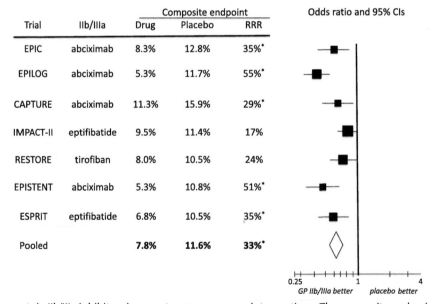

| Trial | IIb/IIIa | Composite endpoint | | | Odds ratio and 95% CIs |
| | | Drug | Placebo | RRR | |
| --- | --- | --- | --- | --- | --- |
| EPIC | abciximab | 8.3% | 12.8% | 35%* | |
| EPILOG | abciximab | 5.3% | 11.7% | 55%* | |
| CAPTURE | abciximab | 11.3% | 15.9% | 29%* | |
| IMPACT-II | eptifibatide | 9.5% | 11.4% | 17% | |
| RESTORE | tirofiban | 8.0% | 10.5% | 24% | |
| EPISTENT | abciximab | 5.3% | 10.8% | 51%* | |
| ESPRIT | eptifibatide | 6.8% | 10.5% | 35%* | |
| Pooled | | **7.8%** | **11.6%** | **33%*** | |

0.25 ————— 1 ————— 4
GP IIb/IIIa better    placebo better

**Fig. 1.** Glycoprotein IIb/IIIa inhibitors in percutaneous coronary interventions. The composite end point is the risk of death, nonfatal myocardial infarction, or urgent revascularization at 30 days. *Statistical significance at *P*<.05. In EPIC, the abciximab bolus plus infusion group was compared with the placebo group. In EPILOG, the abciximab plus low-dose heparin and the abciximab plus standard-dose heparin groups were combined. In IMPACT-II, the low-dose and high-dose eptifibatide groups were combined. In EPISTENT, the stent plus abciximab group was compared with the stent plus placebo group. CIs, confidence intervals; GP, glycoprotein; RRR, relative risk reduction. (*From* Sabatine MS, Jang IK. The use of glycoprotein IIb/IIIa inhibitors in patients with coronary artery disease. Am J Med 2000;109(3):227; with permission.)

**Table 1**
**Recommendations for antithrombin use**

|  | Recommendation | Class of Recommendation | Level of Evidence | Guideline |
|---|---|---|---|---|
| Unfractionated heparin | UFH should not be given to patients already receiving therapeutic SQ enoxaparin | III (Harm) | B | PCI |
|  | For UA/NSTEMI patients in whom an initial conservative strategy is selected, enoxaparin or fondaparinux is preferable to UFH as anticoagulant therapy, unless CABG is planned within 24 h | IIa | B | UA/NSTEMI |
|  | For patients with UA/NSTEMI who are managed conservatively and do not develop an indication for catheterization, continue UFH for 48 h if managed without PCI or CABG; otherwise discontinue | I | A | UA/NSTEMI |
| Enoxaparin | For PCI, additional 0.3 mg/mg IV dose if last SQ dose >8–12 h or <2 doses administered | I | B | PCI |
|  | PCI with enoxaparin may be reasonable in patients either treated with "upstream" SQ enoxaparin for UA/NSTEMI or who have not received prior antithrombin therapy and are administered IV enoxaparin at the time of PCI | IIa | B | PCI |
|  | For UA/NSTEMI patients in whom an initial conservative strategy is selected, enoxaparin or fondaparinux is preferable to UFH as anticoagulant therapy, unless CABG is planned within 24 h | I | A | UA/NSTEMI |
|  | Continue enoxaparin for duration of hospitalization, up to 8 d, if given before diagnostic angiography and no PCI or CABG | I | A | UA/NSTEMI |
| Bivalirudin | For patients undergoing PCI, bivalirudin is useful as an anticoagulant with or without prior treatment with UFH. | I | B | PCI |
|  | Either discontinue bivalirudin or continue at 0.25 mg/kg/h for up to 72 h at the physician's discretion if given before diagnostic angiography and no PCI or CABG | I | B | UA/NSTEMI |
|  | With HIT, it is recommended that bivalirudin or argatroban be used to replace UFH | I | B | PCI |

(continued on next page)

**Table 1**
*(continued)*

| | Recommendation | Class of Recommendation | Level of Evidence | Guideline |
|---|---|---|---|---|
| Fondaparinux | Fondaparinux should not be used as the sole anticoagulant to support PCI | III (Harm) | C | PCI |
| | For UA/NSTEMI patients in whom an initial conservative strategy is selected, enoxaparin or fondaparinux is preferable to UFH as anticoagulant therapy, unless CABG is planned within 24 h | I | A | UA/NSTEMI |
| | Continue fondaparinux for duration of hospitalization, up to 8 d, if given before diagnostic angiography and no PCI or CABG | I | A | UA/NSTEMI |
| | With a conservative strategy, in those patients who have an increased risk of bleeding, fondaparinux is preferable | I | B | UA/NSTEMI |
| Argatroban | With HIT, it is recommended that bivalirudin or argatroban be used to replace UFH | I | B | PCI |
| Glycoprotein IIb/IIIa inhibitors | Elective PCI patients treated with UFH and not pretreated with Clopidogrel, GPI can be used (abciximab, double-bolus eptifibatide, or high-bolus dose of tirofiban). | IIa | B | PCI |
| | If pretreated with clopidogrel, in elective patients using UFH, the level of evidence is less compelling | IIb | B | PCI |

*Abbreviations:* CABG, coronary artery bypass grafting; GPI, glycoprotein IIb/IIIa receptor inhibition; HIT, heparin-induced thrombocytopenia; IV, intravenous; NSTEMI, non–ST-elevation myocardial infarction; SQ, subcutaneous; STEMI, ST-elevation myocardial infarction; UA, unstable angina; UFH, unfractionated heparin.

antiplatelet therapy, or those who have a suboptimal angiographic result or angiographic complications during the procedure, so-called bailout. There is marked variation in opinion regarding the optimal duration of GPI infusion following PCI.

### Abciximab

Abciximab is the Fab fragment of the chimeric human-murine monoclonal antibody 7E3. With intravenous bolus, plasma concentrations decrease rapidly with an initial half-life of less than 10 minutes and second-phase half-life of 30 minutes, likely related to rapid binding to the platelet glycoprotein receptor. At highest dose, 80% of platelet glycoprotein receptors are occupied in 2 hours, and platelet aggregation is completely inhibited. On cessation, free plasma concentrations rapidly decrease over the first 6 hours and thereafter at a slower rate.

When initially studied in ACS, the patients invariably underwent angioplasty without stenting and thienopyridine therapy was not used. Several randomized trials were performed, and in a subsequent meta-analysis including more than 5400 patients from the EPIC,[4–6] EPILOG,[7,8] RAPPORT, EPISTENT,[9] and CAPTURE[10–14] studies who received percutaneous transluminal coronary angioplasty (PTCA), abciximab significantly reduced 30-day mortality and reinfarction (hazard ratio [HR] 0.52, 95% confidence interval [CI] 0.41–0.65).[15] A meta-analysis looking at STEMI patients who underwent PCI with stenting with abciximab or placebo included the RAPPORT,[9] ADMIRAL,[16,17] ISAR-2,[18] CADILLAC,[19] and ACE[20] studies. Abciximab showed a significant reduction in mortality at 30 days (2.4% vs 3.4% with placebo) and at 6 to 12 months (4.4% vs 6.2%), with no increased bleeding seen in these patients.[21]

In terms of patients with stable coronary heart disease undergoing PCI, 2 trials evaluated outcomes comparing abciximab with placebo in predominantly stable patients, and came to differing conclusions. EPISTENT randomized 2399 patients undergoing elective (approximately 40%) or emergent PCI to stenting alone, stenting with abciximab, or PTCA with abciximab.[22,23] All patients who received a stent were given aspirin and ticlopidine. Adverse events (death, myocardial infarction [MI], and urgent revascularization) at 30 days (10.8%, 5.3%, and 6.9%) and 6 months (11.4%, 5.6%, and 7.8%) were significantly lower in the abciximab groups, with the difference largely driven by reduced death and NSTEMI.

The ISAR-REACT study consisted of 2159 patients with stable coronary artery disease undergoing PCI with stenting and treated with aspirin and thienopyridine, who were randomized to abciximab or placebo. The 30-day rates of major adverse cardiac events (MACE) between abciximab and placebo were the same (both 4%), and major bleeding complications were comparable.[2] In the ISAR-REACT 2 trial, abciximab administration, among high-risk NSTEMI patients receiving clopidogrel with a 600 mg loading dose, was associated with a lower incidence of death, MI, or urgent revascularization (8.9% vs 11.9%, $P = .03$; relative risk [RR] 0.75, 95% CI 0.58–0.97), but the benefit was confined to those who with elevated troponin (13.1% vs 18.3%, $P = .02$; RR 0.71, 95% CI 0.54–0.95) compared with those who had a normal troponin level (4.6% vs 4.6%, $P = .98$; RR 0.99, 95% CI 0.56–1.76).[24]

### Tirofiban

Stable patients undergoing PCI were evaluated in the ADVANCE trial, which aimed to assess the potential benefit of using a higher dose of tirofiban than had been used in trials assessing the drug in the setting of ACS (RESTORE, PRISM, and PRISM-PLUS trials).[25–27] A total of 202 patients, pretreated with thienopyridines, were randomized to high-dose bolus tirofiban (25 μg/kg/3 min, and infusion of 0.15 μg/kg/min for 24–48 hours) or to placebo.[28] At 6 months, adverse events (death, MI, target vessel revascularization [TVR], or bailout GPI) were significantly less frequent with tirofiban (20% vs 35%, $P = .01$; HR 0.51, 95% CI 0.29–0.88), a difference driven by the incidence of MI and bailout GPI in the placebo group. In subgroup analysis, the benefit of tirofiban was significant among patients with ACS but not among those with stable angina.

A small study of 96 patients, the TOPSTAR (The Effect of Additional Temporary Glycoprotein IIb/ IIIa Receptor Inhibition on Troponin Release in Elective Percutaneous Coronary Interventions after Pretreatment with Aspirin and Clopidogrel) trial, was a randomized, double-blind, placebo-controlled study, and the first to observe that additional inhibition of platelet aggregation by tirofiban with aspirin and clopidogrel reduced periprocedural troponin release and the composite end point (death, MI, and TVR) after 9 months (2.3% with tirofiban vs 13.0% with placebo, $P<.05$).[29]

### Eptifibatide

Eptifibatide is a heptapeptide of the glycoprotein IIb/IIIa receptor that inhibits platelet aggregation. The plasma half-life is 10 to 15 minutes, and it is predominantly renally excreted (75%) with the remainder via hepatic pathways (25%) (**Table 2**).

More than 4000 patients were enrolled in the IMPACT-II (Integrilin to Minimize Platelet Aggregation and Coronary Thrombosis—II) study (59% with stable coronary disease), which randomized patients to either placebo or 1 of 2 doses of eptifibatide.[30] At 30 days, there was no significant difference in MACE between the groups, and eptifibatide did not increase rates of major bleeding or transfusion. By a treatment-received analysis, the lower dose regimen produced a significant reduction in the composite end point (11.6% vs 9.1%, $P = .035$), with reduced rates of abrupt closure and ischemic events at 30 days, but the higher dose produced a less substantial reduction (11.6% vs 10.0%, $P = .18$). The investigators believed that the doses studied appeared to be at the lower end of the efficacy-response curve, and that further investigation was needed.

The ESPRIT trial randomly assigned 2064 patients to placebo or eptifibatide immediately before elective PCI.[31] The trial was terminated prematurely because eptifibatide reduced the primary end point (48-hour death, MI, urgent revascularization, or bailout GPI) by 37% (6.6% vs 10.5%, $P = .0015$).

## COMPARISONS BETWEEN AGENTS

The TARGET study was designed to test whether tirofiban was not inferior to abciximab in patients undergoing elective PCI, but demonstrated that tirofiban offered less protection from major ischemic events than did abciximab (30-day MACE 7.6% with tirofiban vs 6.0% abciximab; HR 1.26, 95% CI 1.01–1.57, $P = .038$).[32]

The TENACITY (The Tirofiban Evaluation of Novel Dosing vs Abciximab with Clopidogrel and Inhibition of Thrombin) trial randomized patients undergoing elective PCI to abciximab or tirofiban, with all patients receiving aspirin and clopidogrel.

**Table 2**
Overview and dosing for antithrombin agents

| | Dose | Half-Life | Clinical Condition | Note | Trials |
|---|---|---|---|---|---|
| **Heparins** | | | | | |
| Unfractionated heparin | 60 U/kg IV bolus and 12 U/kg infusion adjusted to maintain PTT 50–70 s<br><br>Intermittent bolus dosing during PCI to maintain ACT >200–250 with GPI and >250–300 s for HemoTec or 300–350 s for Hemochron without GPI | — | Stable IHD<br>UA<br>NSTEMI Conservative and invasive<br>STEMI | Contraindicated with HIT<br>Avoid switching to LMWH<br>Continue if planned CABG<br>May use with fibrinolytic therapy although enoxaparin and fondaparinux superior | 6 small randomized studies vs placebo |
| Enoxaparin | 1 mg/kg SQ twice/day up to 100 mg/dose<br>For PCI, additional 0.3 mg/mg IV dose if last SQ dose >8 h or <2 doses administered but prior therapy administered<br>With fibrinolysis and age >75 y, 30 mg IV followed 15 min later by 1 mg/kg SQ every 12 h until hospital discharge for a maximum of 8 d.<br>For age >75 y, eliminate IV bolus and reduce maintenance to 0.75 mg SQ/BID, and if CrCl <30 mL/min reduce SQ dose frequency to daily irrespective of age | 4.5 h | Stable IHD<br>UA<br>NSTEMI<br>STEMI fibrinolysis | Reduce dose (1 mg per kg every 24 h) with renal failure (CrCl <30 mL/min)<br>Avoid switch to UFH<br>Avoid if CABG <24 h.<br>Discontinue 12–24 h before CABG and dose with UFH | ESSENCE/TIMI-11B, SYNERGY, ACUTE-II, INTERACT A to Z, ExTRACT-TIMI 25 |

| | | | | | |
|---|---|---|---|---|---|
| Dalteparin | 120 IU/kg SQ every 12 h (maximum 10,000 IU BID) | Approx. 2–5 h | IV GPI planned: target ACT 200 s using UFH. No IV GPI planned: target ACT 250–300 s for HemoTec; 300–350 s for Hemochron using UFH | — | FRISC, FRIC |
| **Glycoprotein IIb/IIIa inhibitors** | | | | | |
| Abciximab | For PCI, IV 0.25 mg/kg bolus administered 10–60 min before PCI, followed by infusion of 0.125 µg/kg/min (maximum 10 µg/min) for 12 h | Approx. 30 min | UA NSTEMI STEMI | No dose adjustment for renal or hepatic impairment | EPIC, EPILOG, RAPPORT, EPISTENT, CAPTURE, ADMIRAL, ISAR-REACT, ISAR-2, CADILLAC |
| Tirofiban | (Off-label) for PCI: IV loading dose 25 µg/kg over 3 min at time of procedure. Infusion 0.15 µg/kg/min continued for 18–24 h UA/NSTEMI: IV initial rate 0.4 µg/kg/min for 30 min, then continued at 0.1 µg/kg/min. Dosing through procedure and for 12–24 h postintervention | Approx. 2 h | UA/NSTEMI in combination with heparin STEMI (off-label) Elective PCI (off-label) | Reduce dose to 50% normal rate with renal failure (CrCl <30 mL/min) | ADVANCE, TOPSTAR |
| Eptifibatide | PCI: IV bolus 180 µg/kg immediately before PCI, with infusion 2 µg/kg/min. Second bolus 180 µg/kg 10 min after first bolus. Infusion for 18–24 h. Shorter infusion durations can be considered for nonemergent PCI in patients adequately pretreated with clopidogrel | Approx. 2.5 h | Stable IHD UA NSTEMI STEMI in combination with UFH | Heparin infusion after PCI is discouraged Discontinue >2–4 h before CABG Use with caution in renal impairment. Dialysis is a contraindication to use | ESPRIT, IMPACT-II |

(continued on next page)

**Table 2**
*(continued)*

| | Dose | Half-Life | Clinical Condition | Note | Trials |
|---|---|---|---|---|---|
| **Direct thrombin inhibitors** | | | | | |
| Bivalirudin | 0.1 mg/kg IV bolus then 0.25 mg/kg/h IV 0.75 mg per kg IV bolus then 1.75 mg/kg/h for PCI if no prior antithrombotic therapy administered | Approx. 25 min | Stable IHD UA NSTEMI invasive STEMI | Reduced with renal failure (0.25 mg/kg/h IV for hemodialysis) Caution with GFR <30 mL/h Discontinue bivalirudin 3 h before CABG and dose with UFH | REPLACE-2, ISAR-REACT-3, ACUITY, ISAR-REACT-4, HORIZONS-AMI |
| Argatroban | 350 μg/kg IV over 3–5 min then 25 μg/kg/min for PCI | Approx. 50 min | Use in PCI in patients with HIT | Caution with hepatic impairment | — |
| **Parenteral factor Xa inhibitor** | | | | | |
| Fondaparinux | 2.5 mg SQ daily With fibrinolysis, 2.5 mg IV followed 2.5 mg daily until hospital discharge for a maximum of 8 d | 17–21 h | Medical UA/NSTEMI conservative STEMI fibrinolysis | Contraindicated with renal failure (CrCl <30 mL/min) Significantly lower incidence of HIT compared with heparins Discontinue enoxaparin 12–24 h before CABG and dose with UFH | OASIS-5, OASIS-6, PENTUA |

*Abbreviations:* ACT, activated clotting time; BID, twice daily; CrCl, creatinine clearance; GFR, glomerular filtration rate; IHD, ischemic heart disease; LMWH, low molecular weight heparin; PTT, partial thromboplastin time.

Patients were additionally randomized to either unfractionated heparin (UFH) or bivalirudin. For financial reasons the planned enrollment of 8000 reached only 383 patients. Results from this small group suggest that further study is warranted (30-day MACE, 8.8% with abciximab vs 6.9% with tirofiban).[33]

A meta-analysis of 8 prospective trials evaluating 14,644 patients undergoing PCI compared abciximab, tirofiban, and eptifibatide. Certain differences were noted between the agents, but these trials compared each drug with placebo, so conclusions regarding comparative effectiveness based on these studies are limited, especially because these trials largely included patients treated with PTCA only or those who did not receive thienopyridine treatment.[34]

## UNFRACTIONATED HEPARIN

The most commonly used antithrombin agent for PCI has been UFH, which has been the gold standard for many years in the treatment of patients undergoing PCI because of its ease of administration, rapid onset, easily measurable efficacy (monitored by activated clotting time [ACT]), and reversibility. It is a heterogeneous mixture of glycosaminoglycans of varying lengths with a high affinity for antithrombin. The antithrombin activity of UFH depends on antithrombin activation, which subsequently inactivates thrombin, so UFH is considered an indirect antithrombin agent.

Elimination of UFH is initially through a rapid metabolism within the endothelial cells and macrophages (zero-order kinetics), and then by a slower renal clearance (first-order kinetics). Plasma half-life depends on the dose administered but is of the order of 1 hour at doses of 100 U/kg. If necessary, the effects can be reversed with protamine.

UFH remains the mainstay anticoagulant worldwide in patients undergoing PCI. Despite its common use, there have been no prospective randomized comparisons demonstrating efficacy in comparison with placebo for obvious reasons, and the current dosing regimens are empiric because clinical experience and anecdotal evidence demonstrate clearly the need for some degree of anticoagulation with balloon- and stent-mediated vascular wall injury. In a pooled analysis of data from randomized clinical trials using UFH only, there was a gradient of benefit associated with increasing degrees of anticoagulation. At ACT levels greater than 350 seconds there was an association with fewer ischemic events, although bleeding rates increased.[35] The STEEPLE (Safety and Efficacy of Intravenous

Enoxaparin in Elective Percutaneous Coronary Intervention: An International Randomized Evaluation) Study[36] noted that bleeding increased significantly with ACT values greater than 325 seconds, but ischemic events also increased when the ACT value was less than 325 seconds.[36] Available data do not support the use of prolonged heparin infusions after PCI if an excess in bleeding events and accompanying increase in the length of stay without a reduction in ischemic events has been observed with this approach.

Anticoagulation using UFH monotherapy appears to be insufficient to optimally protect against ischemic events such as periprocedural MI in ACS patients. Aggressive antiplatelet therapy is thought to act against embolization of platelet aggregates formed as a result of platelet activation induced by UFH. The use of high-dose clopidogrel or GPI in elective PCI, or the use of both in patients with ACS undergoing PCI, reduces periprocedural ischemic complications with UFH.[22,28,31]

The high ACT levels used in early studies are no longer thought to be required given the high prevalence of stent usage and antiplatelet medications, nearly eliminating the complication of abrupt closure.[37] The optimal dosing regimen is not defined, but most practitioners use regimens of 40 to 60 U/kg for goal ACT of longer than 225 seconds when GPI is used and a goal ACT of longer than 300 seconds when UFH is used alone (see **Table 2**). The optimal dosing regimen with the new oral antiplatelet agents, prasugrel and ticagrelor, remains a matter of debate given variable times of pretreatment and the lack of supportive outcomes studies.

During PCI, major limitations of UFH include the narrow therapeutic window, unpredictable individual antithrombin response across patient populations and disease states, platelet activation, and an inability to bind to clot-bound thrombin. The latter is protected from inhibition by the heparin-antithrombin complex serving to propagate thrombus even while heparin is being administered, and can act as a nidus for further thrombin activation on discontinuation of heparin. There is also a risk of heparin-induced thrombocytopenia (HIT) and thrombosis syndrome (HITTS).[38] The latter is rare in the setting of elective PCI, but can be seen with repeated exposures.[39] To address these limitations, other agents have been developed.

## LOW MOLECULAR WEIGHT HEPARINS

Low molecular weight heparins (LMWHs) are produced by chemical and enzymatic depolymerization of UFH, resulting in fragments with a mean molecular weight of 3000 to 5000 Da. Specifically, these agents have a greater activity against factor Xa than against thrombin, a uniform and predictable anticoagulation action, and lower incidence of HIT, addressing some of the limitations of UFH. LMWHs have a longer half-life than UFH, and clearance is by renal excretion. In patients with severe renal dysfunction (creatinine clearance <30 mL/min), the dosage is typically halved. Because it has greater anti-Xa activity, LMWH dosing cannot be reliably adjusted using the ACT (see **Table 2**).

The most studied of the LMWHs is enoxaparin. An observational study of 803 patients with ACS treated with a twice-daily dose of 1 mg/kg enoxaparin subcutaneously showed that 30-day mortality was closely linked with anti-Xa levels.[40] This study served as the basis of dosing for subsequent PCI studies in which anti-Xa levels greater than 0.5 U/mL are considered therapeutic for enoxaparin.[41] However, anti-Xa levels are not commonly measured during PCI, although they are sometimes measured in medically treated patients.

One aspect of enoxaparin use is that the drug can be administered parenterally or subcutaneously. The subcutaneous route has been used for initial medical management of ACS[42] and the parenteral route is used for PCI.[41,43]

Experience with enoxaparin in PCI included a series of studies performed by the National Investigators Collaborating on Enoxaparin (NICE) group. The NICE-1 registry consisted of 828 patients receiving intravenous enoxaparin before coronary intervention at time of elective or urgent PCI. All patients received aspirin, and clopidogrel pretreatment at that time was left to operator discretion. The composite end point of death, MI, and urgent revascularization at 30 days was seen in 7.7%, with MI in 5.4%.[44]

NICE-4 evaluated PCI with enoxaparin and compared these patients with historical cohorts from the EPILOG and EPISTENT studies in which UFH and GPI (abciximab) were used. NICE-4 adopted a protocol whereby 818 patients received enoxaparin 0.75 mg/kg and abciximab 0.25 mg/kg bolus followed by 0.125 μg/kg/min infusion. The 30-day composite end point of death, MI, or urgent revascularization occurred in 6.8%, suggesting that enoxaparin may confer efficacy and safety similar to that with UFH when used with abciximab.[44]

The SYNERGY (Superior Yield of the New Strategy of Enoxaparin, Revascularization and Glycoprotein IIb/IIIa Inhibitors) trial randomized 10,027 patients with ACS to either subcutaneous enoxaparin or intravenous UFH. Enoxaparin proved noninferior to UFH with the primary end point of death or MI at 30 days. For PCI, there was no difference in rates of unsuccessful PCI, abrupt closure, or emergency coronary artery bypass grafting (CABG) between groups. There was a significantly higher rate of TIMI (Thrombolysis in Myocardial Infarction) major bleeding among patients receiving enoxaparin, but no significant difference in the rate of GUSTO (Global Utilization of Streptokinase and t-PA for Occluded Coronary Arteries) severe bleeding, TIMI minor bleeding, or blood transfusions between enoxaparin or UFH groups.[43] The SYNERGY data were not blinded, and there was significant crossover between UFH and enoxaparin, an occurrence associated with worse bleeding outcomes compared with no crossover.

Though not the primary intent of the study, the ExTRACT-TIMI-25 (Enoxaparin and Thrombolysis Reperfusion for Acute Myocardial Infarction Treatment, Thrombolysis in MI-Study 25) reported on the role of enoxaparin for elective PCI after STEMI. PCI occurred at a median of 109 to 122 hours following fibrinolysis.[45] The 2272 enoxaparin patients undergoing PCI had a significant reduction in 30-day death or MI (10.7% vs 13.8%, P = .001) without an increase in TIMI major bleeding, providing indirect evidence that enoxaparin is superior to UFH in reducing ischemic complications during STEMI and for elective PCI after fibrinolysis.

The CRUISE trial randomized 261 patients undergoing elective or urgent PCI to intravenous enoxaparin 1 mg/kg or UFH, with all patients also receiving eptifibatide. There was no difference in bleeding complications or angiographic complications (6.3% vs 6.2%, not significant) during the procedure, and no differences in ischemic end points at 48 hours or 30 days.

The STEEPLE trial evaluated 3528 PCI patients who were randomized to enoxaparin (0.5 or 0.75 mg/kg) or UFH adjusted according to ACT, and stratified according to the use or nonuse of GPI.[41] GPI and thienopyridines were used in 40% and 95% of patients, respectively, and 16% of cases required multivessel intervention. The lowest rate of non-CABG–related bleeding at 48 hours was seen in the 0.5-mg/kg enoxaparin arm (5.9% vs 8.5%; P = .01), but the 0.75-mg/kg enoxaparin dose was not significantly different (6.5% vs 8.5%, P = .051). Patients in the 0.5-mg/kg group achieved a therapeutic level of anticoagulation 78.8% of the time compared with 91.8% in the 0.75-mg/kg group. Only 19.7% of patients in the UFH arm achieved therapeutic anticoagulation (P<.001 for either enoxaparin dose vs UFH).[16] The trial was not large enough to provide a definitive comparison of efficacy in prevention of ischemic events.

A meta-analysis of 13 trials comparing intravenous LMWH with UFH showed that a strategy of intravenous LMWH was associated with significant reduction in major bleeding (odds ratio 0.57; 95% CI 0.40–0.82), with no difference in death, MI, or TVR.[46] Overall, the use of intravenous enoxaparin during elective PCI is associated with a safety profile better than that of weight-adjusted UFH, with no additional risk of ischemic events. The possibility of improved outcomes compared with UFH among patients undergoing elective PCI with aggressive intravenous or oral antiplatelet therapy remains unproven. Coupled with an inability to easily monitor therapeutic levels during PCI, complex dosing regimens, and the need for dose adjustment among patients with impaired renal function, enoxaparin is not frequently used during elective PCI.

### Dalteparin

Supportive data for the LMWH dalteparin are limited. Although dalteparin was used in 2457 patients undergoing PCI in ACS, the object of this study was to compare an early invasive with a conservative approach to PCI in ACS, not a comparison of anticoagulation strategies.[47] Use of dalteparin in elective PCI has not been adequately studied. A dose-ranging study of 107 patients with all patients receiving aspirin and abciximab led to early unblinding of the study and the decision to terminate the lower-dose 40-U/kg arm. The composite end point of death, MI, and urgent revascularization was observed in 15.5% of patients, and major bleeding and transfusion each occurred in 2.8% of patients. Despite the study being inadequately powered to fully evaluate the agent in this setting, the high rates of clinical events resulted in limited uptake.

### FONDAPARINUX

In the attempt to overcome the limitations of the heparins, newer agents have been developed to specifically inhibit factor Xa. Fondaparinux, a pentasaccharide, is a synthetic indirect inhibitor of factor Xa that mimics the action of heparin through its interaction with antithrombin. Its half-life is approximately 20 hours, allowing once-daily dosing. Action upstream from thrombin in the coagulation cascade is an attractive feature during PCI, and HIT is extremely rare.[48] It is contraindicated with renal insufficiency because of primarily renal excretion (see **Table 2**).

Phase 2 experience proved promising with fondaparinux during PCI in the ASPIRE study (Arixtra Study in Percutaneous Coronary Intervention: A Randomized Evaluation), which randomized 350 patients undergoing elective or urgent PCI to 2 doses intravenously (2.5 and 5.0 mg) or weight-adjusted UFH. There was no difference compared with UFH in terms of total bleeding (7.7% UFH vs 6.4% fondaparinux, P = .61) and the composite of major adverse cardiac events (death, MI, urgent TVR, or use of bailout GPI) (6.0% UFH vs 6.0% fondaparinux, P = .97).[48]

The OASIS-5 (Organization to Assess Strategies in Acute Ischemic Syndromes) trial was the only study to evaluate patients undergoing PCI. More than 20,000 patients with ACS were randomized to enoxaparin or fondaparinux. There were no differences in ischemic complications, but there was benefit in respect of bleeding events with fondaparinux when compared with the LMWH (enoxaparin 8.8% vs fondaparinux 3.3%, P<.001). A substantial number of patients received UFH in both arms of the trial, and the protocol was actually modified during the course of the study to ensure use of UFH with fondaparinux because of a significantly higher rate of catheter-related thrombosis (enoxaparin 0.5% vs fondaparinux 1.3%, P = .001). The concerns of the study were corroborated in the subsequent OASIS-6 trial in patients with STEMI. Primary PCI with fondaparinux resulted in significantly higher 30-day mortality and reinfarction than in patients with UFH.[49] As a result, guidelines recommend the addition of agents with activity against factor IIa during PCI in patients treated with fondaparinux. As such, this medication is suggested for use among patients being treated medically for ACS and has a limited role in elective PCI (see **Table 1**).

### DIRECT ANTITHROMBIN AGENTS

The most studied direct thrombin inhibitor in PCI is bivalirudin. It is a small molecule, consisting of 20 amino acids, and is a bivalent synthetic direct thrombin inhibitor. Bivalirudin binds directly to thrombin in both its fluid phase and its clot-bound form, unlike heparin-based drugs, which bind only to free (unbound) thrombin. Bivalirudin inactivates thrombin directly and does not require laboratory monitoring to assess its effect. Its half-life is approximately 25 minutes and it does not cause HIT. Thrombin-induced platelet aggregation is essentially obliterated by bivalirudin (see **Table 2**).

There is a large body of evidence in support of bivalirudin use in ACS patients, including those with unstable angina, NSTEMI, and STEMI.[50–52] In patients with stable coronary disease undergoing elective PCI there are 2 randomized trials supporting the use of bivalirudin. The REPLACE-2 (Randomized Evaluation of PCI Linking Angiomax to Reduced Clinical Events—2) study was a multicenter, double-blind, triple-dummy randomized trial in patients with a low to moderate risk for ischemic complications undergoing PCI. Patients were randomized to heparin with planned GPI (abciximab or eptifibatide) or bivalirudin with provisional GPI. At 30 days, there was no significant difference in MACE (death, MI, urgent revascularization, or major bleeding) between the groups (9.2% in bivalirudin group vs 10.0% in heparin plus GPI). In-hospital major bleeding rates were significantly reduced by bivalirudin (2.4% vs 4.1%, P<.001).

The ISAR-REACT-3 (Intracoronary Stenting and Antithrombotic Regimen—Rapid Early Action for Coronary Treatment) trial evaluated 4570 troponin-negative patients treated with aspirin and clopidogrel (600 mg loading dose) at least 2 hours before planned PCI. Patients were randomized to 140 U/kg UFH or bivalirudin in what was a placebo-controlled trial. The primary end point of MACE at 30 days (death, MI, urgent TVR, or major bleeding) was not different (UFH 8.7% vs bivalirudin 8.3%; RR 0.94, 95% CI 0.77–1.15, P = .57). There was a significant reduction in major bleeding (4.6% vs 3.1%, P = .008) and minor bleeding (9.9% vs 6.8%, P = .001) with bivalirudin, but one criticism is that UFH dosing was higher than used in contemporary practice.[52,53] Thus, the UFH patients may have had higher bleeding rates, resulting in the apparent advantage for bivalirudin.

Taken together, the REPLACE-2 and ISAR-REACT 3 trials indicate that bivalirudin is a reasonable alternative to UFH alone or in combination with GPI in patients undergoing elective PCI (see **Table 1**). Although not necessarily more efficacious than either UFH strategy in this setting, it is significantly safer.

Of course, bivalirudin has also been extensively studied in pivotal trials assessing its use as an anticoagulant in the setting of NSTEMI and STEMI. Bivalirudin monotherapy in an early invasive PCI strategy in patients with unstable angina and NSTEMI provided superior 30-day clinical outcomes in comparison with a heparin and GPI regimen, and ACUITY scale major bleeding was reduced by 47% with bivalirudin at 30 days (3.0% vs 5.7%; RR 0.53, 95% CI 0.43–0.65, P<.001).[50] The HORIZONS-AMI, the largest trial assessing bivalirudin in STEMI, reported a mortality benefit at 30 days in the bivalirudin monotherapy group on comparison with a heparin plus GPI strategy (cardiac death 1.8% vs 2.9%, P = .03; all-causes death 2.1% vs 3.1%, P = .047). The 30-day rate of net adverse clinical events including a lower rate of major bleeding was lower with bivalirudin alone (4.9% vs 8.3%; RR 0.60, P<.001).[50]

## OTHER AGENTS

Argatroban is a direct thrombin inhibitor approved by the Food and Drug Administration in 2000 for use in prophylaxis or treatment of thrombosis in patients with HIT. In 2002, it was approved for use during PCI in patients who have HIT or are at risk of developing it. Argatroban is given intravenously, has a half-life of 50 minutes, and is metabolized in the liver. It can be used in the setting of renal failure, but not in patients with significant hepatic dysfunction (see **Table 2**). Another direct thrombin inhibitor, lepirudin, had been available for HIT patients. A business decision was made by the manufacturer to discontinue production of this agent in May 2012.

## SUMMARY

Anticoagulation strategies have rapidly evolved over recent decades, and numerous agents are now available. An improved understanding of the coagulation cascade and the interplay between thrombin and platelet activation has led to the development of agents specifically targeting key components of the coagulation cascade. Along with improvements in PCI technique, expanded use of these agents has led to impressive reductions in ischemic outcomes and, more recently, in bleeding events. Although the magnitude of benefit of these agents in clinical trials over UFH is smaller or nonexistent in elective PCI compared with PCI in ACS, there are certainly several patients at high bleeding risk or who have contraindications to UFH who can benefit from these agents.

The mainstay for anticoagulation in PCI for patients with stable disease remains UFH, with selective use of additional intravenous or oral antiplatelet agents, but LMWH and direct thrombin inhibitors, either alone or in combination with heparins, have a variety of benefits. Whether more aggressive dual-antiplatelet therapies, especially prasugrel, ticagrelor, or cangrelor, improve ischemic outcomes with UFH, LMWH, or bivalirudin without an increase in bleeding complications remains unknown, and whether the benefits demonstrated in ACS patients can be generalized to stable patients will remain a matter of debate. Finally, personalizing the optimal antithrombin in combination with the optimal antiplatelet agent for a patient based on individual hematologic, genetic, angiographic, and comorbid factors has the potential to dramatically improve outcomes, but remains an enormously challenging task for future investigation.

# REFERENCES

1. Kandzari DE, Berger PB, Kastrati A, et al. Influence of treatment duration with a 600-mg dose of clopidogrel before percutaneous coronary revascularization. J Am Coll Cardiol 2004;44:2133–6.

2. Kastrati A, Mehilli J, Schuhlen H, et al. A clinical trial of abciximab in elective percutaneous coronary intervention after pretreatment with clopidogrel. N Engl J Med 2004;350:232–8.

3. Puma JA, Banko LT, Pieper KS, et al. Clinical characteristics predict benefits from eptifibatide therapy during coronary stenting: insights from the enhanced suppression of the platelet IIb/IIIa receptor with integrilin therapy (ESPRIT) trial. J Am Coll Cardiol 2006;47:715–8.

4. Use of a monoclonal antibody directed against the platelet glycoprotein IIb/IIIa receptor in high-risk coronary angioplasty. The epic investigation. N Engl J Med 1994;330:956–61.

5. Topol EJ, Califf RM, Weisman HF, et al. Randomised trial of coronary intervention with antibody against platelet IIb/IIIa integrin for reduction of clinical restenosis: results at six months. The EPIC investigators. Lancet 1994;343:881–6.

6. Topol EJ, Ferguson JJ, Weisman HF, et al. Long-term protection from myocardial ischemic events in a randomized trial of brief integrin beta3 blockade with percutaneous coronary intervention. EPIC investigator group. Evaluation of platelet IIb/IIIa inhibition for prevention of ischemic complication. JAMA 1997;278:479–84.

7. Lincoff AM, Tcheng JE, Califf RM, et al. Sustained suppression of ischemic complications of coronary intervention by platelet GP IIb/IIIa blockade with abciximab: one-year outcome in the EPILOG trial. Evaluation in PTCA to improve LOng-term outcome with abciximab GP IIb/IIIa blockade. Circulation 1999;99:1951–8.

8. Platelet glycoprotein IIb/IIIa receptor blockade and low-dose heparin during percutaneous coronary revascularization. The epilog investigators. N Engl J Med 1997;336:1689–96.

9. Brener SJ, Barr LA, Burchenal JE, et al. Randomized, placebo-controlled trial of platelet glycoprotein IIb/IIIa blockade with primary angioplasty for acute myocardial infarction. Reopro and Primary PTCA Organization and Randomized Trial (RAPPORT) investigators. Circulation 1998;98: 734–41.

10. Simoons ML, de Boer MJ, van den Brand MJ, et al. Randomized trial of a GP IIb/IIIa platelet receptor blocker in refractory unstable angina. European Cooperative Study Group. Circulation 1994;89: 596–603.

11. Randomised placebo-controlled trial of abciximab before and during coronary intervention in refractory unstable angina: the CAPTURE study. Lancet 1997;349:1429–35.

12. van den Brand M, Laarman GJ, Steg PG, et al. Assessment of coronary angiograms prior to and after treatment with abciximab, and the outcome of angioplasty in refractory unstable angina patients. Angiographic results from the CAPTURE trial. Eur Heart J 1999;20:1572–8.

13. Klootwijk P, Meij S, Melkert R, et al. Reduction of recurrent ischemia with abciximab during continuous ECG-ischemia monitoring in patients with unstable angina refractory to standard treatment (CAPTURE). Circulation 1998;98:1358–64.

14. Hamm CW, Heeschen C, Goldmann B, et al. Benefit of abciximab in patients with refractory unstable angina in relation to serum troponin t levels. C7e3 fab antiplatelet therapy in unstable refractory angina (CAPTURE) study investigators. N Engl J Med 1999;340:1623–9.

15. Bhatt DL, Lincoff AM, Califf RM, et al. The benefit of abciximab in percutaneous coronary revascularization is not device-specific. Am J Cardiol 2000; 85:1060–4.

16. Montalescot G, Barragan P, Wittenberg O, et al. Platelet glycoprotein IIb/IIIa inhibition with coronary stenting for acute myocardial infarction. N Engl J Med 2001;344:1895–903.

17. Admiral Investigators. Three-year duration of benefit from abciximab in patients receiving stents for acute myocardial infarction in the randomized double-blind ADMIRAL study. Eur Heart J 2005; 26:2520–3.

18. Neumann FJ, Kastrati A, Schmitt C, et al. Effect of glycoprotein IIb/IIIa receptor blockade with abciximab on clinical and angiographic restenosis rate after the placement of coronary stents following acute myocardial infarction. J Am Coll Cardiol 2000;35:915–21.

19. Stone GW, Grines CL, Cox DA, et al. Comparison of angioplasty with stenting, with or without abciximab, in acute myocardial infarction. N Engl J Med 2002;346:957–66.

20. Antoniucci D, Rodriguez A, Hempel A, et al. A randomized trial comparing primary infarct artery stenting with or without abciximab in acute myocardial infarction. J Am Coll Cardiol 2003;42: 1879–85.

21. De Luca G, Suryapranata H, Stone GW, et al. Abciximab as adjunctive therapy to reperfusion in acute ST-segment elevation myocardial infarction: a meta-analysis of randomized trials. JAMA 2005; 293:1759–65.

22. EPISTENT Investigators. Randomised placebo-controlled and balloon-angioplasty-controlled trial to assess safety of coronary stenting with use of platelet glycoprotein-IIb/IIIa blockade. Lancet 1998;352:87–92.

23. Lincoff AM, Califf RM, Moliterno DJ, et al. Complementary clinical benefits of coronary-artery stenting and blockade of platelet glycoprotein IIb/IIIa receptors. Evaluation of Platelet IIb/IIIa Inhibition in Stenting Investigators. N Engl J Med 1999;341: 319–27.

24. Kastrati A, Mehilli J, Neumann FJ, et al. Abciximab in patients with acute coronary syndromes undergoing percutaneous coronary intervention after clopidogrel pretreatment: the ISAR-REACT 2 randomized trial. JAMA 2006;295:1531–8.

25. Effects of platelet glycoprotein IIb/IIIa blockade with tirofiban on adverse cardiac events in patients with unstable angina or acute myocardial infarction undergoing coronary angioplasty. The RESTORE investigators. Randomized efficacy study of tirofiban for outcomes and restenosis. Circulation 1997;96:1445–53.

26. A comparison of aspirin plus tirofiban with aspirin plus heparin for unstable angina. Platelet receptor inhibition in ischemic syndrome management (PRISM) study investigators. N Engl J Med 1998; 338:1498–505.

27. Inhibition of the platelet glycoprotein IIb/IIIa receptor with tirofiban in unstable angina and non-q-wave myocardial infarction. Platelet receptor inhibition in ischemic syndrome management in patients limited by unstable signs and symptoms (PRISM-plus) study investigators. N Engl J Med 1998;338:1488–97.

28. Valgimigli M, Percoco G, Barbieri D, et al. The additive value of tirofiban administered with the high-dose bolus in the prevention of ischemic complications during high-risk coronary angioplasty: the ADVANCE trial. J Am Coll Cardiol 2004;44:14–9.

29. Bonz AW, Lengenfelder B, Strotmann J, et al. Effect of additional temporary glycoprotein IIb/IIIa receptor inhibition on troponin release in elective percutaneous coronary interventions after pretreatment with aspirin and clopidogrel (TOPSTAR trial). J Am Coll Cardiol 2002;40:662–8.

30. Randomised placebo-controlled trial of effect of eptifibatide on complications of percutaneous coronary intervention: impact-II. Integrilin to Minimise Platelet Aggregation and Coronary Thrombosis-II. Lancet 1997;349:1422–8.

31. ESPRIT Investigators. Enhanced Suppression of the Platelet IIb/IIIa Receptor with Integrilin Therapy. Novel dosing regimen of eptifibatide in planned coronary stent implantation (ESPRIT): a randomised, placebo-controlled trial. Lancet 2000;356: 2037–44.

32. Topol EJ, Moliterno DJ, Herrmann HC, et al. Comparison of two platelet glycoprotein IIb/IIIa inhibitors, tirofiban and abciximab, for the prevention of ischemic events with percutaneous coronary revascularization. N Engl J Med 2001;344:1888–94.

33. Moliterno DJ. A randomized two-by-two comparison of high-dose bolus tirofiban versus abciximab and unfractionated heparin versus bivalirudin during percutaneous coronary revascularization and stent placement: the Tirofiban Evaluation of Novel dosing versus Abciximab with Clopidogrel and Inhibition of Thrombin studY (TENACITY) trial. Catheter Cardiovasc Interv 2011;77:1001–9.

34. Brown DL, Fann CS, Chang CJ. Meta-analysis of effectiveness and safety of abciximab versus eptifibatide or tirofiban in percutaneous coronary intervention. Am J Cardiol 2001;87:537–41.

35. Chew DP, Bhatt DL, Lincoff AM, et al. Defining the optimal activated clotting time during percutaneous coronary intervention: aggregate results from 6 randomized, controlled trials. Circulation 2001;103:961–6.

36. Montalescot G, Cohen M, Salette G, et al. Impact of anticoagulation levels on outcomes in patients undergoing elective percutaneous coronary intervention: insights from the STEEPLE trial. Eur Heart J 2008;29:462–71.

37. Brener SJ, Moliterno DJ, Lincoff AM, et al. Relationship between activated clotting time and ischemic or hemorrhagic complications: analysis of 4 recent randomized clinical trials of percutaneous coronary intervention. Circulation 2004;110:994–8.

38. Hirsh J, Fuster V. Guide to anticoagulant therapy. Part 1: heparin. American Heart Association. Circulation 1994;89:1449–68.

39. Warkentin TE. Drug-induced immune-mediated thrombocytopenia—from purpura to thrombosis. N Engl J Med 2007;356:891–3.

40. Montalescot G, Collet JP, Tanguy ML, et al. Anti-Xa activity relates to survival and efficacy in unselected acute coronary syndrome patients treated with enoxaparin. Circulation 2004;110:392–8.

41. Montalescot G, White HD, Gallo R, et al. Enoxaparin versus unfractionated heparin in elective percutaneous coronary intervention. N Engl J Med 2006;355:1006–17.

42. Cohen M, Demers C, Gurfinkel EP, et al. A comparison of low-molecular-weight heparin with unfractionated heparin for unstable coronary artery disease. Efficacy and safety of subcutaneous enoxaparin in non-Q-wave coronary events study group. N Engl J Med 1997;337:447–52.

43. Ferguson JJ, Califf RM, Antman EM, et al. Enoxaparin vs unfractionated heparin in high-risk patients with non-ST-segment elevation acute coronary syndromes managed with an intended early invasive strategy: primary results of the SYNERGY randomized trial. JAMA 2004;292:45–54.

44. Kereiakes DJ, Grines C, Fry E, et al. Enoxaparin and abciximab adjunctive pharmacotherapy during percutaneous coronary intervention. J Invasive Cardiol 2001;13:272–8.

45. Gibson CM, Murphy SA, Montalescot G, et al. Percutaneous coronary intervention in patients receiving enoxaparin or unfractionated heparin after fibrinolytic therapy for ST-segment elevation myocardial infarction in the Extract-TIMI 25 trial. J Am Coll Cardiol 2007;49:2238–46.

46. Dumaine R, Borentain M, Bertel O, et al. Intravenous low-molecular-weight heparins compared with unfractionated heparin in percutaneous coronary intervention: quantitative review of randomized trials. Arch Intern Med 2007;167:2423–30.

47. Invasive compared with non-invasive treatment in unstable coronary-artery disease: FRISC-II prospective randomised multicentre study. Fragmin and fast revascularisation during instability in coronary artery disease investigators. Lancet 1999;354:708–15.

48. Mehta SR, Steg PG, Granger CB, et al. Randomized, blinded trial comparing fondaparinux with unfractionated heparin in patients undergoing contemporary percutaneous coronary intervention: arixtra study in percutaneous coronary intervention: a randomized evaluation (ASPIRE) pilot trial. Circulation 2005;111:1390–7.

49. Yusuf S, Mehta SR, Chrolavicius S, et al. Effects of fondaparinux on mortality and reinfarction in patients with acute ST-segment elevation myocardial infarction: the OASIS-6 randomized trial. JAMA 2006;295:1519–30.

50. Stone GW, McLaurin BT, Cox DA, et al. Bivalirudin for patients with acute coronary syndromes. N Engl J Med 2006;355:2203–16.

51. Lincoff AM, Bittl JA, Harrington RA, et al. Bivalirudin and provisional glycoprotein IIb/IIIa blockade compared with heparin and planned glycoprotein IIb/IIIa blockade during percutaneous coronary intervention: replace-2 randomized trial. JAMA 2003;289:853–63.

52. Stone GW, Witzenbichler B, Guagliumi G, et al. Bivalirudin during primary PCI in acute myocardial infarction. N Engl J Med 2008;358:2218–30.

53. Schulz S, Mehilli J, Ndrepepa G, et al. Bivalirudin vs. unfractionated heparin during percutaneous coronary interventions in patients with stable and unstable angina pectoris: 1-year results of the ISAR-REACT 3 trial. Eur Heart J 2010;31:582–7.

# Combination Antithrombotic Management for Non–ST Segment Elevation Acute Coronary Syndromes

Jayant Bagai, MD[a], Subhash Banerjee, MD[b],
Emmanouil S. Brilakis, MD, PhD[b],*

## KEYWORDS

- Non–ST segment elevation acute coronary syndrome • Anticoagulation • Antiplatelet agents
- Outcomes

## KEY POINTS

- Patients presenting with non–ST segment elevation acute coronary syndromes (NSTEACS) are at high risk for subsequent thrombotic events.
- Combination antithrombotic management with anticoagulant and antiplatelet medications can significantly improve outcomes in this high-risk group of patients.
- In patients with NSTEACS in whom an early invasive strategy is planned, unfractionated heparin or bivalirudin is the anticoagulant of choice; in those in whom an early conservative strategy is planned, unfractionated heparin can be used, but enoxaparin or fondaparinux may be preferred.
- All patients with NSTEACS should receive aspirin and continue it indefinitely unless they cannot tolerate it.
- A second antiplatelet agent should be administered both for an early invasive (ADP P2Y$_{12}$ inhibitor or a glycoprotein IIb/IIIa inhibitor) or early conservative (ADP P2Y$_{12}$ inhibitor) strategy.
- Administration of the ADP P2Y$_{12}$ receptor inhibitor should continue for 12 months, unless the patient is at high risk for bleeding.

Thrombosis is a major pathogenetic mechanism leading to the development of both ST segment elevation acute myocardial infarction (STEMI) and non–ST segment elevation acute coronary syndromes (NSTEACS) and subsequent adverse outcomes.[1–3] Thrombosis is mediated by an intricate interplay between the coagulation system and platelets. Treatments addressing both systems (combination antithrombotic therapy) are needed to optimize clinical outcomes.[4,5] This article summarizes the clinical data on combination antithrombotic therapy along with the current clinical recommendations for use of these agents in patients presenting with NSTEACS.

Conflicts of Interest: J. Bagai, none. S. Banerjee, speaker honoraria from St Jude Medical, Medtronic, and Johnson & Johnson, and research support from Boston Scientific and The Medicines Company. E.S. Brilakis, speaker honoraria from St Jude Medical, Bridgepoint Medical and Terumo, and research support from Guerbet; spouse is employee of Medtronic.

[a] Division of Cardiovascular Medicine, Tennessee Valley VA Healthcare System, Vanderbilt University Medical Center, Nashville, TN, USA; [b] Division of Cardiovascular Medicine, VA North Texas Healthcare System, The University of Texas Southwestern Medical Center at Dallas, Dallas, TX, USA
* Corresponding author.
E-mail address: esbrilakis@yahoo.com

Intervent Cardiol Clin 2 (2013) 553–571
http://dx.doi.org/10.1016/j.iccl.2013.05.002
2211-7458/13/$ – see front matter Published by Elsevier Inc.

interventional.theclinics.com

## ANTICOAGULANT THERAPY

Several anticoagulants are available for treating patients with NSTEACS: unfractionated heparin (UFH), low-molecular-weight heparin (enoxaparin), bivalirudin, and fondaparinux. In patients with NSTEACS in whom an early invasive strategy is planned, UFH or bivalirudin are usually preferred, whereas in those in whom an early conservative strategy is planned UFH can be used but enoxaparin or fondaparinux may be preferred because of easier subcutaneous (instead of intravenous) administration and no need for monitoring of the anticoagulation level.[4,5]

**Table 1**
**Guidelines for the use of UFH in NSTEACS (based on the 2007 ACCF/AHA guidelines for the management of patients with unstable angina/non–ST-elevation MI, incorporating the 2012 focused update)**

| Management Strategy/ Scenario | Recommendation | Class of Recommendation; LOE | Dose |
|---|---|---|---|
| Invasive | Start UFH as soon as diagnosis of ACS (UA/NSTEMI) is definite/likely | Class I; LOE, A | Loading dose of 60 U per kg (max 4000 U) IV bolus. Maintenance IV infusion of 12 U/kg/h (maximum 1000 U per h) to maintain aPTT at 1.5–2.0 times control (approximately 50–70 s) No adjustment in heparin dose is needed for patients with renal failure |
| Conservative | Start UFH as soon as diagnosis of ACS (UA/NSTEMI) is definite/likely | Class I; LOE, A LMWH or fondaparinux are preferred if conservative strategy is chosen (class IIa; LOE, B) | As above |
| During PCI | — | Class I; LOE, B | GPI planned: 50–70 units/kg bolus (ACT of 200–250 s). No GPI planned: 70–100 units/kg bolus (target ACT of 250–300 s for HemoTec or 300–350 s for Hemochron) |
| After uncomplicated PCI | — | Class I; LOE, B | Discontinue heparin |
| Medical management chosen | — | Class I; LOE, A | Discontinue UFH after 48 h |
| CABG chosen | — | Class I; LOE, B | Continue UFH until CABG |

*Abbreviations:* ACT, activated clotting time; aPTT, activated partial thromboplastin time; CABG, coronary artery bypass graft surgery; GPI, glycoprotein IIb/IIIa inhibitor; IV, intravenous; LMWH, low-molecular-weight heparin; NSTEMI, non–ST segment acute MI; PCI, percutaneous coronary intervention; UA, unstable angina.

*Data from* Anderson JL, Adams CD, Antman EM, et al. ACC/AHA 2007 guidelines for the management of patients with unstable angina/non-ST-elevation myocardial infarction: a report of the American College of Cardiology/American Heart Association Task Force on Practice Guidelines (Writing Committee to Revise the 2002 Guidelines for the Management of Patients With Unstable Angina/Non-ST-Elevation Myocardial Infarction) developed in collaboration with the American College of Emergency Physicians, the Society for Cardiovascular Angiography and Interventions, and the Society of Thoracic Surgeons endorsed by the American Association of Cardiovascular and Pulmonary Rehabilitation and the Society for Academic Emergency Medicine. J Am Coll Cardiol 2007;50:e1–157; and Jneid H, Anderson JL, Wright RS, et al. 2012 ACCF/AHA focused update of the guideline for the management of patients with unstable angina/non-ST-elevation myocardial infarction (updating the 2007 guideline and replacing the 2011 focused update): a report of the American College of Cardiology Foundation/American Heart Association Task Force on Practice Guidelines. J Am Coll Cardiol 2012;60:645–81.

## UFH

UFH is an anticoagulant that has been used for many years in patients with acute coronary syndrome (ACS) or patients undergoing percutaneous coronary intervention (PCI). The first randomized evaluation of UFH in unstable angina compared outcomes in patients who were randomized to placebo, aspirin alone, heparin alone, and aspirin and heparin in combination.[6] UFH alone (5000-unit bolus, followed by 1000 units/h) reduced the incidence of refractory angina, myocardial infarction (MI), and death compared with placebo. Similar reductions were noted with aspirin alone and the combination of aspirin and heparin. Heparin was noted to be particularly effective in reducing the incidence of MI: 0.8% compared with 11.9% in the placebo group. The current guidelines for using UFH in NSTEACS are summarized in **Table 1**.[4,5]

## Enoxaparin

Enoxaparin is the most widely studied low-molecular-weight heparin in patients with NSTEACS and has been shown to be superior to UFH in patients treated with an early conservative approach.[7–10] However, in the Superior Yield of the New Strategy of Enoxaparin, Revascularization and Glycoprotein IIb/IIIa Inhibitors (SYNERGY) trial, enoxaparin-treated high-risk patients managed with an early invasive strategy had a similar incidence of death or MI compared with those treated with UFH, with a higher incidence of major bleeding (**Fig. 1**).[10] In a meta-analysis of 6 trials including 22,000 patients comparing enoxaparin with UFH, enoxaparin reduced the risk of death or MI at 30 days (10.1% vs 11.0%; odds ratio [OR], 0.91; 95% confidence interval [CI], 0.83–0.99; number needed to treat, 107).[11] The reduction was more significant in patients receiving no prerandomization antithrombin therapy (8.0% vs 9.4%; OR, 0.81; 95% CI, 0.70–0.94; number needed to treat, 72), without significant difference in the rate of blood transfusion or major bleeding.[11] The results of the SYNERGY trial along with the difficulties associated with managing the patient during PCI (need for additional intravenous bolus in some patients, inability to monitor anticoagulation level in the cardiac catheterization laboratory,

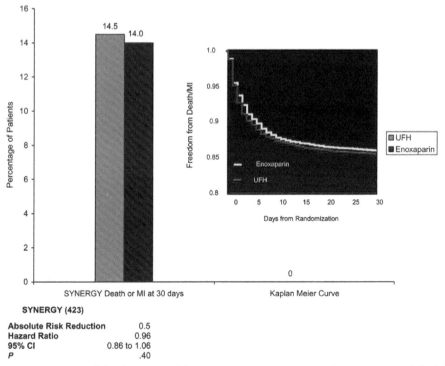

Fig. 1. Thirty-day incidence of death or MI with heparin versus enoxaparin in the SYNERGY trial.[10] Although no overall difference was noted, enoxaparin was superior to heparin in the group of patients who did not receive prerandomization antithrombotic or who received prerandomization therapy that was the same as the randomly assigned therapy. CI, confidence interval. (*From* Anderson JL, Adams CD, Antman EM, et al. ACC/AHA 2007 Guidelines for the management of patients with unstable angina/non-ST-elevation myocardial infarction-executive summary: a report of the American College of Cardiology/American Heart Association Task Force on Practice Guidelines. J Am Coll Cardiol 2007;50:690; with permission.)

**Table 2**
**Guidelines for the use of enoxaparin in NSTEACS (based on the 2007 ACCF/AHA guidelines for the management of patients with unstable angina/non–ST elevation MI incorporating the 2012 focused update)**

| Management Strategy/ Scenario | Recommendation | Class of Recommendation; LOE | Dose |
|---|---|---|---|
| Early invasive | Start enoxaparin as soon as diagnosis of UA/NSTEMI is definite/likely | Class I; LOE, A | Loading dose of 30 mg IV bolus may be given. Maintenance dose 1 mg per kg SC every 12 h; extend dosing interval to 1 mg/kg every 24 h if estimated Ccr<30 mL per min |
| Initial conservative | Start enoxaparin as soon as diagnosis of UA/NSTEMI is definite/likely | Class I; LOE, A Preferential use of enoxaparin instead of UFH preferred if initial conservative strategy is chosen unless CABG planned within 24 h (class IIa; LOE, B) | As above |
| During PCI | — | Class IIb; LOE, B | If last SC dose was administered <8 h before PCI and at least 2 doses were given before PCI: no additional therapy<br>If last SC dose was administered >8 h but <12 h before PCI or fewer than 2 doses were given before PCI: 0.3 mg per kg IV bolus is recommended (class I recommendation; LOE, B)<br>If last SC dose was administered >12 h before PCI, then full-dose de novo anticoagulation using an established regimen (full-dose UFH or bivalirudin) should be given[18]<br>No prior enoxaparin administered: 0.5–0.75 mg per kg IV bolus in catheter laboratory |
| | | Class III; LOE, B | UFH should not be given to patients already receiving therapeutic subcutaneous enoxaparin. This practice, known as stacking, resulted in greater bleeding in the SYNERGY trial |
| After uncomplicated PCI | Discontinue enoxaparin | Class I; LOE, B | — |
| Medical management chosen (with or without angiography/ stress testing) | Continue enoxaparin for the duration of hospitalization, up to 8 d | Class I; LOE, A | — |

(continued on next page)

| Table 2 (continued) | | | |
|---|---|---|---|
| **Management Strategy/ Scenario** | **Recommendation** | **Class of Recommendation; LOE** | **Dose** |
| CABG chosen | Discontinue enoxaparin 12–24 h before CABG, and dose with UFH per institutional practice | Class I; LOE, B | — |

*Abbreviations:* Ccr, creatinine clearance; SC, subcutaneous.

*Data from* Anderson JL, Adams CD, Antman EM, et al. ACC/AHA 2007 guidelines for the management of patients with unstable angina/non-ST-elevation myocardial infarction: a report of the American College of Cardiology/American Heart Association Task Force on Practice Guidelines (Writing Committee to Revise the 2002 Guidelines for the Management of Patients With Unstable Angina/Non-ST-Elevation Myocardial Infarction) developed in collaboration with the American College of Emergency Physicians, the Society for Cardiovascular Angiography and Interventions, and the Society of Thoracic Surgeons endorsed by the American Association of Cardiovascular and Pulmonary Rehabilitation and the Society for Academic Emergency Medicine. J Am Coll Cardiol 2007;50:e1–157; and Jneid H, Anderson JL, Wright RS, et al. 2012 ACCF/AHA focused update of the guideline for the management of patients with unstable angina/non-ST-elevation myocardial infarction (updating the 2007 guideline and replacing the 2011 focused update): a report of the American College of Cardiology Foundation/American Heart Association Task Force on Practice Guidelines. J Am Coll Cardiol 2012;60:645–81.

and delays in removal of the femoral sheath [until 6–8 hours after the last subcutaneous dose and 4–6 hours after the last intravenous dose]) limit the enthusiasm for using enoxaparin in patients with NSTEACS, in whom an early invasive approach is planned. The current guidelines for using enoxaparin in NSTEACS are summarized in **Table 2**.

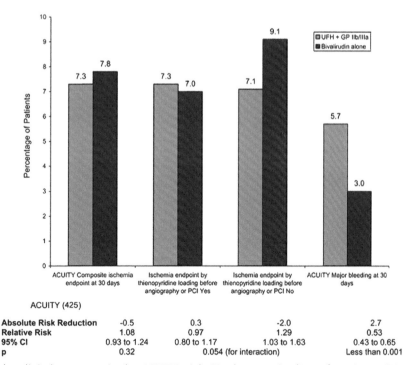

Fig. 2. Thirty-day clinical outcomes in the ACUITY trial. GP, glycoprotein. (*Data from* Stone GW, McLaurin BT, Cox DA, et al. Bivalirudin for patients with acute coronary syndromes. N Engl J Med 2006;355:2203–16; and *From* Anderson JL, Adams CD, Antman EM, et al. ACC/AHA 2007 Guidelines for the management of patients with unstable angina/non-ST-elevation myocardial infarction-executive summary: a report of the American College of Cardiology/American Heart Association Task Force on Practice Guidelines. J Am Coll Cardiol 2007;50:691; with permission.)

## Bivalirudin

Bivalirudin is a direct thrombin inhibitor that has been evaluated in the setting of NSTEACS in several studies.[12–15] The largest study was the Acute Catheterization and Urgent Intervention Triage Strategy (ACUITY) trial, which compared bivalirudin monotherapy with combinations of bivalirudin plus glycoprotein IIa/IIIa inhibitor (GPI) and UFH plus GPI.[14,15] Bivalirudin alone was associated with a noninferior rate of the composite ischemia end point (death, MI, or unplanned revascularization) (7.8% and 7.3%, respectively; $P$ = .32) and significantly reduced the rates of major bleeding (3.0% vs 5.7%; $P<.001$) (**Fig. 2**). In patients not pretreated with clopidogrel before angiography or PCI, the composite ischemic event rate was higher in the bivalirudin group (9.1% vs 7.1%; relative risk, 1.29; $P$ = .054 for interaction).[14] The ACUITY trial excluded patients with ACS who

**Table 3**
**Guidelines for the use of bivalirudin in NSTEACS (based on the 2007 ACCF/AHA guidelines for the management of patients with unstable angina/non–ST elevation MI incorporating the 2012 focused update)**

| Management Strategy/Scenario | Recommendation | Recommendation Class; LOE | Dose |
|---|---|---|---|
| Invasive | Start bivalirudin as soon as diagnosis of UA/NSTEMI is definite/likely | Class I; LOE, B | 0.1 mg per kg bolus followed by 0.25 mg per kg per h infusion |
| Initial conservative | Not recommended (not evaluated in clinical trials) | — | — |
| During PCI | — | Class I; LOE, B | If already on bivalirudin infusion, give additional 0.5 mg per kg bolus and increase infusion to 1.75 mg per kg per h. If not on infusion, administer 0.75 mg per kg bolus followed by 1.75 mg per kg per h infusion |
| After PCI | — | — | No additional treatment or continue infusion for up to 4 h |
| Medical management chosen after coronary artery disease noted on angiography | Either discontinue bivalirudin or continue at low dose for up to 72 h at the physician's discretion, if given before diagnostic angiography | Class I; LOE, B | 0.25 mg/kg per h |
| CABG chosen | Discontinue bivalirudin until 3 h before CABG and dose with UFH per institutional practice | Class I; LOE, B | — |

*Data from* Anderson JL, Adams CD, Antman EM, et al. ACC/AHA 2007 guidelines for the management of patients with unstable angina/non-ST-elevation myocardial infarction: a report of the American College of Cardiology/American Heart Association Task Force on Practice Guidelines (Writing Committee to Revise the 2002 Guidelines for the Management of Patients With Unstable Angina/Non-ST-Elevation Myocardial Infarction) developed in collaboration with the American College of Emergency Physicians, the Society for Cardiovascular Angiography and Interventions, and the Society of Thoracic Surgeons endorsed by the American Association of Cardiovascular and Pulmonary Rehabilitation and the Society for Academic Emergency Medicine. J Am Coll Cardiol 2007;50:e1–157; and Jneid H, Anderson JL, Wright RS, et al. 2012 ACCF/AHA focused update of the guideline for the management of patients with unstable angina/non-ST-elevation myocardial infarction (updating the 2007 guideline and replacing the 2011 focused update): a report of the American College of Cardiology Foundation/American Heart Association Task Force on Practice Guidelines. J Am Coll Cardiol 2012;60:645–81.

received angiography after 72 hours or were managed conservatively; hence bivalirudin is not approved for use in either of these clinical scenarios. Bivalirudin or argatroban can also be used for PCI in patients with heparin-induced thrombocytopenia. The current guidelines for using bivalirudin in NSTEACS are summarized in **Table 3**.

## Fondaparinux

Fondaparinux is a factor Xa inhibitor that was compared with enoxaparin in the Fifth Organization to Assess Strategies in Acute Ischemic Syndromes (OASIS 5) trial that enrolled 20,078 patients with NSTEACS.[16] Patient receiving fondaparinux had lower 30-day mortality compared with those receiving enoxaparin (2.9% vs 3.5%; hazard ratio, 0.83; 95% CI, 0.71–0.97; $P$ = .02), likely related to the lower risk for major bleeding (2.2% vs 4.1% at 9 days; $P<.001$) (**Fig. 3**). However, patients undergoing PCI on fondaparinux had a 3-fold higher rate of guide catheter thrombus (0.9% vs 0.3%).[16] As a result, it is currently

recommended that intravenous (IV) UFH (85 units/kg without GPI and 60 units/kg with GPI) be administered to patients on fondaparinux who require PCI (**Table 4**).[17,18]

## ANTIPLATELET THERAPY
### Aspirin

Aspirin has been an integral part of medical therapy in ACS since initial randomized trials showed that it reduced the incidence of MI in patients with unstable angina compared with placebo[19] and reduced vascular death in patients with STEMI.[20] Aspirin should be administered as soon as the diagnosis of ACS is suspected and continued indefinitely. In the Antithrombotics Trialists' Collaboration meta-analysis, the minimal effective dose of aspirin was 75 mg daily, which resulted in a 22% reduction in vascular death, MI, and stroke.[21] Higher doses are associated with increased risk of bleeding without reduction in ischemic events.[22,23] Hence, it is reasonable to use low-dose (81 mg) aspirin rather than high-dose aspirin after PCI (class IIa recommendation).[8]

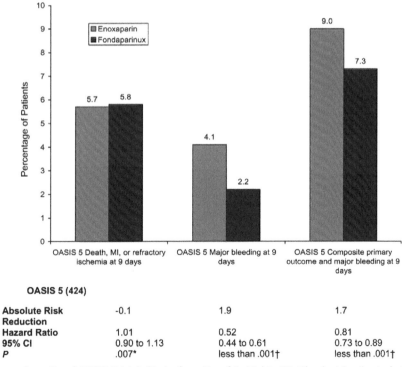

| OASIS 5 (424) | | | |
|---|---|---|---|
| Absolute Risk Reduction | -0.1 | 1.9 | 1.7 |
| Hazard Ratio | 1.01 | 0.52 | 0.81 |
| 95% CI | 0.90 to 1.13 | 0.44 to 0.61 | 0.73 to 0.89 |
| P | .007* | less than .001† | less than .001† |

**Fig. 3.** Summary of results of OASIS 5 trial. (*Data from* Yusuf S, Mehta SR, Chrolavicius S, et al. Comparison of fondaparinux and enoxaparin in acute coronary syndromes. N Engl J Med 2006;354:1464–76; and *From* Anderson JL, Adams CD, Antman EM, et al. ACC/AHA 2007 Guidelines for the management of patients with unstable angina/non-ST-elevation myocardial infarction-executive summary: a report of the American College of Cardiology/American Heart Association Task Force on Practice Guidelines. J Am Coll Cardiol 2007;50:692; with permission.)

**Table 4**
**Guidelines for the use of fondaparinux in NSTEACS (based on the 2007 ACCF/AHA guidelines for the management of patients with unstable angina/non–ST elevation MI incorporating the 2012 focused update)**

| Management Strategy/Scenario | Recommendation | Recommendation Class; LOE | Dose |
|---|---|---|---|
| Invasive | Start fondaparinux as soon as diagnosis of UA/NSTEMI is definite/likely | Class I; LOE, B | 2.5 mg subcutaneously once daily. Avoid for Ccr<30 mL/min |
| Initial conservative | Start fondaparinux as soon as diagnosis of UA/NSTEMI is definite/likely | Class I; LOE, B | As above |
| | Use is preferred rather than other agents if bleeding risk is high | Class I; LOE, B | |
| | Preferred use rather than UFH, unless CABG planned within 24 h | Class IIa; LOE, B | |
| During PCI | Fondaparinux should not be used as the sole anticoagulant to support PCI. An additional anticoagulant with anti-IIa activity should be administered because of the risk of catheter thrombosis | Class III; LOE, C | No additional fondaparinux (with GPI) and 2.5 mg IV (without GPI) if time to last dose <6 h<br>2.5 mg IV (with GPI) and 5 mg IV (without GPI) if time to last dose >6 h<br>Supplemental 50–60 U/kg IV bolus of UFH was recommended by the OASIS 5 Investigators. Another study recommended a standard dose of UFH (85 U/kg, 60 U/kg with GPI) rather than by a low dose of UFH (50 U/kg)[17] |
| Medical management chosen (with or without angiography/stress testing) | Continue fondaparinux for the duration of hospitalization, up to 8 d | Class I; LOE, B | 2.5 mg subcutaneously once daily. Avoid for Ccr<30 mL/min |
| CABG chosen | Discontinue fondaparinux 24 h before CABG and dose with UFH per institutional practice | Class I; LOE, B | — |

Data from Anderson JL, Adams CD, Antman EM, et al. ACC/AHA 2007 guidelines for the management of patients with unstable angina/non-ST-elevation myocardial infarction: a report of the American College of Cardiology/American Heart Association Task Force on Practice Guidelines (Writing Committee to Revise the 2002 Guidelines for the Management of Patients With Unstable Angina/Non-ST-Elevation Myocardial Infarction) developed in collaboration with the American College of Emergency Physicians, the Society for Cardiovascular Angiography and Interventions, and the Society of Thoracic Surgeons endorsed by the American Association of Cardiovascular and Pulmonary Rehabilitation and the Society for Academic Emergency Medicine. J Am Coll Cardiol 2007;50:e1–157; and Jneid H, Anderson JL, Wright RS, et al. 2012 ACCF/AHA focused update of the guideline for the management of patients with unstable angina/non-ST-elevation myocardial infarction (updating the 2007 guideline and replacing the 2011 focused update): a report of the American College of Cardiology Foundation/American Heart Association Task Force on Practice Guidelines. J Am Coll Cardiol 2012;60:645–81.

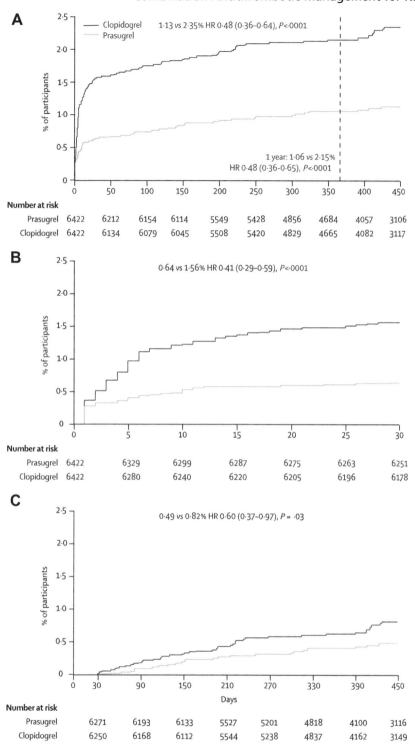

**Fig. 4.** Incidence of the Academic Research Consortium definite or probable stent thrombosis for all patients receiving at least one intracoronary stent in the Trial to Assess Improvement in Therapeutic Outcomes by Optimizing Platelet Inhibition with Prasugrel–Thrombolysis in Myocardial Infarction (TRITON–TIMI) 38 trial. (*A*) Kaplan-Meier curves of stent thrombosis from randomization (day 0) to day 450 after randomization; (*B*) Kaplan-Meier curves of early stent thrombosis from 0 to 30 days. (*C*) Kaplan-Meier curves for late stent thrombosis using landmark analysis for all patients alive at 30 days, with events occurring from 0 to 30 days censored from the analysis. (*From* Wiviott SD, Braunwald E, McCabe CH, et al, TRITON-TIMI 38 Investigators. Intensive oral antiplatelet therapy for reduction of ischaemic events including stent thrombosis in patients with acute coronary syndromes treated with percutaneous coronary intervention and stenting in the TRITON-TIMI 38 trial: a subanalysis of a randomized trial. Lancet 2008;371(9621):1358; with permission.)

## ADP P2Y$_{12}$ Inhibitors

Three ADP P2Y$_{12}$ inhibitors are currently used in patients with NSTEACS: clopidogrel, prasugrel, and ticagrelor. Ticlopidine is another ADP P2Y$_{12}$ inhibitor but is almost never currently used because of the risk of serious hematologic side effects. Clopidogrel is the most widely used ADP P2Y$_{12}$ inhibitor and a loading dose (usually 600 mg) should be administered as soon as possible after diagnosis. The pivotal Clopidogrel in Unstable Angina to Prevent Recurrent Events (CURE) trial, by showing a 20% reduction in the composite end point of cardiovascular death, MI, or stroke compared with placebo in medically and invasively managed patients with NSTEACS, established a firm role for the continuation of clopidogrel for 12 months after NSTEACS.[23,24]

However, there is significant interpatient variability in the response to clopidogrel, explained in part by genetic polymorphism of the CYP 2C 19 gene.

Carriers of reduced function *2 and *3 alleles have high on-treatment platelet reactivity (HTPR) and an increased risk of MI and stent thrombosis after PCI.[25] Unlike clopidogrel, agents such as prasugrel and ticagrelor result in predictable and high levels of platelet inhibition with unaltered pharmacodynamics even in carriers of loss-of-function CYP 2C19 alleles. These agents have shown improved outcomes compared with clopidogrel in patients with ACS.

Prasugrel reduced the incidence of cardiovascular death, MI, or stroke and stent thrombosis when compared with clopidogrel in patients with NSTEACS undergoing PCI (**Fig. 4**).[26,27] Prasugrel was associated with harm among patients with

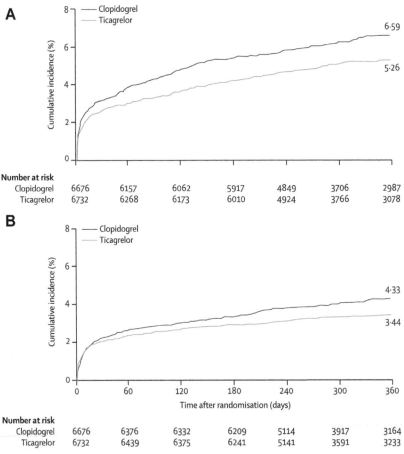

**Fig. 5.** Kaplan-Meier curves of the incidence of (A) MI or (B) cardiovascular death with clopidogrel versus ticagrelor among patients in whom an early invasive strategy was planned in the Study of Platelet Inhibition and Patient Outcomes (PLATO) trial. (*From* Cannon CP, Harrington RA, James S, et al. PLATelet Inhibition and Patient Outcomes Investigators. Comparison of ticagrelor with clopidogrel in patients with a planned invasive strategy for acute coronary syndromes (PLATO): a randomized double-blind study. Lancet 2010;375(9711):286; with permission.)

**Table 5**
**Guidelines for the use of ADP P2Y$_{12}$ inhibitors in NSTEACS (based on the 2007 ACCF/AHA guidelines for the management of patients with unstable angina/non–ST elevation MI incorporating the 2012 focused update)**

| Management Strategy/Scenario | Recommendation | Class of Recommendation; LOE | Dose |
|---|---|---|---|
| Aspirin allergy (hypersensitivity or major GI intolerance) | Clopidogrel or | Class I; LOE, B | — |
| | Prasugrel (only if PCI performed) or | Class I; LOE, C | |
| | Ticagrelor Only 1 agent should be used | Class I; LOE, C | |
| Early invasive, before PCI | Clopidogrel or | Class I; LOE, B | 300–600 mg loading dose, 75 mg daily maintenance dose |
| | Ticagrelor As soon as diagnosis of medium to high-risk UA/NSTEMI is definite and before diagnostic angiography | Class I; LOE, B | 180 mg loading dose, 90 mg twice daily maintenance dose |
| | Prasugrel before definition of coronary anatomy, if both the risk for bleeding is low and the need for CABG is considered unlikely | Class IIb; LOE, C | — |
| Initial conservative | Clopidogrel or | Class I; LOE, A | As above |
| | Ticagrelor As soon as diagnosis of UA/NSTEMI is definite/ likely | Class I; LOE, B | |
| PCI planned after angiography | Clopidogrel as early as possible before PCI or at time of PCI, if not given before angiography or | Class I; LOE, A | 600 mg loading dose 300 mg supplemental loading dose, if 300 mg had been given before angiography |
| | Ticagrelor as early as possible before PCI or at time of PCI (if not given before angiography) or | Class I; LOE, B | 180 mg loading dose |
| | Prasugrel promptly and no later than 1 h after PCI, once coronary anatomy defined and suitable for PCI | Class I; LOE, B | 60 mg loading dose |
| | Use of prasugrel in patients with prior stroke/transient ischemic attack | Class III (harm: not recommended) | — |

*(continued on next page)*

**Table 5**
*(continued)*

| Management Strategy/Scenario | Recommendation | Class of Recommendation; LOE | Dose |
|---|---|---|---|
| After PCI | Clopidogrel × 12 mo or | Class I; LOE, A | 75 mg daily |
| | Ticagrelor × 12 mo or | Class I; LOE, B | 90 mg twice daily |
| | Prasugrel × 12 mo Duration of 12 mo recommended regardless of BMS or DES | Class I; LOE, B | 10 mg daily |
| | Higher early clopidogrel maintenance dose, if patient not at high risk for bleeding | Class IIb; LOE, B | 75 mg twice daily × 6 d, then 75 mg daily for the following 12 mo |
| | Earlier than 12 mo discontinuation if risk of bleeding outweighs benefit | Class I; LOE, C | — |
| Medical management chosen (with or without angiography/ stress testing) | Clopidogrel or Ticagrelor Duration of therapy: 1 mo minimum, ideally 12 mo | Class I; LOE, A for clopidogrel Class I; LOE, B for both — | As above |
| CABG chosen | Discontinue Clopidogrel ≥ 5 d Prasugrel ≥ 7 d Ticagrelor ≥ 5 d | — Class I; LOE, B Class I; LOE, C Class I; LOE, C | — |

*Abbreviations:* BMS, bare metal stent; DES, drug-eluting stent; GI, gastrointestinal.

*Data from* Anderson JL, Adams CD, Antman EM, et al. ACC/AHA 2007 guidelines for the management of patients with unstable angina/non-ST-elevation myocardial infarction: a report of the American College of Cardiology/American Heart Association Task Force on Practice Guidelines (Writing Committee to Revise the 2002 Guidelines for the Management of Patients With Unstable Angina/Non-ST-Elevation Myocardial Infarction) developed in collaboration with the American College of Emergency Physicians, the Society for Cardiovascular Angiography and Interventions, and the Society of Thoracic Surgeons endorsed by the American Association of Cardiovascular and Pulmonary Rehabilitation and the Society for Academic Emergency Medicine. J Am Coll Cardiol 2007;50:e1–e157; and Jneid H, Anderson JL, Wright RS, et al. 2012 ACCF/AHA focused update of the guideline for the management of patients with unstable angina/non-ST-elevation myocardial infarction (updating the 2007 guideline and replacing the 2011 focused update): a report of the American College of Cardiology Foundation/American Heart Association Task Force on Practice Guidelines. J Am Coll Cardiol 2012;60:645–81.

prior transient ischemic attack or stroke and no benefit among patients 75 years of age or older or less than 60 kg body weight. Further, prasugrel should only be administered after coronary anatomy is defined and deemed suitable for PCI. There is no role for prasugrel in medically managed patients with NSTEACS.

Ticagrelor reduced the 12-month incidence of vascular death, MI, or stroke as well as all-cause mortality, compared with clopidogrel, in a large trial that included patients with NSTEACS treated with either an early invasive (**Fig. 5**) or early conservative strategy.[28,29] Ticagrelor was associated with a higher rate of non–coronary artery bypass graft (CABG)–related major bleeding, dyspnea and ventricular pauses lasting 3 seconds or longer. Significant geographic differences in the effect of ticagrelor (no benefit in North American patients) were observed and were likely caused by coadministration of a daily dose of greater than or equal to 100 mg of aspirin.[30] A lower aspirin dose of 81 mg is therefore recommended with ticagrelor.

Cangrelor is a reversible intravenous ADP P2Y$_{12}$ inhibitor with a short half-life of 3 to 6 minutes. Randomized controlled trials of cangrelor, compared with clopidogrel, during PCI have shown mixed results. Although the Cangrelor versus

Standard Therapy to Achieve Optimal Management of Platelet Inhibition (CHAMPION) PCI[31] trial showed no benefit of a peri-PCI cangrelor infusion compared with a loading dose of clopidogrel given before PCI, the CHAMPION PLATFORM[32] trial showed a reduction in death and stent thrombosis with cangrelor compared with clopidogrel given after PCI. The recently reported CHAMPION PHOENIX trial showed a consistent benefit of cangrelor in the prevention of ischemic complications such as death, MI, and stent thrombosis, compared with clopidogrel given just before or after PCI.[33] Cangrelor effectively suppressed platelets ($P2Y_{12}$ Reaction Units <240) compared with placebo (99% vs 19%) after discontinuation of thienopyridine before CABG without excessive surgical bleeding in the Maintenance of Platelet inihiBition With cangRelor After dIscontinuation of Thienopyr-iDines in Patients Undergoing surGEry (BRIDGE) trial.[34] Approximately one-third of the patients had NSTEACS, and the median duration of cangrelor infusion was 3.4 days. Cangrelor is not currently approved for clinical use in the United States.

A summary of guidelines for the use of $P2Y_{12}$ inhibitors in NSTEACS is presented in **Table 5**.

### GPIs

The favorable outcomes of the ACUITY trial have led to a significant reduction in GPI use in contemporary practice. Despite this, GPIs still have a role in high-risk patients with NSTEACS, such as those who have an increased troponin and are managed with PCI (**Fig. 6**).[35] Administration of abciximab for 48 hours in patients with NSTEACS in whom coronary revascularization is not planned, and upstream administration of eptifibatide in patients who are either low risk or have high risk of bleeding are not recommended.[36,37] Current guidelines for GPI use in NSTEACS are summarized in **Table 6**.

### COMBINATION ANTITHROMBOTIC THERAPY

Given the pivotal role played by both platelets and the coagulation cascade in the pathogenesis and adverse outcomes in NSTEACS, a combination of antiplatelet and anticoagulant therapy is recommended for initial management. **Table 7** summarizes combination antithrombotic therapy based on the 2007 ACC/AHA guidelines with changes from the 2012 focused update incorporated.

### SPECIAL GROUPS OF PATIENTS

The optimal antithrombotic therapy among patients with NSTEACS who undergo PCI with coronary stents and subsequently need noncardiac surgery remains controversial, because discontinuation of

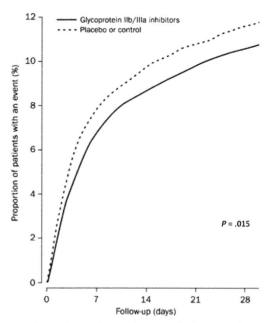

**Fig. 6.** Kaplan-Meier estimates of the cumulative occurrence of death or MI within 30 days from randomization in patients who received a glycoprotein IIb/IIIa inhibitor versus those who did not. (*From* Boersma E, Harrington RA, Moliterno DJ, et al. Platelet glycoprotein IIb/IIIa inhibitors in acute coronary syndromes: a meta-analysis of all major randomised clinical trials. Lancet 2002;359(9302):192; with permission.)

aspirin and clopidogrel carries an increased risk for perioperative stent thrombosis, a potentially catastrophic complication.[38] Approximately 5% of patients require noncardiac surgery within 12 months of ACS or PCI. A bare metal stent approach should be used in patients at high risk of bleeding or with anticipated need for surgery in the near future. After bare metal stenting, the risk of major adverse cardiac events in the perioperative period decreases significantly after 6 weeks.[39] After 6 weeks, clopidogrel can be interrupted with continuation of aspirin if possible. In the case of drug-eluting stents, noncardiac surgery should be postponed until after completion of a 12-month course of dual antiplatelet therapy with aspirin and clopidogrel. However, if surgery needs to be performed earlier, continuation of dual (or at least single) oral antiplatelet therapy may help minimize the stent thrombosis risk.[40] Close collaboration between the surgeon, cardiologist, and anesthesiologist is the best way to optimize the management of such patients. Cangrelor, which showed ability to bridge patients in need of continued antiplatelet effect leading up to CABG surgery, needs to be studied in the setting of noncardiac surgery.

In patients with NSTEACS who receive a ADP $P2Y_{12}$ inhibitor and subsequently require CABG,

**Table 6**
Guidelines for the use of glycoprotein IIb/IIIa inhibitors in NSTEACS (based on the 2007 ACCF/AHA guidelines for the management of patients with unstable angina/non–ST elevation MI incorporating the 2012 focused update)

| Management Strategy/Scenario | Recommendation | Recommendation Class; LOE | Dose |
|---|---|---|---|
| Invasive | Start GPI, as an alternative to clopidogrel or ticagrelor, before PCI, in medium-risk to high-risk patients with definite UA/NSTEMI | Class I; LOE, A | Eptifibatide<br>Before PCI, loading dose, 180 µg/kg IV; maintenance dose, 2 µg/kg/min IV infusion |
| | IV eptifibatide or tirofiban are preferred, if GPI started before PCI | Class I; LOE, B | If started during PCI, loading dose of 180 µg/kg followed 10 min later by second IV bolus of 180 µg/kg. Maintenance dose, 2 µg/kg/min |
| | Upstream use of GPI in addition to aspirin and clopidogrel/ticagrelor can be considered for high-risk patients (diabetes, ST depression, increased troponin) and not at high risk for bleeding | Class IIb; LOE, B | Reduce infusion rate by 50% if estimated Ccr<50 mL/min<br>Tirofiban (high dose) |
| | Upstream use of GPI in addition to aspirin and clopidogrel/ticagrelor should be avoided for low risk ACS (TIMI risk score <2) or high risk of bleeding | Class III | Loading dose of 0.25 µg/kg IV bolus followed by maintenance infusion of 0.15 µg/kg/min<br>Reduce infusion rate by 50% if estimated Ccr<50 mL/min |
| Initial conservative | Routine use of upstream GPI in addition to antiplatelet and anticoagulant therapy | Class IIb; LOE, B | Eptifibatide<br>Same as above |
| | Abciximab should not be administered to patients in whom PCI is not planned | Class III | Tirofiban<br>Loading dose of 0.4 µg per kg per min for 30 min IV. Maintenance dose 0.1 µg/kg/min<br>Reduce rate of infusion by 50% if estimated Ccr <30 mL/min |

| Scenario | Recommendation | Class; LOE | Dose |
|---|---|---|---|
| Initial conservative with recurrent symptoms/ischemia, congestive heart failure or arrhythmias and change to invasive strategy | Eptifibatide or tirofiban as an alternative to clopidogrel or ticagrelor, should be added to aspirin and anticoagulant before angiography | Class I; LOE, A | Same as initial conservative strategy dose above |
| | GPI can be administered in addition to aspirin, clopidogrel/ticagrelor, and anticoagulant, before angiography | Class IIa; LOE, C | |
| During PCI | Start GPI, as an alternative to clopidogrel or ticagrelor, during PCI, in medium-risk to high-risk definite UA/NSTEMI | Class I; LOE, A | Same as dose during PCI for eptifibatide and tirofiban<br>Abciximab can also be used during PCI: loading dose of 0.25 mg/kg IV bolus, maintenance dose of 0.125 µg/kg/min (max 10 µg per min) for 12 h after PCI |
| After PCI | — | — | Continue maintenance dose for 18–24 h after PCI for both eptifibatide and tirofiban |
| Medical management chosen after coronary artery disease noted on angiography or if low-risk stress test | Discontinue GPI | Class I; LOE, B | — |
| CABG chosen | Discontinue GPI (eptifibatide or tirofiban) 4 h before CABG | Class I; LOE, B | — |

*Abbreviation:* TIMI, thrombolysis in myocardial infarction.

*Data from* Anderson JL, Adams CD, Antman EM, et al. ACC/AHA 2007 guidelines for the management of patients with unstable angina/non-ST-elevation myocardial infarction: a report of the American College of Cardiology/American Heart Association Task Force on Practice Guidelines (Writing Committee to Revise the 2002 Guidelines for the Management of Patients With Unstable Angina/Non-ST-Elevation Myocardial Infarction) developed in collaboration with the American College of Emergency Physicians, the Society for Cardiovascular Angiography and Interventions, and the Society of Thoracic Surgeons endorsed by the American Association of Cardiovascular and Pulmonary Rehabilitation and the Society for Academic Emergency Medicine. J Am Coll Cardiol 2007;50:e1–e157; and Jneid H, Anderson JL, Wright RS, et al. 2012 ACCF/AHA focused update of the guideline for the management of patients with unstable angina/non-ST-elevation myocardial infarction (updating the 2007 guideline and replacing the 2011 focused update): a report of the American College of Cardiology Foundation/American Heart Association Task Force on Practice Guidelines. J Am Coll Cardiol 2012;60:645–81.

**Table 7**
Summary of combination regimens for initial management of NSTEACS

| Scenario | Early Invasive | Conservative | Conservative Changed to Early Invasive Because of Refractory Ischemia | PCI |
|---|---|---|---|---|
| Preferred regimen | Aspirin 162–325 mg + either clopidogrel (600 mg) or ticagrelor (90 mg) or GPI (eptifibatide or tirofiban) + UFH or bivalirudin | Aspirin 162–325 mg + either clopidogrel (600 mg LD) or ticagrelor (90 mg LD) + enoxaparin or UFH or fondaparinux (fondaparinux preferred if patient is at high risk of bleeding) | One of the following is added: Clopidogrel LD (if not given previously) Or Ticagrelor LD (if not given previously) Or GPI (eptifibatide or tirofiban) | PCI planned Clopidogrel LD (if not given previously) Or Ticagrelor LD (if not given previously) Or GPI (eptifibatide or tirofiban if not given previously) PCI started Prasugrel (60 mg LD) just before or within 1 h of PCI |
| Alternatives | Enoxaparin or fondaparinux may be used for anticoagulation if a delay in coronary angiography is anticipated | — | — | — |

the ADP $P2Y_{12}$ inhibitor should be discontinued for at least 5 days (for aspirin and ticagrelor) or 7 days (for prasugrel) before CABG to minimize the risk for perioperative bleeding.[5]

Patients who require long-term oral anticoagulation and also undergo PCI for NSTEACS are at increased risk of bleeding if they receive triple therapy with aspirin, clopidogrel, and warfarin.[5] To decrease the risk of bleeding, such patients should receive low-dose aspirin (81 mg daily) and possibly aim for an International Normalization Ratio between 2.0 and 2.5.[5] A novel alternative approach is to discontinue aspirin and continue with warfarin and clopidogrel. In the What is the Optimal Antiplatelet and Anticoagulant Therapy in Patients with Oral Anticoagulation and Coronary Stenting (WOEST) trial, patients in need of oral anticoagulation who underwent stenting were randomized to open-label dual therapy (warfarin and clopidogrel) versus triple therapy (aspirin, clopidogrel, and warfarin).[41] Patients receiving dual therapy had lower incidence of bleeding and lower mortality compared with patients receiving triple therapy. However, more studies are needed to confirm these findings.

## SUMMARY

Combining anticoagulant and antiplatelet medications can significantly improve outcomes in patients with NSTEACS.[4,5] At present, the combination is only administered during the initial hospitalization and patients are dismissed on antiplatelet treatment only with aspirin and an ADP $P2Y_{12}$ inhibitor.[4,5] The Anti-Xa Therapy to Lower Cardiovascular Events in Addition to Standard Therapy in Subjects with Acute Coronary Syndrome 2 –Thrombolysis in Myocardial Infarction 51 (ATLAS ACS 2 –TIMI 51) trial showed that post-dismissal anticoagulation with a direct factor Xa inhibitor (rivaroxaban) at low doses (2.5 mg twice daily) improved outcomes and reduced mortality when administered in addition to aspirin and clopidogrel.[42] Whether dual long-term therapy with aspirin and ticagrelor or prasugrel is similar or superior to triple therapy with aspirin, clopidogrel, and rivaroxaban remains to be determined.

## REFERENCES

1. Jackson SP. Arterial thrombosis–insidious, unpredictable and deadly. Nat Med 2011;17:1423–36.
2. DeWood MA, Spores J, Notske R, et al. Prevalence of total coronary occlusion during the early hours of transmural myocardial infarction. N Engl J Med 1980;303:897–902.
3. DeWood MA, Stifter WF, Simpson CS, et al. Coronary arteriographic findings soon after non-Q-wave myocardial infarction. N Engl J Med 1986;315:417–23.
4. Anderson JL, Adams CD, Antman EM, et al. ACC/AHA 2007 guidelines for the management of patients with unstable angina/non-ST-elevation myocardial infarction: a report of the American College of Cardiology/American Heart Association Task Force on Practice Guidelines (writing committee to revise the 2002 guidelines for the management of patients with unstable angina/non-ST-elevation myocardial infarction) developed in collaboration with the American College of Emergency Physicians, the Society for Cardiovascular Angiography and Interventions, and the Society of Thoracic Surgeons endorsed by the American Association of Cardiovascular and Pulmonary Rehabilitation and the Society for Academic Emergency Medicine. J Am Coll Cardiol 2007;50:e1–157.
5. Jneid H, Anderson JL, Wright RS, et al. 2012 ACCF/AHA focused update of the guideline for the management of patients with unstable angina/non-ST-elevation myocardial infarction (updating the 2007 guideline and replacing the 2011 focused update): a report of the American College of Cardiology Foundation/American Heart Association Task Force on Practice Guidelines. J Am Coll Cardiol 2012;60:645–81.
6. Theroux P, Ouimet H, McCans J, et al. Aspirin, heparin, or both to treat acute unstable angina. N Engl J Med 1988;319:1105–11.
7. Cohen M, Demers C, Gurfinkel EP, et al. A comparison of low-molecular-weight heparin with unfractionated heparin for unstable coronary artery disease. efficacy and safety of subcutaneous enoxaparin in Non-Q-Wave Coronary Events Study Group. N Engl J Med 1997;337:447–52.
8. Antman EM, McCabe CH, Gurfinkel EP, et al. Enoxaparin prevents death and cardiac ischemic events in unstable angina/non–Q-wave myocardial infarction: results of the Thrombolysis in Myocardial Infarction (TIMI) 11B trial. Circulation 1999;100:1593–601.
9. Blazing MA, de Lemos JA, White HD, et al. Safety and efficacy of enoxaparin vs unfractionated heparin in patients with non-ST-segment elevation acute coronary syndromes who receive tirofiban and aspirin: a randomized controlled trial. JAMA 2004;292:55–64.
10. Ferguson JJ, Califf RM, Antman EM, et al. Enoxaparin vs unfractionated heparin in high-risk patients with non–ST-segment elevation acute coronary syndromes managed with an intended early invasive strategy: primary results of the synergy randomized trial. JAMA 2004;292:45–54.
11. Petersen JL, Mahaffey KW, Hasselblad V, et al. Efficacy and bleeding complications among patients

randomized to enoxaparin or unfractionated heparin for antithrombin therapy in non-ST-segment elevation acute coronary syndromes: a systematic overview. JAMA 2004;292:89–96.

12. Lincoff AM, Bittl JA, Harrington RA, et al. Bivalirudin and provisional glycoprotein IIb/IIIa blockade compared with heparin and planned glycoprotein IIb/IIIa blockade during percutaneous coronary intervention: REPLACE-2 randomized trial. JAMA 2003;289:853–63.

13. Lincoff AM, Kleiman NS, Kereiakes DJ, et al. Long-term efficacy of bivalirudin and provisional glycoprotein IIb/IIIa blockade vs heparin and planned glycoprotein IIb/IIIa blockade during percutaneous coronary revascularization: REPLACE-2 randomized trial. JAMA 2004;292:696–703.

14. Stone GW, McLaurin BT, Cox DA, et al. Bivalirudin for patients with acute coronary syndromes. N Engl J Med 2006;355:2203–16.

15. Stone GW, White HD, Ohman EM, et al. Bivalirudin in patients with acute coronary syndromes undergoing percutaneous coronary intervention: a subgroup analysis from the Acute Catheterization and Urgent Intervention Triage strategy (ACUITY) trial. Lancet 2007;369:907–19.

16. Yusuf S, Mehta SR, Chrolavicius S, et al. Comparison of fondaparinux and enoxaparin in acute coronary syndromes. N Engl J Med 2006;354:1464–76.

17. Steg PG, Jolly SS, Mehta SR, et al. Low-dose vs standard-dose unfractionated heparin for percutaneous coronary intervention in acute coronary syndromes treated with fondaparinux: the FUTURA/OASIS-8 randomized trial. JAMA 2010;304:1339–49.

18. Levine GN, Bates ER, Blankenship JC, et al. 2011 ACCF/AHA/SCAI guideline for percutaneous coronary intervention. A report of the American College of Cardiology Foundation/American Heart Association Task Force on Practice Guidelines and the Society for Cardiovascular Angiography and Interventions. J Am Coll Cardiol 2011;58:e44–122.

19. Lewis HD Jr, Davis JW, Archibald DG, et al. Protective effects of aspirin against acute myocardial infarction and death in men with unstable angina. Results of a Veterans Administration cooperative study. N Engl J Med 1983;309:396–403.

20. Randomised trial of intravenous streptokinase, oral aspirin, both, or neither among 17,187 cases of suspected acute myocardial infarction: ISIS-2. ISIS-2 (Second International Study of Infarct Survival) Collaborative Group. Lancet 1988;2:349–60.

21. Antithrombotics Trialists' Collaboration. Collaborative meta-analysis of randomised trials of antiplatelet therapy for prevention of death, myocardial infarction, and stroke in high risk patients. BMJ 2002;324:71–86.

22. Mehta SR, Bassand JP, Chrolavicius S, et al. Dose comparisons of clopidogrel and aspirin in acute coronary syndromes. N Engl J Med 2010;363:930–42.

23. Yusuf S, Zhao F, Mehta SR, et al. Effects of clopidogrel in addition to aspirin in patients with acute coronary syndromes without ST-segment elevation. N Engl J Med 2001;345:494–502.

24. Mehta SR, Yusuf S, Peters RJ, et al. Effects of pretreatment with clopidogrel and aspirin followed by long-term therapy in patients undergoing percutaneous coronary intervention: the PCI-CURE study. Lancet 2001;358:527–33.

25. Holmes DR Jr, Dehmer GJ, Kaul S, et al. ACCF/AHA clopidogrel clinical alert: approaches to the FDA "boxed warning": a report of the American College of Cardiology Foundation Task Force on Clinical Expert Consensus Documents and the American Heart Association endorsed by the Society for Cardiovascular Angiography and Interventions and the Society of Thoracic Surgeons. J Am Coll Cardiol 2010;56:321–41.

26. Wiviott SD, Braunwald E, McCabe CH, et al. Prasugrel versus clopidogrel in patients with acute coronary syndromes. N Engl J Med 2007;357:2001–15.

27. Wiviott SD, Braunwald E, McCabe CH, et al. Intensive oral antiplatelet therapy for reduction of ischaemic events including stent thrombosis in patients with acute coronary syndromes treated with percutaneous coronary intervention and stenting in the TRITON-TIMI 38 trial: a subanalysis of a randomised trial. Lancet 2008;371:1353–63.

28. Wallentin L, Becker RC, Budaj A, et al. Ticagrelor versus clopidogrel in patients with acute coronary syndromes. N Engl J Med 2009;361:1045–57.

29. Cannon CP, Harrington RA, James S, et al. Comparison of ticagrelor with clopidogrel in patients with a planned invasive strategy for acute coronary syndromes (PLATO): a randomised double-blind study. Lancet 2010;375:283–93.

30. Mahaffey KW, Wojdyla DM, Carroll K, et al. Ticagrelor compared with clopidogrel by geographic region in the platelet inhibition and patient outcomes (PLATO) trial. Circulation 2011;124:544–54.

31. Harrington RA, Stone GW, McNulty S, et al. Platelet inhibition with cangrelor in patients undergoing PCI. N Engl J Med 2009;361:2318–29.

32. Bhatt DL, Lincoff AM, Gibson CM, et al. Intravenous platelet blockade with cangrelor during PCI. N Engl J Med 2009;361:2330–41.

33. Bhatt DL, Stone GW, Mahaffey KW, et al. Effect of platelet inhibition with cangrelor during PCI on ischemic events. N Engl J Med 2013;368:1303–13.

34. Angiolillo DJ, Firstenberg MS, Price MJ, et al. Bridging antiplatelet therapy with cangrelor in

patients undergoing cardiac surgery: a randomized controlled trial. JAMA 2012;307(3):265–74.

35. Boersma E, Harrington RA, Moliterno DJ, et al. Platelet glycoprotein IIb/IIIa inhibitors in acute coronary syndromes: a meta-analysis of all major randomised clinical trials. Lancet 2002;359:189–98.

36. Simoons ML. Effect of glycoprotein IIb/IIIa receptor blocker abciximab on outcome in patients with acute coronary syndromes without early coronary revascularisation: the GUSTO IV-ACS randomised trial. Lancet 2001;357:1915–24.

37. Giugliano RP, White JA, Bode C, et al. Early versus delayed, provisional eptifibatide in acute coronary syndromes. N Engl J Med 2009;360:2176–90.

38. Alshawabkeh LI, Banerjee S, Brilakis ES. Systematic review of the frequency and outcomes of non-

cardiac surgery after drug-eluting stent implantation. Hellenic J Cardiol 2011;52:141–8.

39. Reddy PR, Vaitkus PT. Risks of noncardiac surgery after coronary stenting. Am J Cardiol 2005;95(6):755–7.

40. Brilakis ES, Banerjee S, Berger PB. Perioperative management of patients with coronary stents. J Am Coll Cardiol 2007;49:2145–50.

41. Dewilde WJ, Oirbans T, Verheugt FW, et al. Use of clopidogrel with or without aspirin in patients taking oral anticoagulant therapy and undergoing percutaneous coronary intervention: an open-label, randomised, controlled trial. Lancet 2013;381(9872):1107–15.

42. Mega JL, Braunwald E, Wiviott SD, et al. Rivaroxaban in patients with a recent acute coronary syndrome. N Engl J Med 2012;366:9–19.

# Combination Antithrombotic Management of STEMI with Pharmacoinvasive Strategy, Primary PCI, or Rescue PCI

Piera Capranzano, MD[a],*, Corrado Tamburino, MD, PhD[a],
George D. Dangas, MD, PhD[b]

## KEYWORDS

- STEMI • PCI • Fibrinolysis • Antithrombotic therapy

## KEY POINTS

- In STEMI patients, primary percutaneous coronary intervention (PPCI) remains the preferred reperfusion strategy if it is performed within guideline-mandated time targets.
- Fibrinolysis remains a common reperfusion therapy for ST segment elevation myocardial infarction (STEMI), because a considerable proportion of patients is not able to receive PPCI within guideline-recommended benchmarks.
- Several transfer strategies after fibrinolysis have been elaborated, including urgent transfer for rescue percutaneous coronary intervention (PCI) and immediate transfer for routine early angiography (pharmacoinvasive strategy).
- The pharmacoinvasive strategy seems an effective option for early presenters who cannot undergo PPCI within 1 hour.
- Combinations of antiplatelet and anticoagulant agents are key to achieving and sustaining reperfusion. Currently, several effective combinations are possible and the best antithrombotic regimen remains unknown.

The mainstay of acute STEMI emergent management consists of reperfusion therapy in combination with antithrombotic treatment. Coronary reperfusion can be achieved mechanically by PCI or pharmacologically by fibrinolysis. According to contemporary guidelines, PPCI, that is, emergent PCI without previous administration of fibrinolytic therapy or platelet glycoprotein IIb/IIIa inhibitors (GPIs), is the preferred reperfusion strategy for STEMI.[1,2] The choice of PPCI of the infarct artery is contingent, however, on performing PCI in a timely fashion.[1,2] Because a considerable proportion of STEMI patients who present to non-PCI facilities do not subsequently receive PPCI within guideline-recommended benchmarks, and delays to PCI increase morbidity and mortality, alternative reperfusion strategies are needed.[3–5] Given this background, in recent years there has been interest and progress in the elaboration of several triage and transfer strategies. Facilitated PCI is a strategy consisting of administration of pharmacologic agents, including GPIs or fibrinolysis (full dose or half dose), with or without GPIs, followed by immediate transfer for PCI within 2 hours. Two large trials failed to show a net clinical benefit with this strategy compared with PPCI.[6,7] Rescue PCI is a strategy

Disclosures: G.D. Dangas has received speaker honoraria from Astra Zeneca, Bristol-Meiers Squibb, The Medicines Company, Sanofi Aventis, and Abbott Vascular. The other authors have no conflicts of interest to declare.
[a] Cardiovascular Department, Ferrarotto Hospital, University of Catania, Citelli 1, Catania 95124, Italy; [b] Icahn School of Medicine at Mount Sinai, One Gustave L. Levy Place, Box 1030, New York, NY 10029, USA
* Corresponding author.
E-mail address: pcapranzano@gmail.com

Intervent Cardiol Clin 2 (2013) 573–583
http://dx.doi.org/10.1016/j.iccl.2013.05.004
2211-7458/13/$ – see front matter © 2013 Elsevier Inc. All rights reserved.

consisting of the administration of fibrinolysis with subsequent urgent transfer for PCI only of patients who demonstrate findings of failed reperfusion. Finally, the pharmacoinvasive strategy consists of administration of fibrinolytic therapy either in a pre-hospital setting or at a non–PCI-capable hospital, followed by immediate transfer to a PCI-capable hospital for routine early coronary angiography and eventually PCI. Adjunctive antithrombotic regimens, including an array of combinations of anti-platelet and anticoagulant agents, are essential to support these reperfusion approaches and vary dependent on the selected strategy.

This article provides an overview of data and recommendations on PPCI, rescue PCI, and pharmacoinvasive strategy as well as of the antithrombotic regimens used to support these STEMI reperfusion approaches.

## PRIMARY PCI

PPCI is the preferred reperfusion strategy provided it is performed expeditiously in a high-volume center with an experienced team, including both skilled interventional cardiologists and support staff. PPCI compared with fibrinolytic therapy yields: higher rates of infarct-related artery patency and Thrombolysis in Myocardial Infarction (TIMI) 3 grade flow; lower rates of recurrent ischemia, reinfarction, emergency repeat revascularization, intracranial hemorrhage (ICH); and, finally, improved survival.[8] Current indications for PPCI are summarized in **Table 1**. In hemodynamically stable patients, only the infarct-related artery should be treated during the primary procedure. Single multivesssel PCI of culprit and nonculprit lesions has been associated with worse clinical outcomes in several studies, thus is not recommended, unless localization of the infarct is ambiguous, cardiogenic shock is present, or highly unstable lesions are found.[9,10]

### Adjunctive Antiplatelet Therapy for PPCI

Antiplatelet drugs currently recommended for PPCI include[1,2]

- Aspirin
- Adenosine diphosphate (ADP) platelet receptor (P2Y$_{12}$) antagonists (clopidogrel, prasugrel, and ticagrelor), which are orally administered
- GPIs, which are intravenous agents

### Aspirin

Aspirin should be given immediately after presentation at an initial dose of 162 mg to 325 mg.

After PPCI, aspirin should be continued indefinitely, and a maintenance dose of 81 mg daily is preferred to higher maintenance doses.

**Table 1**
**Recommendations for PPCI according to the American and European guidelines**

| Recommendation | American Class[a]/LOE | European Class[a]/LOE |
|---|---|---|
| Ischemic symptoms <12 h if PCI is performed by an experienced team within 120 min of FMC | I/A | I/A |
| Ischemic symptoms <12 h and contraindications to fibrinolysis irrespective of time delay from FMC | I/A | I/A |
| Cardiogenic shock or acute severe HF irrespective of time delay from symptom onset | I/B | NA |
| Cardiogenic shock or acute severe HF unless the expected PCI related delay is excessive and the patient presents early after symptom onset | NA | I/B |
| Evidence of ongoing ischemia 12–24 h after symptom onset | IIa/B | I/C |
| In stable patients presenting 12–24 h after symptom onset | NA | IIb/B |

[a] Class of recommendation; FMC, first medical contact; HF, heart failure; LOE, level of evidence; NA, not applicable (recommendation not stated).

### P2Y$_{12}$ receptor antagonists

Clopidogrel (300-mg or 600-mg loading dose and 75-mg once-daily maintenance dose) has been for years the standard antithrombotic treatment recommended on top of aspirin in overall patients with acute coronary syndrome (ACS) and/or undergoing PCI, including PPCI, although clopidogrel has not been evaluated against placebo in any large-outcome study in the setting of PPCI.[11,12] For PPCI, a 600-mg loading dose of clopidogrel is preferred to a 300-mg loading dose, given the enhanced and more rapid platelet inhibition achieved with the higher dose as well as the reported beneficial effects in STEMI patients.[13,14]

Large evidence has demonstrated a wide response variability to clopidogrel.[15] This clopidogrel limitation is relevant, given that inadequate inhibition of the ADP platelet activation pathway has been demonstrated to increase the risk for thrombotic events, prompting the development of novel antiplatelet agents.[15]

Prasugrel, a third-generation thienopyridine, was shown to provide a more rapid, enhanced, and consistent antiplatelet effect than clopidogrel, even compared with higher clopidogrel doses in a non-STEMI setting.[16] The clinical efficacy and safety of prasugrel (60-mg loading dose followed by a 10-mg maintenance dose) compared with clopidogrel (300-mg loading dose followed by 75-mg daily maintenance dose) has been evaluated in the large-scale phase III TRITON-TIMI 38 enrolling patients (n = 13,608) with moderate- to high-risk ACS and planned PCI.[17] In the overall population of the TRITON-TIMI 38 trial, over a follow-up period of 14.5 months, a significant 19% relative reduction of the primary efficacy endpoint (composite of cardiovascular death, nonfatal myocardial infarction [MI], or nonfatal stroke) was observed with prasugrel compared with clopidogrel. Prasugrel provided, however, a 32% relative increase in non–coronary artery bypass grafting (CABG)-related TIMI major bleeding. Prasugrel was associated with no net clinical benefit in the elderly patients ($\geq$75 years) and in those weighing less than 60 kg, with a net clinical harm in patients with prior cerebrovascular events. In the prespecified TRITON-TIMI 38 subgroup analysis focusing on STEMI patients (those within 12 hours after symptoms onset if PPCI was planned or within 14 days after receiving medical treatment), prasugrel compared with clopidogrel provided reductions in ischemic events, without increasing bleeding (**Table 2**).[18]

Ticagrelor, a cyclopentyl-triazolo-pyrimidine, has a more rapid onset and offset of action, and provides a greater and more consistent platelet inhibition than the standard clopidogrel dose.[19] The clinical effectiveness and safety of ticagrelor (180-mg loading dose followed by 90 mg twice daily) compared with clopidogrel (300-mg to 600-mg loading dose followed by 75 mg daily) has been evaluated in the large-scale phase III PLATO trial enrolling patients (n = 18,624) with moderate-risk to high-risk ACS (non–ST elevation ACS invasively or medically managed or STEMI managed with PPCI).[20] In the overall population of the PLATO trial, over a follow-up period of 12 months, a significant 16% relative reduction of the primary efficacy endpoint (composite of cardiovascular death, nonfatal MI, or nonfatal stroke) was observed with ticagrelor compared with clopidogrel. A significantly lower rate of cardiovascular death was observed in the ticagrelor group. Ticagrelor was associated with a 31% relative increase of non–CABG-related TIMI major bleeding. In the prespecified PLATO subgroup analysis focusing on STEMI

**Table 2**
**Rates and hazard ratios for the efficacy and safety endpoints within the STEMI cohorts of the TRITON-TIMI 38 and PLATO studies during 15 and 12 months of follow-up, respectively**

| Recommendation | TRITON-TIMI 38 (n = 3534) Rates and HR for Prasugrel vs Clopidogrel | PLATO (n = 7544) Rates and HR for Ticagrelor vs Clopidogrel |
|---|---|---|
| Cardiovascular death, nonfatal MI or nonfatal stroke | 10.0% vs 12.4% HR 0.79; 95% CI, 0.65–0.97 | 9.4% vs 10.8% HR 0.87; 95% CI, 0.75–1.01 |
| Cardiovascular death | 2.4% vs 3.4% HR 0.74; 95% CI, 0.50–1.09 | 4.5% vs 5.5% HR 0.83; 95% CI, 0.67–1.02 |
| All-cause death | 3.3 vs 4.3% HR 0.76; 95% CI, 0.54–1.07 | 5.0% vs 6.1% HR 0.82; 95% CI, 0.67–1.00 |
| MI | 6.8% vs 9.0% HR 0.75; 95% CI, 0.59–0.95 | 4.7% vs 5.8% HR 0.80; 95% CI, 0.65–0.98 |
| Stroke | 1.6% vs 1.5% HR 1.03; 95% CI, 0.60–1.79 | 1.7% vs 1.0% HR 1.63; 95% CI, 1.07–2.48 |
| Stent thrombosis[a] | 1.6% vs 2.8% HR 0.58; 95% CI, 0.36–0.93 | 2.6% vs 3.4% HR 0.74; 95% CI, 0.55–1.00 |
| Non–CABG-related TIMI major bleeding | 2.4% vs 2.1% HR 1.11; 95% CI, 0.70–1.77 | 2.5% vs 2.2% HR 1.09; 95% CI, 0.80–1.48 |

*Abbreviation:* CABG: coronary artery by-pass grafting; CI, confidence interval; HR, hazard ratio; MI, myocardial infarction; TIMI, Thrombolysis in Myocardial Infarction.
[a] Definite and probable stent thrombosis.

patients (n = 7544), ticagrelor was associated with lower rates of the primary endpoint, MI and all-cause mortality, and higher rates of stroke, with no differences in bleeding (see **Table 2**).[21]

Based on these data, approved options for STEMI patients undergoing PPCI include[1,2]

- Clopidogrel (600-mg loading dose and 75-mg once-daily maintenance dose)
- Prasugrel (60-mg loading dose and 10-mg once-daily maintenance dose)
- Ticagrelor (180-mg loading dose and 90-mg twice-daily maintenance dose)

The loading dose should be given as early as possible and the maintenance dose should be continued for 1 year.[1,2] Prasugrel is contraindicated in patients with prior stroke or transient ischemic attack. Also, the European guidelines recommend avoiding prasugrel in patients aged greater than or equal to 75 years.[1]

Current American guidelines do not endorse 1 of these 3 antiplatelet therapeutic options over another, acknowledging the superior effectiveness of new agents but also emphasizing the increased risk of bleeding associated with the use of the novel antiplatelet drugs.[2] In contrast, European guidelines recommend considering ticagrelor or prasugrel use before clopidogrel in patients with ACS and restricting the use of clopidogrel in patients with contraindications to the other 2 agents.[1]

A novel P2Y$_{12}$ inhibitor, cangrelor, has undergone phase III investigation in patients with ACS, including STEMI. Cangrelor is an intravenous, immediate-acting, potent, and direct-acting agent that has rapidly reversible effects (platelet function is restored within 1 hour after cessation of the infusion).[22] The pharmacologic profiles of cangrelor make it an attractive strategy for patients with STEMI, in which a rapid antiplatelet inhibition is desirable. A recent trial (CHAMPION-PHOENIX) has shown that cangrelor compared with clopidogrel significantly reduced the primary endpoint (death from any cause, MI, ischemia-driven revascularization, or stent thrombosis [ST]) at 48 hours and 30 days in 11,000 patients undergoing PCI, including stable coronary artery disease and ACS patients (18% with STEMI).[23] From subgroup analyses, it seems that reductions in the primary endpoint with cangrelor were similar among patients with STEMI, non-STEMI, and stable angina (interaction $P = .98$).[23]

### GPIs

The clinical benefits of GPIs (abciximab) in the setting of PPCI for STEMI have been shown in several trials predating the routine use of oral dual antiplatelet therapy (DAPT).[24]

Studies on GPIs in the setting of PPCI performed in the recent era of DAPT have evaluated the following:

- The additional benefits of GPIs given before PCI (prehospital on in-hospital) on top of clopidogrel loading versus placebo or no-GPIs in patients treated with heparin (BRAVE-3 and On-TIME 2 trials)[25,26]
- The impact of prehospital versus in-cathlab routine administration of GPIs (FINESSE trial)[7]
- The impact of intravenous GPIs plus unfractionated heparin (UFH) versus bivalirudin (HORIZONS-AMI)[27]
- The adjunctive benefit of intracoronary GPI bolus on top of bivalirudin versus no-GPI (INFUSE-AMI)[28]
- The effects of intracoronary versus intravenous administration of GPIs (several small studies and the AIDA-4 trial)[29,30]
- The differential impact of GPI types (MULTI-STRATEGY trial and a subanalysis from the SCAAR [Swedish Coronary Angiography and Angioplasty Registry])[31,32]

All these studies evaluating the different aspects regarding GPI use on top of DAPT in the setting of PPCI are outlined later.

The issue of whether abciximab (bolus plus continuous infusion for 12 hours) remains beneficial after pretreatment with high-dose clopidogrel loading (600-mg) in STEMI patients undergoing PPCI and receiving heparin was tested in the BRAVE-3 trial, in which patients were randomly assigned within 24 hours from symptoms onset to receive either abciximab (n = 401) or placebo (n = 399) in an ICU before catheterization.[25] The BRAVE-3 trial showed no benefits in terms of reduction in infarct size prior to discharge and in the 30-day rate of ischemic events. The adjunctive impact of GPIs on top of clopidogrel (600 mg) has been also evaluated in 1398 patients enrolled in the On-TIME 2 trial, which found improvements in markers of reperfusion and reduction in ischemic outcomes with prehospital initiation of high-bolus dose tirofiban compared with only provisional use in a catheterization laboratory.[26]

The optimal timing of GPI administration has been evaluated in the FINESSE trial, which showed that routine upstream use of abciximab before PPCI in a prehospital setting did not yield superior efficacy but increased bleeding risk compared with routine use in a catheterization laboratory.[7] A post hoc subset analysis of the FINESSE trial, however, focusing on patients presenting early within 4 hours of symptom onset to non-PCI hospitals and requiring transfer, suggested they might derive a survival benefit from upstream use of abciximab.[33]

In the large HORIZONS-AMI trial, there was no superior clinical efficacy associated with the combination of GPI continuous infusion on top of UFH compared with bivalirudin in patients with STEMI undergoing PPCI and pretreated with clopidogrel (600 mg).[27]

In the INFUSE-AMI trial, which randomized 452 patients to local delivery of abciximab versus no abciximab, intracoronary abciximab reduced the 30-day infarct size, evaluated by MRI, but did not improve abnormal wall motion score, ST segment resolution, post-PCI coronary flow, or myocardial perfusion.[28]

Several small studies have suggested the potential benefits of intracoronary over intravenous administration of abciximab.[29] The AIDA-4 trial, which randomized 2065 patients with recent STEMI (<24 hours) to intracoronary versus intravenous abciximab bolus during PCI with a subsequent infusion for 12 hours, showed similar efficacy and safety at 90 days between the 3 administration routes, with a borderline reduction in heart failure in the intracoronary group.[30]

Finally, the different GPI agents have been compared in the setting of PPCI, showing noninferiority of eptifibatide and tirofiban versus abciximab.[31,32]

From overall available data, it seems that in the era of DAPT, especially with the more potent agents, a clear clinical role of GPIs remains unsettled. In addition, there are no definitive answers.

Regarding the use of GPIs for PPCI, based on available data in aggregate, current guidelines suggest that[1,2]

- Adjunctive use of intravenous GPIs at the time of PCI performed with heparin can be considered in selected case (ie, for large thrombus burden or inadequate $P2Y_{12}$ receptor antagonist loading).
- Upstream administration of GPIs in a prehospital setting may be considered in high-risk patients who presented early after symptoms onset and are transferred for PPCI.
- For patients receiving bivalirudin, routine adjunctive use of GPIs is not recommended but may be considered as adjunctive or bailout therapy in selected cases.
- It may be reasonable to administer intracoronary abciximab.

## Adjunctive Anticoagulant Therapy for PPCI

Anticoagulant drugs currently recommended for PPCI include[1,2]

- UFH
- Low-molecular-weight heparin
- Bivalirudin

Use of fondaparinux in the context of PPCI was associated with potential harm in the OASIS-6 trial and is, therefore, not recommended for PPCI.[34]

Intravenous UFH titrated to an appropriate activated clotting time is a familiar and well-established anticoagulant to support PCI for STEMI.

Enoxaparin has been less extensively studied in the setting of PPCI. In the ATOLL trial comparing intravenous enoxaparin with UFH for PPCI, the 30-day primary composite endpoint of death, complication of MI, procedural failure, and major bleeding was not significantly reduced (17% reduction, $P = .063$) with enoxaparin, although there were reductions in the composite main secondary endpoint of death, recurrent MI or ACS, or urgent revascularization and in other secondary composite endpoints, such as death, resuscitated cardiac arrest and death, or complication of MI.[35] Importantly, there was no increased bleeding with enoxaparin over UFH.[35] Based on the finding of this study and on the considerable clinical experience with enoxaparin in other PCI settings, the European guidelines suggest that enoxaparin may be preferred over UFH.[1] Differently, the American guidelines do not make any recommendation regarding enoxaparin.[2]

Bivalirudin has been compared with a combination of UFH and GPIs for the treatment of STEMI patients undergoing PPCI, in the HORIZONS-AMI trial.[27] This trial showed the superiority of bivalirudin driven by a marked reduction in bleeding. A higher rate of acute (within 24 hours) ST with bivalirudin was observed (1% excess), which disappeared at 30 days. Significant interactions between prerandomization use of UFH, use of a loading dose of clopidogrel (600 mg), and reduced risk of ST were observed.[36] The excess of ST in the bivalirudin-treated patients was limited to the first 5 hours after PCI. This suggests that a treatment gap may exist in the initial hours after PCI, which was probably due to the combination of bivalirudin's short half-life and the delayed onset of adequate $P2Y_{12}$ inhibition after clopidogrel loading (even at 600 mg) in the setting of STEMI.[37] Possible alternative strategies to minimize the risk of these early thrombotic events include an early UFH bolus, prolonged infusion of bivalirudin after PCI, and/or the use of a more rapid onset $P2Y_{12}$ inhibitor. Bivalirudin significantly reduced overall and cardiac at 30 days, 1 year, and 3 years.[27] Based on findings of the HORIZONS-AMI, trial, both the American and European guidelines recommend bivalirudin as a reasonable anticoagulant alternative for PPCI in STEMI (class IB).[1,2] Current American guidelines, however, do not endorse one option over another (bivalirudin and UFH are in class IB and class IC, respectively), whereas European guidelines recommend considering bivalirudin over UFH and restricting UFH use in patients not receiving bivalirudin or enoxaparin (recommendation in class IC).

## PCI AFTER FIBRINOLYSIS

In the absence of contraindications, fibrinolytic therapy should be given to patients with STEMI when it is anticipated that PPCI cannot be performed within 120 minutes of first medical contact.[1,2] In cases of evidence of failed reperfusion (lack of resolution of ST elevation by at least 50% in the worst lead at 60 to 90 minutes) or reocclusion after fibrinolysis, a decision to proceed with urgent coronary angiography and rescue PCI has to be considered. In the so-called pharmacoinvasive strategy, fibrinolytic therapy can be given at a non-PCI hospital to establish reperfusion and is followed by nonurgent transfer to a PCI-capable hospital for routine early coronary angiography.

### Rescue PCI

Several trials in the stent era and meta-analyses have examined the impact of rescue PCI after failed fibrinolysis compared with conservative therapy, defined as no additional immediate reperfusion treatment.[38–41] Overall, these studies showed that rescue PCI compared with a watchful waiting strategy is associated with a trend toward a lower mortality rate and significantly lower rates of recurrent MI and HF. Higher rates of periprocedural major bleeding and stroke have been reported, however, in patients undergoing rescue PCI than in patients treated conservatively.[40,41] Major bleeding in the rescue PCI has been associated with the femoral access for catheterization and with the concomitant use of abciximab.[41] Therefore, a large proportion of bleeding events after rescue PCI could be avoided, with a larger use of the radial approach and perhaps also with a more restricted use of GPIs in this setting. In addition, a conservative treatment might be reasonable in patients with improving symptoms and a limited infarction despite persistence of ST elevation, in which benefits of rescue PCI may not justify the risks. Based on the evidence consistently showing the benefits in terms of mortality and reinfarction associated with rescue PCI, this strategy is endorsed by current guidelines (class I and class IIa in the European and American

guidelines, respectively).[1,2] An emergency angiography after fibrinolysis is indicated for cardiogenic shock or severe acute HF irrespective of time delay from MI onset (class I recommendation in both guidelines).[1,2]

### Pharmacoinvasive Strategy

Several randomized clinical trials have compared routine early versus routine delayed or ischemia-driven catheterization and PCI after fibrinolytic therapy.[42–50] The TRANSFER-AMI trial was the largest of these randomized clinical trials, which evaluated a pharmacoinvasive strategy of immediate transfer for early catheterization after fibrinolysis versus a conservative approach.[49] In this trial, 1059 STEMI patients with high risk receiving fibrinolytic therapy with tenecteplase at non-PCI centers were randomized either to an immediate transfer to a PCI-capable hospital (with the goal of performing coronary angiography and target revascularization within 6 hours after fibrinolysis) or standard treatment, including clinically indicated rescue PCI. PCI was performed in 84.9% of the patients in the immediate-transfer group at a median of 3.2 hours after randomization and 67.4% of the patients in the standard-treatment group at a median of 21.9 hours after randomization. The TRANSFER-AMI trial showed a significant reduction in the primary composite endpoint of death, reinfarction, recurrent ischemia, new or worsening congestive heart failure, or shock within 30 days in the immediate-transfer group, with no significant differences in the rates of TIMI major or minor bleeding, transfusions, or ICHs. Overall, the results of this and the other smaller studies suggest that STEMI patients benefit more from immediate transfer for early catheterization compared with either an ischemia-guided approach or delayed routine catheterization. A larger proportional benefit with early catheterization and PCI was found among patients with higher risk.[51] Based on these observations, the guidelines recommend the strategy of early transfer to a PCI-capable center after fibrinolysis, even in patients hemodynamically stable and with clinical evidence of successful reperfusion (class IA and class IIaB in the European and American guidelines, respectively).[1,2] Angiography should be performed within 3 to 24 hours after fibrinolysis. Because of the associated increased bleeding risk, early (<2–3 hours), catheterization after fibrinolysis should be reserved for patients with failed fibrinolysis and significant myocardial jeopardy, for whom rescue PCI would be appropriate.

The pharmacoinvasive strategy has been also compared with PPCI in 2 previous small studies (WEST and GRACIA-2) and in a recent large

STREAM trial.[47,52,53] The WEST and GRACIA-2 studies, although not adequately sized, generated the hypothesis that a strategy of early routine post-fibrinolysis PCI may be equivalent to PPCI.[47,52] In the recent STREAM trial, STEMI patients (n = 1892) who presented within 3 hours after symptom onset and who were unable to undergo PPCI within 1 hour, were randomly assigned to undergo either PPCI or fibrinolytic therapy with bolus tenecteplase plus contemporary antithrombotic therapy (clopidogrel and enoxaparin) before transport to a PCI-capable hospital to undergo angiography—urgently if fibrinolysis failed, otherwise 6 to 24 hours after randomization.[53] Emergency angiography was required in 36.3% of patients in the fibrinolysis group, whereas the remainder of patients underwent angiography at a median of 17 hours after randomization. Therefore, this trial resembles the design of the TRANSFER-AMI study, in that after fibrinolysis is given, patients are transferred to a PCI center without the decision made for automatic immediate PCI on arrival; rather, PCI represents an invasive backup. This is different from facilitated PCI, where the decision to perform PCI is made before the additional pharmacologic reperfusion treatment is given. In the STREAM trial, the 30-day clinical efficacy endpoints were found similar between the 2 groups (**Fig. 1**). There was a significant increase, however, in ICH in the pharmacoinvasive group (see **Fig. 1**), which led to the dose of tenecteplase halved in the elderly (≥75 years) after 20% of planned recruitment, after which 2 ICH rate in the fibrinolysis group was reduced to 0.5%, with no significant differences between the 2 groups.[53]

## Adjunctive Antiplatelet Therapy After Fibrinolysis

Antiplatelet drugs that are currently recommended as adjunctive therapy coadministered with fibrinolysis (given before or with the fibrinolytic) include[1,2]

- Aspirin (162-mg to 325-mg loading dose, followed by a maintenance dose of 81 mg to 100 mg, continued indefinitely)
- Clopidogrel (300-mg loading dose only if aged ≤75 years, followed by a maintenance dose of 75 mg/d continued for at least 14 days and up to 1 year in absence of bleeding risk)

The coadministration of prasugrel and ticagrelor with fibrinolytic therapy has not been prospectively studied.

Antiplatelet regimens currently recommended to support PCI after fibrinolytic therapy include[1,2]

- Clopidogrel (75 mg/d) without an additional loading dose for patients who received a loading dose of clopidogrel with fibrinolytic therapy (class IC)
- Clopidogrel (300-mg loading dose) before or at the time of PCI for patients who have not received a loading dose of clopidogrel and PCI is performed less than or equal to 24 hours after fibrinolysis (class IC)
- Clopidogrel (600-mg loading dose) before or at the time of PCI for patients who have not received a loading dose of clopidogrel and PCI is performed more than 24 hours after fibrinolysis (class IC)

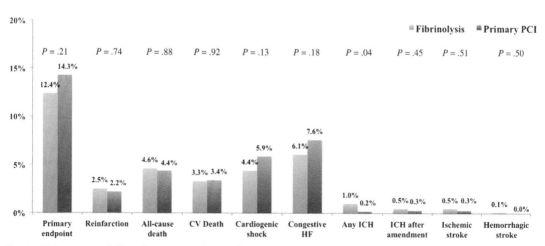

**Fig. 1.** 30-Day rates of clinical outcomes observed in the STREAM trial. The primary efficacy endpoint was a composite of death, shock, congestive heart failure, or reinfarction up to 30 days. CV, cardiovascular mortality; HF, heart failure.

- Prasugrel (60-mg loading dose) before or at the time of PCI for patients who have not received a loading dose of clopidogrel and PCI is performed more than 24 hours after treatment with a fibrin-specific agent or more than 48 hours after a non–fibrin-specific agent (class IIaB)

The recommendation of prasugrel as an alternative to clopidogrel in patients with STEMI who undergo delayed PCI after fibrinolysis is based on data from a TRITON-TIMI 38 subset of patients with STEMI who received fibrinolytic therapy more than 24 hours (for fibrin-specific agents) or more than 48 hours (for non–fibrin-specific agents) before PCI. In this subset, the use of prasugrel compared with clopidogrel was associated with a significantly lower rate of the primary composite endpoint (hazard ratio 0.65; 95% CI, 0.54–0.87; $P = .002$), with no differences in non–CABG-related TIMI major bleeding.

### Adjunctive Anticoagulant Therapy After Fibrinolysis

In patients with STEMI treated with fibrinolysis, parenteral anticoagulation should preferably be given until revascularization. Otherwise, it should be given for at least 48 hours or for the duration of hospital stay, up to 8 days. Anticoagulant drugs currently recommended as adjunctive therapy coadministered with fibrinolysis (given before or with the fibrinolytic) include[1,2]

- UFH, 60 U/kg intravenous bolus (maximum 4000 U) followed by an infusion of 12 U/kg/h (maximum 1000 U/h) initially, adjusted to maintain activated partial thromboplastin time at 1.5 to 2.0 times control (approximately 50–70 s) (class IC) for maximum 48 hours
- Enoxaparin, 30-mg intravenous bolus, followed 15 minutes later by 1 mg/kg subcutaneously every 12 hours (maximum 100 mg for the first 2 doses) if age less than 75 years; no bolus, start with 0.75 mg/kg subcutaneously every 12 hours (maximum 75 mg for the first 2 doses) if age greater than or equal to 75 years; 1 mg/kg subcutaneously every 24 hours regardless of age, if creatinine clearance less than 30 mL/min (class IA)
- Fondaparinux, initial 2.5-mg intravenous dose, then 2.5 mg subcutaneously once daily (class IB)

Based on findings from the ExTRACT-TIMI 25 trial, in which the net clinical benefit (absence of death, nonfatal infarction, and ICH) favored enoxaparin over UFH in patients with STEMI treated with fibrinolysis, the European guidelines endorse enoxaparin over UFH in this setting.[54]

Fondaparinux was shown superior to UFH in preventing death and reinfarction, especially in patients who received streptokinase, in the large OASIS-6 trial.[34]

Anticoagulants regimens currently recommended to support PCI after fibrinolytic therapy include[1,2]

- UFH continued through PCI, administering additional IV boluses as needed to maintain therapeutic activated clotting time, depending on use of GPIs
- Enoxaparin continued through PCI with no additional drug if last dose was within previous 8 hours or 0.3-mg/kg intravenous bolus if last dose was 8 to 12 hours earlier

Fondaparinux is contraindicated as a sole anticoagulant for PCI.

### REFERENCES

1. Steg PG, James SK, Atar D, et al. ESC Guidelines for the management of acute myocardial infarction in patients presenting with ST-segment elevation. Task Force on the management of ST-segment elevation acute myocardial infarction of the European Society of Cardiology (ESC). Eur Heart J 2012;33:2569–619.
2. O'Gara PT, Kushner FG, Ascheim DD, et al, American College of Cardiology Foundation/American Heart Association Task Force on Practice Guidelines. 2013 ACCF/AHA guideline for the management of ST-elevation myocardial infarction: a report of the American College of Cardiology Foundation/American Heart Association Task Force on Practice Guidelines. Circulation 2013;127:e362–425.
3. Nallamothu BK, Bates ER, Herrin J, et al, NRMI Investigators. Times to treatment in transfer patients undergoing primary percutaneous coronary intervention in the United States: National Registry of Myocardial Infarction (NRMI)-3/4 analysis. Circulation 2005;111:761–7.
4. Roe MT, Messenger JC, Weintraub WS, et al. Treatments, trends, and outcomes of acute myocardial infarction and percutaneous coronary intervention. J Am Coll Cardiol 2010;56:254–63.
5. Terkelsen CJ, Sørensen JT, Maeng M, et al. System delay and mortality among patients with STEMI treated with primary percutaneous coronary intervention. JAMA 2010;304:763–71.
6. Assessment of the Safety and Efficacy of a New Treatment Strategy with Percutaneous Coronary Intervention (ASSENT-4 PCI) Investigators. Primary versus tenecteplase-facilitated percutaneous coronary intervention in patients with ST-segment

elevation acute myocardial infarction (ASSENT-4 PCI): randomised trial. Lancet 2006;367:569–78.

7. Ellis SG, Tendera M, de Belder MA, et al. Facilitated PCI in patients with ST-elevation myocardial infarction. N Engl J Med 2008;358:2205–17.

8. Keeley EC, Boura JA, Grines CL. Primary angioplasty versus intravenous thrombolytic therapy for acute myocardial infarction: a quantitative review of 23 randomised trials. Lancet 2003;361:13–20.

9. Kornowski R, Mehran R, Dangas G, et al. Prognostic impact of staged versus "one-time" multivessel percutaneous intervention in acute myocardial infarction: analysis from the HORIZONS-AMI (Harmonizing Outcomes With Revascularization and Stents in Acute Myocardial Infarction) trial. J Am Coll Cardiol 2011;58:704–11.

10. Vlaar PJ, Mahmoud KD, Holmes DR Jr, et al. Culprit vessel only versus multivessel and staged percutaneous coronary intervention for multivessel disease in patients presenting with ST-segment elevation myocardial infarction: a pairwise and network meta-analysis. J Am Coll Cardiol 2011;58:692–703.

11. Wijns W, Kolh P, Danchin N, et al, Task Force on Myocardial Revascularization of the European Society of Cardiology (ESC) and the European Association for Cardio-Thoracic Surgery (EACTS), European Association for Percutaneous Cardiovascular Interventions (EAPCI). Guidelines on myocardial revascularization. Eur Heart J 2010;31:2501–55.

12. Levine GN, Bates ER, Blankenship JC, et al, American College of Cardiology Foundation; American Heart Association Task Force on Practice Guidelines, Society for Cardiovascular Angiography and Interventions. 2011 ACCF/AHA/SCAI Guideline for Percutaneous Coronary Intervention. A report of the American College of Cardiology Foundation/American Heart Association Task Force on Practice Guidelines and the Society for Cardiovascular Angiography and Interventions. J Am Coll Cardiol 2011;58:e44–122.

13. Dangas G, Mehran R, Guagliumi G, et al, HORIZONS-AMI Trial Investigators. Role of clopidogrel loading dose in patients with ST-segment elevation myocardial infarction undergoing primary angioplasty: results from the HORIZONS-AMI (harmonizing outcomes with revascularization and stents in acute myocardial infarction) trial. J Am Coll Cardiol 2009;54:1438–46.

14. CURRENT-OASIS 7 Investigators, Mehta SR, Bassand JP, Chrolavicius S, et al. Dose comparisons of clopidogrel and aspirin in acute coronary syndromes. N Engl J Med 2010;363:930–42.

15. Ferreiro JL, Angiolillo DJ. Clopidogrel response variability: current status and future directions. Thromb Haemost 2009;102:7–14.

16. Capranzano P, Ferreiro JL, Angiolillo DJ. Prasugrel in acute coronary syndrome patients undergoing percutaneous coronary intervention. Expert Rev Cardiovasc Ther 2009;7:361–9.

17. Wiviott SD, Braunwald E, McCabe CH, et al. Prasugrel versus clopidogrel in patients with acute coronary syndromes. N Engl J Med 2007;357:2001–15.

18. Montalescot G, Wiviott SD, Braunwald E, et al, TRITON-TIMI 38 investigators. Prasugrel compared with clopidogrel in patients undergoing percutaneous coronary intervention for ST-elevation myocardial infarction (TRITON-TIMI 38): double-blind, randomized controlled trial. Lancet 2009;373:723–31.

19. Gurbel PA, Bliden KP, Butler K, et al. Randomized double-blind assessment of the ONSET and OFFSET of the antiplatelet effects of ticagrelor versus clopidogrel in patients with stable coronary artery disease: the ONSET/OFFSET study. Circulation 2009;120:2577–85.

20. Wallentin L, Becker RC, Budaj A, et al. Ticagrelor versus clopidogrel in patients with acute coronary syndromes. N Engl J Med 2009;361:1045–57.

21. Steg PG, James S, Harrington RA, et al, PLATO Study Group. Ticagrelor versus clopidogrel in patients with ST-elevation acute coronary syndromes intended for reperfusion with primary percutaneous coronary intervention: a Platelet Inhibition and Patient Outcomes (PLATO) trial subgroup analysis. Circulation 2010;122:2131–41.

22. Ferreiro JL, Ueno M, Angiolillo DJ. Cangrelor: a review on its mechanism of action and clinical development. Expert Rev Cardiovasc Ther 2009;7:1195–201.

23. Bhatt DL, Stone GW, Mahaffey KW, et al, the CHAMPION PHOENIX Investigators. Effect of Platelet Inhibition with Cangrelor during PCI on Ischemic Events. N Engl J Med 2013;368(14):1303–13.

24. De Luca G, Suryapranata H, Stone GW, et al. Abciximab as adjunctive therapy to reperfusion in acute ST-segment elevation myocardial infarction: a meta-analysis of randomized trials. JAMA 2005;293:1759–65.

25. Mehilli J, Kastrati A, Schulz S, et al, Bavarian Reperfusion Alternatives Evaluation-3 (BRAVE-3) Study Investigators. Abciximab in patients with acute ST-segment-elevation myocardial infarction undergoing primary percutaneous coronary intervention after clopidogrel loading: a randomized double-blind trial. Circulation 2009;119:1933–40.

26. Van't Hof AW, Ten Berg J, Heestermans T, et al. Pre-hospital initiation of tirofiban in patients with ST-elevation myocardial infarction undergoing primary angioplasty (On-TIME 2): a multicentre, double-blind, randomised controlled trial. Lancet 2008;372:537–46.

27. Stone GW, Witzenbichler B, Guagliumi G, et al. Bivalirudin during primary PCI in acute myocardial infarction. N Engl J Med 2008;358:2218–30.

28. Stone GW, Maehara A, Witzenbichler B, et al, INFUSE-AMI Investigators. Intracoronary abciximab and aspiration thrombectomy in patients with large anterior myocardial infarction: the INFUSE-AMI randomized trial. JAMA 2012;307:1817–26.

29. Friedland S, Eisenberg MJ, Shimony A. Meta-analysis of randomized controlled trials of intracoronary versus intravenous administration of glycoprotein IIb/IIIa inhibitors during percutaneous coronary intervention for acute coronary syndrome. Am J Cardiol 2011;108:1244–51.

30. Thiele H, Wohrle J, Hambrecht R, et al. Intracoronary versus intravenous bolus abciximab during primary percutaneous coronary intervention in patients with acute ST-elevation myocardial infarction: a randomised trial. Lancet 2012;379:923–31.

31. Valgimigli M, Campo G, Percoco G, et al. Comparison of angioplasty with infusion of tirofiban or abciximab and with implantation of sirolimus-eluting or uncoated stents for acute myocardial infarction: the MULTISTRATEGY randomized trial. JAMA 2008;299:1788–99.

32. Akerblom A, James SK, Koutouzis M, et al. Eptifibatide is noninferior to abciximab in primary percutaneous coronary intervention: results from the SCAAR (Swedish Coronary Angiography and Angioplasty Registry). J Am Coll Cardiol 2010;56:470–5.

33. Herrmann HC, Lu J, Brodie BR, et al. Benefit of facilitated percutaneous coronary intervention in high-risk ST-segment elevation myocardial infarction patients presenting to nonpercutaneous coronary intervention hospitals. JACC Cardiovasc Interv 2009;2:917–24.

34. Yusuf S, Mehta SR, Chrolavicius S, et al. Effects of fondaparinux on mortality and reinfarction in patients with acute ST-segment elevation myocardial infarction: the OASIS-6 randomized trial. JAMA 2006;295:1519–30.

35. Montalescot G, Zeymer U, Silvain J, et al. Intravenous enoxaparin or unfractionated heparin in primary percutaneous coronary intervention for ST-elevation myocardial infarction: the international randomised open-label ATOLL trial. Lancet 2011;378:693–703.

36. Dangas GD, Caixeta A, Mehran R, et al. Frequency and predictors of stent thrombosis after percutaneous coronary intervention in acute myocardial infarction. Circulation 2011;123:1745–56.

37. Capranzano P, Dangas G. Bivalirudin for primary percutaneous coronary intervention in acute myocardial infarction: the HORIZONS-AMI trial. Expert Rev Cardiovasc Ther 2012;10:411–22.

38. Sutton AG, Campbell PG, Graham R, et al. A randomized trial of rescue angioplasty vs a conservative approach for failed fibrinolysis in ST-segment elevation myocardial infarction: the Middlesbrough Early Revascularization to Limit INfarction (MERLIN) trial. J Am Coll Cardiol 2004;44:287–96.

39. Gershlick AH, Stephens-Lloyd A, Hughes S, et al. Rescue angioplasty after failed thrombolytic therapy for acute myocardial infarction. N Engl J Med 2005;353:2758–68.

40. Wijeysundera HC, Vijayaraghavan R, Nallamothu BK, et al. Rescue angioplasty or repeat fibrinolysis after failed fibrinolytic therapy for ST-segment myocardial infarction: a meta-analysis of randomized trials. J Am Coll Cardiol 2007;49:422–30.

41. Collet JP, Montalescot G, Le MM, et al. Percutaneous coronary intervention after fibrinolysis: a multiple meta-analyses approach according to the type of strategy. J Am Coll Cardiol 2006;48:1326–35.

42. Scheller B, Hennen B, Hammer B, et al. Beneficial effects of immediate stenting after thrombolysis in acute myocardial infarction. J Am Coll Cardiol 2003;42:634–41.

43. Fernandez-Aviles F, Alonso JJ, Castro-Beiras A, et al. Routine invasive strategy within 24 hours of thrombolysis vs ischaemia-guided conservative approach for acute myocardial infarction with ST-segment elevation (GRACIA-1): a randomised controlled trial. Lancet 2004;364:1045–53.

44. Thiele H, Engelmann L, Elsner K, et al. Comparison of pre-hospital combination-fibrinolysis plus conventional care with pre-hospital combination-fibrinolysis plus facilitated percutaneous coronary intervention in acute myocardial infarction. Eur Heart J 2005;26:1956–63.

45. Le May MR, Wells GA, Labinaz M, et al. Combined angioplasty and pharmacological intervention vs thrombolysis alone in acute myocardial infarction (CAPITAL AMI study). J Am Coll Cardiol 2005;46:417–24.

46. Di Pasquale P, Cannizzaro S, Parrinello G, et al. Is delayed facilitated percutaneous coronary intervention better than immediate in reperfused myocardial infarction? Six months follow up findings. J Thromb Thrombolysis 2006;21:147–57.

47. Armstrong PW. A comparison of pharmacologic therapy with/without timely coronary intervention vs primary percutaneous intervention early after ST-elevation myocardial infarction: the WEST (Which Early ST-elevation myocardial infarction Therapy) study. Eur Heart J 2006;27:1530–8.

48. Di Mario C, Dudek D, Piscione F, et al. Immediate angioplasty vs standard therapy with rescue angioplasty after thrombolysis in the Combined

Abciximab REteplase Stent Study in Acute Myocardial Infarction (CARESS-in-AMI): an open, prospective, randomised, multicentre trial. Lancet 2008;371:559–68.

49. Cantor WJ, Fitchett D, Borgundvaag B, et al. Routine early angioplasty after fibrinolysis for acute myocardial infarction. N Engl J Med 2009;360: 2705–18.

50. Bohmer E, Hoffmann P, Abdelnoor M, et al. Efficacy and safety of immediate angioplasty vs ischemia-guided management after thrombolysis in acute myocardial infarction in areas with very long transfer distances results of the NORDISTEMI (NORwegian study on DIstrict treatment of ST-elevation myocardial infarction). J Am Coll Cardiol 2010;55: 102–10.

51. Borgia F, Goodman SG, Halvorsen S, et al. Early routine percutaneous coronary intervention after fibrinolysis vs. standard therapy in ST-segment elevation myocardial infarction: a meta-analysis. Eur Heart J 2010;31:2156–69.

52. Fernández-Avilés F, Alonso JJ, Peña G, et al, GRACIA-2 (Groupo de Análisis de Cardiopatía Isquémica Aguda) Investigators. Primary angioplasty vs. early routine post-fibrinolysis angioplasty for acute myocardial infarction with ST-segment elevation: the GRACIA-2 non-inferiority, randomized, controlled trial. Eur Heart J 2007;28:949–60.

53. Armstrong PW, Gershlick AH, Goldstein P, et al, the STREAM Investigative Team. Fibrinolysis or Primary PCI in ST-Segment Elevation Myocardial Infarction. N Engl J Med 2013;368(15):1379–87.

54. Giraldez RR, Nicolau JC, Corbalan R, et al. Enoxaparin is superior to unfractionated heparin in patients with ST elevation myocardial infarction undergoing fibrinolysis regardless of the choice of lytic: an ExTRACT-TIMI 25 analysis. Eur Heart J 2007;28:1566–73.

# The Optimal Duration of Dual Combination Antiplatelet Therapy After Stent Implantation and Perioperative Management Issues

Nisharahmed Kherada, MD[a], Roxana Mehran, MD[b,c],
George D. Dangas, MD, PhD[d],*

## KEYWORDS

- Drug-eluting stents • Thrombosis • Percutaneous coronary intervention • Noncardiac surgery

## KEY POINTS

- Dual antiplatelet therapy (DAPT) is essential to prevent stent thrombosis.
- The optimal duration of DAPT is still uncertain.
- Balancing the risk of stent thrombosis (ST) and bleeding is crucial.
- Studies on prolonged (>12 months) DAPT have shown mixed results.
- Improvements in stent technologies and coronary intervention strategies have contributed to a reduction of ST and have opened up the possibilities of shorter durations of DAPT.
- Perioperative DAPT management has been a crucial topic owing to concerns about bleeding related to the surgery and at the same time worries of ST related to stopping DAPT.
- Many factors should be considered in deciding and the perioperative management of DAPT.

## INTRODUCTION

Percutaneous coronary intervention (PCI) with stent implantation is a cornerstone therapy for symptomatic coronary artery disease. Although there have been many improvements in coronary intervention and stent technology, the risk of stent thrombosis (ST) remains a concern. Since the introduction and widespread use of drug-eluting stents (DES), the risk of restenosis was reduced but the risk of late ST has emerged. Drug-eluting stent–induced thrombogenicity can be due to (1) inhibition of endothelial cell proliferation, leading to diminished endothelial coverage and deferred local healing; (2) tissue factor induction by the eluted drug (**Fig. 1**); (3) a hypersensitive local reaction to the drug or polymer-coating; and (4) patient

Disclosures: NK, None; RM, Institutional Research Grant Support: The Medicines Company, BMS/Sanofi, and Lilly/DSI. Consulting: Abbott Vascular, Astra Zeneca, Janssen (J+J), Regado Biosciences, The Medicines Company, BMS/Sanofi, and Merck; GD, Institutional Research Grant Support: The Medicines Company, BMS/Sanofi, and Lilly/DSI. Consulting: Abbott Vascular, Astra Zeneca, Janssen (J+J), Regado Biosciences, The Medicines Company, BMS/Sanofi, and Merck.
[a] Hypertension Section, The Icahn School of Medicine at Mount Sinai, One Gustave L. Levy Place, Box 1030, New York, NY 10029, USA; [b] Department of Cardiology, The Icahn School of Medicine at Mount Sinai, One Gustave L. Levy Place, Box 1030, New York, NY 10029, USA; [c] Cardiovascular Research Foundation, 111 East 59th Street, New York, NY 10022-1202, USA; [d] Department of Cardiology, The Zena and Michael A. Wiener Cardiovascular Institute, The Icahn School of Medicine at Mount Sinai, One Gustave L. Levy Place, Box 1030, New York, NY 10029, USA
* Corresponding author. The Zena and Michael A. Wiener Cardiovascular Institute, The Icahn School of Medicine at Mount Sinai, One Gustave L. Levy Place, Box 1030, New York, NY 10029.
E-mail address: george.dangas@mssm.edu

Intervent Cardiol Clin 2 (2013) 585–594
http://dx.doi.org/10.1016/j.iccl.2013.05.003
2211-7458/13/$ – see front matter © 2013 Elsevier Inc. All rights reserved.

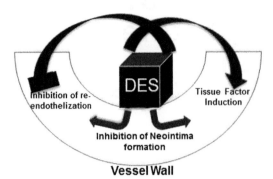

**Fig. 1.** DES action on vessel wall and thrombogenicity. DES, drug eluting stent.

nonadherence to antiplatelet therapy or drug resistance.[1–3] In addition, stent underexpansion and malapposition (from either the time of implantation or "late" acquired) are mechanical risks for stent restenosis and thrombosis.[4]

It is noteworthy that the rate of early ST (within 30 days) is similar between DES and bare metal stent (BMS).[5] The risk of late and very late ST in DES patients led to the obligatory use of dual antiplatelet therapy (DAPT) with aspirin and a $P2Y_{12}$ receptor inhibitor, including clopidogrel, prasugrel, and ticagrelor. These antiplatelet agents act on multiple steps of the complex thrombus formation process (**Fig. 2**).[6]

The outcomes of ST also vary: subacute stent thrombosis has a more severe clinical course and bears a higher association with mortality than late or very late stent thrombosis.[7] Clinical and angiographic risk factors can be used to risk-stratify individual patient risk for ST, and the high-risk group was reported to have ST risk up

to 9%.[8] The additional impact of genetic risk factors related to clopidogrel resistance (either delayed absorption or conversion to its active metabolite) has also been proposed for inclusion in such a risk assessment.[9] The latter implies that DAPT nonadherence against medical advice would also be a major risk to be considered.

Although the use of DES is widespread, the optimal duration of DAPT still remains unknown. The association between ST and DAPT nonadherence varies over time after stenting: strongest in the first month, important for 6 months, and not as strong afterward. Interestingly, very late ST was shown association with cessation of DAPT or aspirin alone but not with the cessation of a $P2Y_{12}$ inhibitor alone,[10] creating an uncertainty regarding the optimal DAPT duration, which is echoed by the differing guidelines by the American College of Cardiology (ACC)/American Heart Association (AHA) and European Society of Cardiology (ESC). Premature discontinuation of DAPT due to various clinical and sociodemographic factors[11] is considered a significant risk for ST and subsequent death and myocardial infarction (MI),[12] whereas prolonged DAPT use can put the patient at greater risk for bleeding.[13] Several studies have produced a variety of conflicting results, indicating the controversial nature of this issue. The decision for optimal use of DAPT is multifactorial, including baseline characteristics (low vs high risk) and clinical status (acute coronary syndrome [ACS] vs non-ACS), stent properties (BMS, first-generation or second-generation DES), and procedural characteristics (bifurcation or more complex cases).

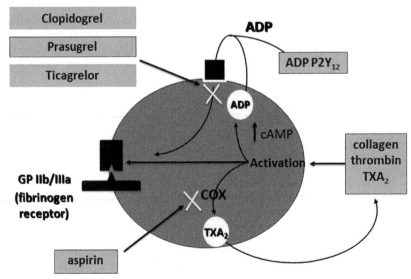

**Fig. 2.** Oral antiplatelet therapies mechanisms of action. ADP, adenosine diphosphate; COX, cyclooxygenase; $TXA_2$, thromboxane $A_2$.

In patients on DAPT poststenting who are undergoing planned or emergent noncardiac or cardiac surgical procedure, there is a concern for platelet dysfunction-related surgical site bleeding. On the other hand, surgery is a thrombogenic event because it causes tissue damage, increased platelet aggregation, higher fibrinogen, temporary shutdown of fibrinolysis, inflammation, and homeostatic disturbance.[14,15] Thus, interruption of DAPT before the procedure increases the risk for stent thrombosis and recurrent cardiovascular events. Approximately 4% to 11% of patients in 1 year and 22% of patients within 3 years of coronary stent placement may require noncardiac surgery.[14] Most of these procedures are not true surgical emergencies and were not known or scheduled ahead of the time of coronary stent implantation. Initial reports indicated that ST can occur in up to 40% of patients perioperatively when DAPT was suspended without careful consideration.[16] The expert consensus on this subject is to delay elective or nonurgent surgery for at least 12 months in case of DES implantation, or 30 to 45 days for BMS or balloon angioplasty. If antiplatelet therapy must be stopped before major surgery, aspirin should be continued (except for the neurosurgery) and the $P2Y_{12}$ inhibitor should be restarted as soon as possible after the procedure.[17] A consideration has been given lately for only a 6-month delay after an uncomplicated PCI procedure with a secnd-generation DES.

## CURRENT PRACTICE GUIDELINES AND PHARMACOLOGIC STRATEGIES

ACC/AHA guidelines for post-PCI DAPT
- Dosage of DAPT after stenting
  - Combination of aspirin 81 mg daily and one of the $P2Y_{12}$ inhibitors, including
    - Clopidogrel 75 mg daily
    - Prasugrel 10 mg daily (5 mg for patients with high bleeding risk), or
    - Ticagrelor 90 mg twice daily for ACS patients
  - Combination of aspirin and clopidogrel for non-ACS patients with significant coronary artery disease
- Patients with DES implantation
  - Aspirin indefinitely (class I, level B)
  - $P2Y_{12}$ inhibitor for at least 12 months (class I, level B) regardless of the patient's clinical status (ACS or non-ACS), with the exception of non-ACS patients with high risk of bleeding
- In patients receiving BMS
  - Aspirin indefinitely (class I, level B)

  - $P2Y_{12}$ inhibitor for ACS patients for at least 12 months and for non-ACS patients a minimum of 1 month and up to 12 months unless the patient is at high risk of bleeding, in whom it should be given for a minimum of 2 weeks (class I, level B)[18–20]

ESC guidelines for post-PCI DAPT
- For ST segment elevation MI:
  - DAPT for up to 12 months (class I, level C) with a strict minimum of $P2Y_{12}$ inhibitor
    - 1 month for patients with BMS (class I, level C), and
    - 6 months for patients with DES (class IIb, level B)[21]
- For non-ST segment elevation ACS:
  - DAPT for 12 months unless contraindications such as high risk of bleeding (class I, level A)[22,23]

It is important to understand that these are general guidelines and physicians should tailor therapy to each patient by carefully stratifying risk and using the 12-month DAPT recommendation as a default strategy after stenting.

General guidelines for perioperative DAPT management (**Table 1**)
- A considerable number of patients may require PCI who are scheduled for elective noncardiac surgery in the following 12 months; this scenario should drive the decision-making in type of PCI procedure that requires short duration of mandatory DAPT therapy.
- Similarly, some PCI patients may need noncardiac surgery while still on obligatory DAPT regimen. It is important to be aware of how long to withhold antiplatelet therapy perioperatively as well as the appropriate amount of time to delay the surgical procedure.

ESC perioperative management guidelines (**Table 2**):
- Continue aspirin in patients previously treated with aspirin
- Discontinue aspirin in those with difficult-to-control hemostasis during noncardiac surgery (class IIa, level B)
- If clopidogrel interruption is necessary before a noncardiac surgery
  - Stop at least 5 days to as much as 10 days before surgery
  - Resume approximately 24 hours after surgery with adequate hemostasis[24]

**Table 1**
**ACCF/AHA/SCAI guideline for revascularization before noncardiac surgery and perioperative DAPT management**

| Recommendation | Class | Level of Evidence |
|---|---|---|
| For patients who require PCI and are scheduled for elective noncardiac surgery in the subsequent 12 mo, a strategy of balloon angioplasty or BMS implantation followed by 4–6 wk of DAPT is reasonable | IIa (benefit ≫ risk, additional studies with focused objective needed) (It is reasonable to proceed) | B (limited population evaluated; data derived from a single randomized trial or nonrandomized studies) |
| For patients with DES who must undergo urgent surgical procedures that mandate the discontinuation of DAPT, it is reasonable to continue aspirin if possible and restart the $P2Y_{12}$ inhibitor as soon as possible in the immediate postoperative period | IIa | C (very limited populations evaluated; consensus expert opinion, case studies, or standard of care) |
| Routine prophylactic coronary revascularization should not be performed in patients with stable coronary artery disease before noncardiac surgery | III (harm; indicated procedure is of no benefit or has potential for harm) | B |
| Elective noncardiac surgery should not be performed in the 4–6 wk after balloon angioplasty or BMS implantation or the 12 mo after DES implantation in patients in whom the $P2Y_{12}$ inhibitor will need to be discontinued perioperatively | III | B |

*Adapted from* Levine GN, Bates ER, Blankenship JC, et al. 2011 ACCF/AHA/SCAI Guideline for Percutaneous Coronary Intervention: a report of the American College of Cardiology Foundation/American Heart Association Task Force on Practice Guidelines and the Society for Cardiovascular Angiography and Interventions. Circulation 2011;124:e574–651; with permission.

ACC/AHA guidelines for cardiac surgery:
- Coronary artery bypass graft surgery (CABG) patients (class I, level B) preoperatively
  - Aspirin 81 mg to 325 mg daily
- For elective CABG
  - Discontinue clopidogrel and ticagrelor for at least 5 days before surgery (class I, level B)
  - Discontinue prasugrel for at least 7 days (class I, level C) to limit blood transfusions
- For urgent CABG indication
  - Discontinue clopidogrel and ticagrelor at least 24 hours preprocedure to reduce major bleeding complications (class I, level B)[23,25]

The decision to discontinue antiplatelet therapy in the perioperative period should be made after an informed discussion among the surgeon, managing cardiologist, hematologist, anesthesiologist, and the patient.

## OUTCOMES OF LONG-TERM POST-STENTING DAPT

Several studies highlight the beneficial effect of the longer than 12 months' use of DAPT on major adverse cardiac events (MACE),[26,27] whereas other studies fail to show significant differences in rates of MI and death in 12 versus 24 months of DAPT.[28,29]

Studies with positive outcome with long-term DAPT
- A study by Ho and colleagues,[26] of 1455 ACS patients treated by 65.8% BMS and 34.2% DES showed higher mortality risk

**Table 2**
**ESC Guideline on timing of noncardiac surgery in patients with prior PCI**

| Recommendation | Class | Level of Evidence |
|---|---|---|
| Patients with previous CABG within last 5 y should be sent for noncardiac surgery without further delay | I (evidence that a procedure is beneficial and effective) | C (consensus of opinion of the expert, small studies, registries) |
| Noncardiac surgery should be performed in patients with recent BMS after a minimum 6 wk and optimally 3 mo following the intervention | I | B (data derived from single randomized trial or large nonrandomized studies) |
| Noncardiac surgery should be performed in patients with recent DES no sooner than 12 mo following the intervention | I | B |
| Consideration should be given to postponing noncardiac surgery in patients with recent balloon angioplasty until at least 2 wk following the intervention | IIa (weight of evidence in favor of usefulness) | B |

*Adapted from* Poldermans D, Bax JJ, Boersma E, et al. Guidelines for pre-operative cardiac risk assessment and perioperative cardiac management in non-cardiac surgery. Eur Heart J 2009;30:2769–812; with permission.

with clopidogrel withdrawal up to 18 months, especially with DES use after ACS and indicated extended clopidogrel therapy after ACS PCI.

- Another single-center cohort study of 4666 patients by Eisenstein and colleagues[27] showed that in the patients with DES use who were event-free at 6 months and 12 months, clopidogrel use predicted lower rates of death (3.1% vs 7.2%, $P = .02$) and MI (0% vs 4.5%, $P<.001$) at 24 months, and similar end points were not different in BMS patients.

Long-term DAPT increases bleeding risk
- A retrospective study of 9256 patients by Petersen and colleagues[30] showed, at 18-months analysis, compared with clopidogrel high use group (n = 3102, defined as ≥490 days' supply), higher death or nonfatal MI found in medium use group (n = 3069, <490, and ≥305 days' supply of clopidogrel, hazard ratio [HR] 1.46, 95% CI 1.09–1.99, $P = .01$) and lower use group (n = 3085, <305, and ≥90 days' supply of clopidogrel, HR 1.59, 95% CI 1.18–2.14, $P = .002$); but the bleeding risk was lower in latter 2 groups (HR 0.84, 95% CI 0.71–0.98, $P = .03$) and (HR 0.77, 95% CI 0.65–0.90, $P = .002$), respectively.
- Similarly, the HMO Research Network–Stent registry by Tsai and colleagues[13] showed

that clopidogrel treatment increased in major bleeding at 13 to 18 months (relative risk = 2.34, 95% CI = 1.26–4.34) compared with patients not on clopidogrel (but on aspirin alone), but at the same time also showed decreased MI risk (relative risk = 0.53, 95% CI = 0.29–0.99).
- The randomized PRODIGY trial (Prolonging Dual antiplatelet treatment after grading stent-induced Intimal hyperplasia study) of 2013 all-comer patients who were implanted with a balanced mixture of BMS or DES showed significantly high risk of type 2, 3, or 5 BARC (Bleeding Academic Research Consortium) bleeding in 24 months of DAPT population compared with 6 months (7.4% vs 3.5%, $P<.001$).[31]

Long-term DAPT studies with unfavorable outcomes
- A merged analysis of 2 prospective randomized trials REAL-LATE (Correlation of Clopidogrel Therapy Discontinuation in Real-World Patients Treated with Drug-Eluting Stent Implantation and Late Coronary Arterial Thrombotic Events, n = 2000) and ZEST-LATE (Evaluation of the Long-Term Safety after Zotarolimus–Eluting Stent [ZES], Sirolimus-Eluting Stent [SES], or Paclitaxel-Eluting Stent Implantation for Coronary Lesions—Late Coronary Arterial Thrombotic

Events, n = 2000) trials done by Park and colleagues[29] did not show any significant benefit associated with clopidogrel continuation beyond 12 months compared with discontinuation in reducing the incidence of cardiac death or MI in patients with DES implantation. However, the study had insufficient power to make conclusions regarding the safety of clopidogrel discontinuation after 12 months.

- The Guthrie PCI Registry showed that beyond 12 months DAPT was not associated with lower incidence of death or MI than 12 months of DAPT (adjusted HR = 1.01; 95% CI 0.74 to 1.37, $P$ = .95).[28]
- A recent report on 2997 patients from the large-scale HORIZONS-AMI (Harmonizing Outcomes with Revascularization and Stents in Acute Myocardial Infarction) trial studying ST risk after ST-segment elevation MI PCI suggested declining benefit of DAPT over time, beginning at 6 months. Essentially, beyond 1 year from initial stenting, aspirin-alone therapy was more important than DAPT for the prevention of definite/probable ST.[32]

It will be interesting to follow the results of the ongoing, large multicenter, randomized-controlled DAPT (The Dual Antiplatelet Therapy Study) trial that definitely assesses the safety and efficacy of 12 versus 30 months of DAPT in subjects undergoing PCI with either DES or BMS for further conclusive insight on the subject of long-term DAPT after PCI and stenting. Until further data are obtained regarding the optimal duration of DAPT, the incremental risk of bleeding complications with prolonged DAPT therapy must be balanced against the potential decrement of ST. Utilization of bleeding risk assessment tools in clinical practice can be useful in evaluating the early as well as the long-term clinical outcomes.[33,34]

## OUTCOMES OF SHORT-TERM DAPT AFTER CORONARY STENT IMPLANTATION

The advent of newer generation of DES achieved lower stent thrombosis[35,36] and enabled the conduct of many clinical studies investigating short-term DAPT treatment. Indeed, careful insights from several registry studies indicated that short term, less than 12 months of DAPT, does not increase MACE and there is no obvious clinical advantage of greater than 6 months of DAPT.

- Specifically, a Japanese observational study of 10,778 patients showed the rates of MI or death at 6 months of DAPT after SES

implantation was 4.1% and at 24 months was 4.1% ($P$ = .99).[37]
- The DATE (Duration of Dual Antiplatelet Therapy After Implantation of Endeavor Stent) registry of 823 patients proposed the possibility of 3 months of DAPT after ZES implantation by showing the failure of increase in death, MI, or any revascularization (HR 0.89; 95% CI, 0.48–1.67) at 1-year follow-up after propensity score matching.[38]
- Another trial assessing the shorter 3 months' duration was the randomized RESET (REal Safety and Efficacy of 3-month dual antiplatelet Therapy following Endeavor zotarolimus-eluting stent implantation) trial. The trial showed noninferiority of 3 months of DAPT after ZES versus standard 12 months DAPT after other DES in composite rates of any death, MI, or ST (0.8% vs 1.3%, 95% CI −1.5–0.5; $P$ = .48).[39]
- The randomized, multicenter EXCELLENT (The Efficacy of Xience/Promus vs Cypher to Reduce Late Loss After Stenting) study of 1443 patients compared 6-month versus 12-month DAPT after DES implantation. The rate of target vessel failure at 6 months did not increase compared with 12-month DAPT, particularly in the everolimus-eluting stent subset. On the other hand, the overall short DAPT result was not as favorable in the diabetic subgroup. Unfortunately, this randomized study was underpowered for outcomes of death and MI with wide noninferiority margin to adapt the result into current practice without the subsequent larger trial.[40]
- As mentioned previously, the multicenter PRODIGY trial studied 2013 all-comer patients for the effect of 6 months versus 24 months of DAPT on clinical outcome. The composite risk of death of any cause, MI, or stroke at 2 years was 10.0%, which was identical in both groups assigned to 6 and 24 months DAPT regimen.[31]

It is also important to assess the short-term DAPT and risk of ST with early discontinuation of DAPT because it was shown to be a strong predictor of ST.[41]

- A prospective study by Airoldi and colleagues,[42] of 3021 patients with 5389 lesions treated with SES or Paclitaxel-eluting stent showed early within 6 months discontinuation of $P2Y_{12}$ inhibitor was strongly associated with ST risk compared at 18 months follow-up (HR, 13.74; 95% CI, 4.04 to 46.68; $P$<.001) and later than 6 months discontinuation failed to show any predictive value for ST (HR, 0.94; 95% CI, 0.30 to 2.98; $P = .92$).

- Conversely, the short-term DAPT study by Kimura and colleagues[37] suggested that discontinuation of both aspirin and $P2Y_{12}$ inhibitor was related to high ST risk compared with $P2Y_{12}$ inhibitor therapy alone outside 1 month of SES implantation. The study concluded that whenever DAPT therapy was clinically irrelevant for long-term continuation, then it is reasonable to discontinue $P2Y_{12}$ inhibitor with continuation of aspirin.
- Again, the EXCELLENT trial showed ST risk after everolimus eluting Xience stent was higher at 6 months (0.6%) compared with 12 months (0.2%) of DAPT groups (HR 3.00; 95% CI, 0.31–28.84; $P = .34$), but no relevant difference in composite safety endpoints of death, MI, stroke, ST, or TIMI (Thrombolysis in Myocardial Infarction) major bleeding risk between 2 groups (3.0% vs 3.0%; HR 1.00; 95% CI, 0.50–2.00; $P = .99$).[40]

More evidence regarding the safety of 6-month DAPT can be expected from the ongoing randomized trial, such as the Safety and Efficacy of Six Months DAPT After Drug-Eluting Stenting (ISAR-SAFE) trial. However, a large adequately powered randomized trial will be needed to ultimately answer this question.

## ROLE OF INTRAVASCULAR ULTRASOUND–GUIDED PCI ON DAPT DURATION DECISION-MAKING

Advancement in PCI techniques, such as intravascular ultrasound (IVUS) -guided DES implantation, has shown promising results in terms of reducing ST, death, and MI, which may potentially help clinicians to decide on the appropriate duration of DAPT after stenting. The IVUS substudy of ADAPT-DES (Assessment of Dual-Antiplatelet Therapy With Drug-Eluting Stents) demonstrated 50% reduction in incidence of ST and 33% reduction in MI starting 30 days postprocedure up to 12 months after IVUS-guided DES implantation. The study by Roy and colleagues[43] showed IVUS-guided DES implantation reduced ST in 30 days (0.5% in IVUS vs 1.4% in angiographic-guided group) and 12-months (0.7% in IVUS vs 2.0% in angiographic-guided group), and also reduced revascularization and MACE in 30 days. Furthermore, the MATRIX (Comprehensive Assessment of Sirolimus-Eluting Stents in Complex Lesions) registry showed a reduction in death, MI, and MACE at 30-day, 1-year, and 2-year

follow-up with IVUS-guided PCI.[44] Thus, a shorter duration of DAPT after newer generation DES implantation may be possible with IVUS-guided PCI and stenting.

## PERIOPERATIVE DAPT MANAGEMENT

Cessation of DAPT in patients with DES implantation is the dominant risk factor for the occurrence of late ST and very late ST in addition to early ST.[45] In the perioperative period the risk of ST worsens with DAPT discontinuation and can lead to catastrophic complications like ST-elevation MI (2%–28%), malignant arrhythmias, or death (3%–20%).[46–48] In addition, Schouten and colleagues[43] also indicated that delay in noncardiac surgery for at least 6 weeks should be considered in patients with PCI and stenting and mandatory DAPT for this duration reduces the mortality. It has also shown no difference between SES and paclitaxel-eluting stent for higher MACE with early noncardiac surgery than late. Thus, based on observational evidence, guidelines are consistent with the deferral of the noncardiac surgery for 4 to 6 weeks for BMS and 12 months for DES.[49,50]

Due to synergistic antiplatelet effects of DAPT agents, risk of surgical bleeding, blood transfusion, and length of stay in the hospital increases with continual DAPT use perioperatively. Approximate increase in surgical blood loss with aspirin is 2.5% to 20% and with DAPT (aspirin and clopidogrel) it further worsens to 30% to 50% without any translation into surgical mortality with the exception of neurosurgery.[51] The current data on periprocedural bleeding on prasugrel and ticagrelor are limited. As the DAPT cessation is the single most prominent risk factor for ST, it is vital to keep the balance between the risk of bleeding and ST in these patients.[52] A meta-analysis of 49,590 patients by Burger and colleagues[53] showed that doing noncardiac surgery on aspirin alone can lead to a 1.5 times increase in bleeding risk but without any critical bleeding complication or fatal bleed except for transurethral prostatectomy and neurosurgery, respectively. Thus, it showed the feasibility and safety to complete essentially all noncardiac surgeries on 81 mg of aspirin with the above exceptions.

Eisenberg and colleagues[54] evaluated the safety of short-term DAPT discontinuation in patients with DES. Interestingly, the study found that the median time to event was 7 days with both DAPT agent discontinuation, whereas 122 days if $P2Y_{12}$ inhibitor only was stopped. It was concluded that the short-term discontinuation of $P2Y_{12}$ inhibitor may be relatively safe in patients with DES if aspirin therapy was maintained, or it DAPT can be reinstituted within 7 days. Data from the multi-center PARIS (Patterns of Non-Adherence to Anti-Platelet Regimens in Stented Patients) Registry were presented at the Transcatheter Cardiovascular Therapeutics 2012 conference and showed of the rate of 1-year major adverse cardiac events were higher in DAPT nonadherent patients compared with the patient who discontinued DAPT on physician recommendation (13.7% vs 6.5%, $P<.001$). Thus, supervised discontinuation including verifying patient condition, stent specification, and an agreement from a cardiologist have favorable results on post-PCI DAPT management.

In the case of unavoidable noncardiac surgery to allow completion of mandatory DAPT therapy for recommended duration, vigilant assessment of the patient and procedural risk profile are required.[55] The role of bridging therapy with intravenous glycoprotein IIb/IIIa inhibitors and unfractionated or low molecular weight heparin (enoxaparin 1 mg/kg subcutaneously twice daily with adjustment for impaired renal function) is unclear in the perioperative period for the patients after stenting. However, it will be interesting to evaluate the role of reversible $P2Y_{12}$ inhibitor ticagrelor as bridging therapy in this clinical setting due to its short half-life and quick onset of action. The randomized BRIDGE (Maintenance of Platelet inhiBition With cangRelor After dIscontinuation of ThienopyriDines in Patients Undergoing surGEry) trial on the use of another reversible, intravenous $P2Y_{12}$ inhibitor Cangrelor for bridging in patients undergoing cardiac surgery was able to gain and sustain the target platelet inhibition level with low risk of thrombosis and bleeding complication.[56] New studies are necessary to improve current guidelines on the perioperative management of DAPT. At this point, no clear bridging therapy is recommended by any professional society guidelines until further data on short-acting antithrombotic therapies are available.

## SUMMARY

Determination of the optimal duration of DAPT after stenting and management decisions regarding periprocedural DAPT require taking into account characteristics of the patient (low or high risk), the clinical status (ACS vs non-ACS), the type of interventional procedure (bifurcation, total occlusion, or more complex cases), the stent properties (BMS, first-generation DES, or second-generation DES), the surgical procedure (territory, bleeding risk, ability to take and absorb oral medications), and overall bleeding risk. After coronary revascularization with DES, the appropriate duration of aspirin and $P2Y_{12}$ inhibitor therapy remains

undefined and 1-year duration is prescribed by consensus. Multiple studies have demonstrated that DAPT reduces MI and death risk but not late or very late ST; however, empiric data on extended DAPT therapy are still conflicting, leaving unanswered the question of whether indefinite or less than 12 months of DAPT can be adequate or beneficial. The improvements in stent technologies (second-generation DES) and coronary intervention strategies (IVUS-guided PCI) may indeed make shorter DAPT durations feasible. New study data should be incorporated to improve the existing guidelines and recommendations accordingly.

## REFERENCES

1. Stone GW, Moses JW, Ellis SG, et al. Safety and efficacy of sirolimus- and paclitaxel-eluting coronary stents. N Engl J Med 2007;356:998–1008.
2. Joner M, Finn AV, Farb A, et al. Pathology of drug-eluting stents in humans: delayed healing and late thrombotic risk. J Am Coll Cardiol 2006;48:193–202.
3. Luscher TF, Steffel J, Eberli FR, et al. Drug-eluting stent and coronary thrombosis: biological mechanisms and clinical implications. Circulation 2007; 115:1051–8.
4. Liu X, Doi H, Maehara A, et al. A volumetric intravascular ultrasound comparison of early drug-eluting stent thrombosis versus restenosis. JACC Cardiovasc Interv 2009;2:428–34.
5. Bavry AA, Kumbhani DJ, Helton TJ, et al. Late thrombosis of drug-eluting stents: a meta-analysis of randomized clinical trials. Am J Med 2006;119: 1056–61.
6. Schafer AI. Antiplatelet therapy. Am J Med 1996; 101:199–209.
7. Dangas GD, Claessen BE, Mehran R, et al. Clinical outcomes following stent thrombosis occurring in-hospital versus out-of-hospital: results from the HORIZONS-AMI (Harmonizing Outcomes with Revascularization and Stents in Acute Myocardial Infarction) trial. J Am Coll Cardiol 2012;59:1752–9.
8. Dangas GD, Claessen BE, Mehran R, et al. Development and validation of a stent thrombosis risk score in patients with acute coronary syndromes. JACC Cardiovasc Interv 2012;5:1097–105.
9. Cayla G, Hulot JS, O'Connor SA, et al. Clinical, angiographic, and genetic factors associated with early coronary stent thrombosis. JAMA 2011;306: 1765–74.
10. Tamburino C, Capranzano P, Capodanno D, et al. Plaque distribution patterns in distal left main coronary artery to predict outcomes after stent implantation. JACC Cardiovasc Interv 2010;3:624–31.
11. Spertus JA, Kettelkamp R, Vance C, et al. Prevalence, predictors, and outcomes of premature discontinuation of thienopyridine therapy after

drug-eluting stent placement: results from the PREMIER registry. Circulation 2006;113:2803–9.

12. Rossini R, Capodanno D, Lettieri C, et al. Prevalence, predictors, and long-term prognosis of premature discontinuation of oral antiplatelet therapy after drug eluting stent implantation. Am J Cardiol 2011;107:186–94.

13. Tsai TT, Ho PM, Xu S, et al. Increased risk of bleeding in patients on clopidogrel therapy after drug-eluting stents implantation: insights from the HMO Research Network-Stent Registry (HMORN-stent). Circ Cardiovasc Interv 2010;3:230–5.

14. Huang PH, Croce KJ, Bhatt DL, et al. Recommendations for management of antiplatelet therapy in patients undergoing elective noncardiac surgery after coronary stent implantation. Crit Pathw Cardiol 2012;11:177–85.

15. Samama CM, Thiry D, Elalamy I, et al. Perioperative activation of hemostasis in vascular surgery patients. Anesthesiology 2001;94:74–8.

16. Bell B, Layland J, Poon K, et al. Focused clinical review: periprocedural management of antiplatelet therapy in patients with coronary stents. Heart Lung Circ 2011;20:438–45.

17. Fleisher LA, Beckman JA, Brown KA, et al. ACC/AHA 2007 guidelines on perioperative cardiovascular evaluation and care for noncardiac surgery: a report of the American College of Cardiology/American Heart Association Task Force on Practice Guidelines (Writing Committee to Revise the 2002 Guidelines on Perioperative Cardiovascular Evaluation for Noncardiac Surgery): developed in collaboration with the American Society of Echocardiography, American Society of Nuclear Cardiology, Heart Rhythm Society, Society of Cardiovascular Anesthesiologists, Society for Cardiovascular Angiography and Interventions, Society for Vascular Medicine and Biology, and Society for Vascular Surgery. Circulation 2007; 116:e418–99.

18. O'Gara PT, Kushner FG, Ascheim DD, et al. 2013 ACCF/AHA Guideline for the Management of ST-Elevation Myocardial Infarction: Executive Summary: a Report of the American College of Cardiology Foundation/American Heart Association Task Force on Practice Guidelines. Circulation 2013;127:529–55.

19. Jneid H, Anderson JL, Wright RS, et al. 2012 ACCF/AHA focused update of the guideline for the management of patients with unstable angina/non-ST-elevation myocardial infarction (updating the 2007 guideline and replacing the 2011 focused update): a report of the American College of Cardiology Foundation/American Heart Association Task Force on practice guidelines. Circulation 2012;126: 875–910.

20. Levine GN, Bates ER, Blankenship JC, et al. 2011 ACCF/AHA/SCAI Guideline for Percutaneous Coronary Intervention: a report of the American College of Cardiology Foundation/American Heart Association Task Force on Practice Guidelines and the Society for Cardiovascular Angiography and Interventions. Circulation 2011;124:e574–651.

21. Steg PG, James SK, Atar D, et al. ESC guidelines for the management of acute myocardial infarction in patients presenting with ST-segment elevation. Eur Heart J 2012;33:2569–619.

22. Hamm CW, Bassand JP, Agewall S, et al. ESC guidelines for the management of acute coronary syndromes in patients presenting without persistent ST-segment elevation: the Task Force for the management of acute coronary syndromes (ACS) in patients presenting without persistent ST-segment elevation of the European Society of Cardiology (ESC). Eur Heart J 2011;32:2999–3054.

23. Wijns W, Kolh P, Danchin N, et al. Guidelines on myocardial revascularization. Eur Heart J 2010; 31:2501–55.

24. Poldermans D, Bax JJ, Boersma E, et al. Guidelines for pre-operative cardiac risk assessment and perioperative cardiac management in noncardiac surgery. Eur Heart J 2009;30:2769–812.

25. Hillis LD, Smith PK, Anderson JL, et al. 2011 ACCF/AHA guideline for coronary artery bypass graft surgery: a report of the American College of Cardiology Foundation/American Heart Association Task Force on Practice Guidelines. Circulation 2011; 124:e652–735.

26. Ho PM, Fihn SD, Wang L, et al. Clopidogrel and long-term outcomes after stent implantation for acute coronary syndrome. Am Heart J 2007;154: 846–51.

27. Eisenstein EL, Anstrom KJ, Kong DF, et al. Clopidogrel use and long-term clinical outcomes after drug-eluting stent implantation. JAMA 2007;297: 159–68.

28. Harjai KJ, Shenoy C, Orshaw P, et al. Dual antiplatelet therapy for more than 12 months after percutaneous coronary intervention: insights from the Guthrie PCI Registry. Heart 2009;95:1579–86.

29. Park SJ, Park DW, Kim YH, et al. Duration of dual antiplatelet therapy after implantation of drug-eluting stents. N Engl J Med 2010;362:1374–82.

30. Petersen JL, Barron JJ, Hammill BG, et al. Clopidogrel use and clinical events after drug-eluting stent implantation: findings from the HealthCore Integrated Research Database. Am Heart J 2010; 159:462–470.e1.

31. Valgimigli M, Campo G, Monti M, et al. Short-versus long-term duration of dual-antiplatelet therapy after coronary stenting: a randomized multicenter trial. Circulation 2012;125:2015–26.

32. Dangas GD, Claessen BE, Mehran R, et al. Stent thrombosis after primary angioplasty for STEMI in relation to non-adherence to dual antiplatelet

therapy over time: results of the HORIZONS-AMI trial. EuroIntervention 2013;8:1033–9.

33. Mehran R, Pocock SJ, Nikolsky E, et al. A risk score to predict bleeding in patients with acute coronary syndromes. J Am Coll Cardiol 2010;55:2556–66.

34. Pisters R, Lane DA, Nieuwlaat R, et al. A novel user-friendly score (HAS-BLED) to assess 1-year risk of major bleeding in patients with atrial fibrillation: the Euro Heart Survey. Chest 2010;138:1093–100.

35. Baber U, Mehran R, Sharma SK, et al. Impact of the everolimus-eluting stent on stent thrombosis: a meta-analysis of 13 randomized trials. J Am Coll Cardiol 2011;58:1569–77.

36. Palmerini T, Kirtane AJ, Serruys PW, et al. Stent thrombosis with everolimus-eluting stents: meta-analysis of comparative randomized controlled trials. Circ Cardiovasc Interv 2012;5:357–64.

37. Kimura T, Morimoto T, Nakagawa Y, et al. Antiplatelet therapy and stent thrombosis after sirolimus-eluting stent implantation. Circulation 2009;119:987–95.

38. Hahn JY, Song YB, Choi JH, et al. Three-month dual antiplatelet therapy after implantation of zotarolimus-eluting stents: the DATE (Duration of Dual Antiplatelet Therapy AfterImplantation of Endeavor Stent) registry. Circ J 2010;74:2314–21.

39. Kim BK, Hong MK, Shin DH, et al. A new strategy for discontinuation of dual antiplatelet therapy: the RESET Trial (REal Safety and Efficacy of 3-month dual antiplatelet Therapy following Endeavor zotarolimus-eluting stent implantation). J Am Coll Cardiol 2012;60:1340–8.

40. Gwon HC, Hahn JY, Park KW, et al. Six-month versus 12-month dual antiplatelet therapy after implantation of drug-eluting stents: the Efficacy of Xience/Promus Versus Cypher to Reduce Late Loss After Stenting (EXCELLENT) randomized, multicenter study. Circulation 2012;125:505–13.

41. Iakovou I, Schmidt T, Bonizzoni E, et al. Incidence, predictors, and outcome of thrombosis after successful implantation of drug-eluting stents. JAMA 2005;293:2126–30.

42. Airoldi F, Colombo A, Morici N, et al. Incidence and predictors of drug-eluting stent thrombosis during and after discontinuation of thienopyridine treatment. Circulation 2007;116:745–54.

43. Roy P, Steinberg DH, Waksman R, et al. The potential clinical utility of intravascular ultrasound guidance in patients undergoing percutaneous coronary intervention with drug-eluting stents. Eur Heart J 2008;29(15):1851–7.

44. Ge L, Airoldi F, Iakovou I, et al. Clinical and angiographic outcome after implantation of drug-eluting stents in bifurcation lesions with the crush stent technique: importance of final kissing balloon post-dilation. J Am Coll Cardiol 2005;46:613–20.

45. Park DW, Park SW, Park KH, et al. Frequency of and risk factors for stent thrombosis after drug-eluting stent implantation during long-term follow-up. Am J Cardiol 2006;98:352–6.

46. Ong AT, McFadden EP, Regar E, et al. Late angiographic stent thrombosis (LAST) events with drug-eluting stents. J Am Coll Cardiol 2005; 45:2088–92.

47. McFadden EP, Stabile E, Regar E, et al. Late thrombosis in drug-eluting coronary stents after discontinuation of antiplatelet therapy. Lancet 2004;364: 1519–21.

48. Schouten O, Bax JJ, Damen J, et al. Coronary artery stent placement immediately before noncardiac surgery: a potential risk? Anesthesiology 2007;106:1067–9.

49. Nuttall GA, Brown MJ, Stombaugh JW, et al. Time and cardiac risk of surgery after bare-metal stent percutaneous coronary intervention. Anesthesiology 2008;109:588–95.

50. Anwaruddin S, Askari AT, Saudye H, et al. Characterization of post-operative risk associated with prior drug-eluting stent use. JACC Cardiovasc Interv 2009;2:542–9.

51. Chassot PG, Delabays A, Spahn DR. Perioperative antiplatelet therapy: the case for continuing therapy in patients at risk of myocardial infarction. Br J Anaesth 2007;99:316–28.

52. Abualsaud AO, Eisenberg MJ. Perioperative management of patients with drug-eluting stents. JACC Cardiovasc Interv 2010;3:131–42.

53. Burger W, Chemnitius JM, Kneissl GD, et al. Low-dose aspirin for secondary cardiovascular prevention—cardiovascular risks after its perioperative withdrawal versus bleeding risks with its continuation—review and meta-analysis. J Intern Med 2005;257:399–414.

54. Eisenberg MJ, Richard PR, Libersan D, et al. Safety of short-term discontinuation of antiplatelet therapy in patients with drug-eluting stents. Circulation 2009;119:1634–42.

55. Dweck MR, Cruden NL. Noncardiac surgery in patients with coronary artery stents. Arch Intern Med 2012;172:1054–5.

56. Gwon HC, Hahn JY, Koo BK, et al. Final kissing ballooning and long-term clinical outcomes in coronary bifurcation lesions treated with 1-stent technique: results from the COBIS registry. Heart 2012;98:225–31.

# Triple Antiplatelet Therapy and Combinations with Oral Anticoagulants After Stent Implantation

Vijay Kunadian, MBBS, MD, FRCP, FESC[a,b,*],
Joseph Robert Dunford[a,b], Daniel Swarbrick, MBBS[a,b],
Rim Halaby, BS[c], Ogheneochuko Ajari, MS, MBBS[c],
Madeleine Cochet, BS[c], Kristin Feeney, BS[c],
Emily Larkin, BS[c], Gonzalo Romero Gonzalez, MBBS[c],
Aditya Govindavarjhulla, MBBS[c], Daniel Nethala, BS[c],
Hardik Patel, MBBS[c], Raviteja Reddy Guddeti, MBBS[c],
Farman Khan, MBBS[c], Shankar Kumar, MBBS[c],
Sapan Patel, MBBS[c], Prashanth Saddala, MBBS[c],
Vishnu Vardhan Serla, MBBS[c], Marcelo Zacarkim, MD[c],
Divya Yadav, MD[c], C. Michael Gibson, MS, MD[c]

## KEYWORDS

- Triple therapy • Acute coronary syndrome • Percutaneous coronary intervention
- Stent implantation • Novel anticoagulants

## KEY POINTS

- Dual antiplatelet therapy (DAPT) plays a major role in the management of patients with coronary artery disease following stenting.
- Triple therapy with the addition of an anticoagulant, such as rivaroxaban or apixaban, to DAPT has been evaluated in clinical trials to improve clinical outcomes following an acute coronary syndrome.
- Studies have evaluated the use of anticoagulants (warfarin, dabigatran) in addition to DAPT following stenting for coexisting conditions such as atrial fibrillation, mechanical valves, left ventricular thrombus, or other thromboembolic events.
- The benefit of such triple therapy (ie, DAPT) with another antiplatelet agent or with an anticoagulant in special circumstances must be weighed very carefully against the potential risk of severe bleeding events.

Disclosures: The authors have nothing to disclose.
[a] Institute of Cellular Medicine, Faculty of Medical Sciences, Newcastle University, Newcastle upon Tyne, UK; [b] Cardiothoracic Centre, Freeman Hospital, Newcastle upon Tyne Hospitals NHS Foundation Trust, Newcastle upon Tyne, UK; [c] Cardiovascular Division, Department of Medicine, Beth Israel Deaconess Medical Center, Harvard Medical School, Boston, MA 02215, USA
* Corresponding author. Institute of Cellular Medicine, Faculty of Medical Sciences, Newcastle University, 3rd Floor William Leech Building, Newcastle upon Tyne NE2 4HH, UK.
*E-mail address:* vijay.kunadian@ncl.ac.uk

interventional.theclinics.com

## INTRODUCTION

Dual antiplatelet therapy (DAPT) is indicated following the implantation of a stent in the management of coronary artery disease.[1,2] Antiplatelet therapy has been demonstrated to produce a significantly improved prognosis in terms of reduced rates of subsequent myocardial infarction (MI) or death following percutaneous coronary intervention (PCI).[3] Triple antiplatelet therapy (TAPT) has previously been evaluated with agents such as cilostazol[4] or glycoprotein IIb/IIIa inhibitors[5] as the third agent. Among patients at greater risk of a major adverse cardiac event (MACE) following an acute coronary syndrome (ACS), the use of novel anticoagulant drugs such as rivaroxaban, apixaban, or dabigatran may be desirable in addition to DAPT.[6] Oral anticoagulation therapy (OAT) is administered to patients with atrial fibrillation (AF) or other prothromboembolic conditions to reduce the likelihood of thrombotic emboli forming and causing strokes or other events.[7] There are many cases in which DAPT plus OAT is indicated. It is estimated that 5% to 7% of patients undergoing PCI have indications for OAT in addition to DAPT.[8] Although this may significantly reduce patient's risks of embolic events, DAPT plus OAT can lead to a range of further hemorrhagic consequences. It is, therefore, imperative that any decision to commence DAPT plus OAT involves careful consideration of the potential risks and evaluation of the evidence base regarding its suitability.[9]

This article evaluates the benefits and risks associated with the use of TAPT and dual antiplatelet therapy combinations with oral anticoagulants following stent implantation.

## METHODS

A series of database searches using MEDLINE, EMBASE, and PubMed were performed using the keywords triple therapy, ACS, percutaneous coronary intervention, stent implantation, and novel anticoagulants.

### Pathophysiology of Arterial Thrombosis

Formation of intraarterial thrombus is usually associated with the rupture of an atherosclerotic plaque and is an interaction between platelet reactivity and the sequential activation of blood clotting factors. Rupture of an atherosclerotic plaque results in platelet activation by collagen via platelet glycoprotein VI and von Willebrand factor, causing a conformational change in the platelet membrane and the exposure of acidic phospholipids. At the same time, a cocktail of mediators is released from granules within the platelets, including thromboxane-$A_2$ and adenosine diphosphate, which causes further platelet activation and aggregation. Simultaneously, tissue factor exposed by the denuded plaque initiates activation of the clotting cascade by activation of factor VII. This, in turn, acts to activate factor X, the final common pathway of blood coagulation and the main enzyme for conversion of prothrombin (factor II) to the active enzyme thrombin. Thrombin cleaves soluble fibrinogen to fibrin monomers, which polymerize to form an insoluble meshwork in which platelets and red blood cells become trapped, forming a thrombus. The acidic phospholipids on the surface of activated platelets catalyze the reactions in several steps of the coagulation cascade, while both thrombin and fibrinogen interact with platelets to enhance further their aggregation. Activation of both platelets and of the clotting cascade is important in the pathophysiology of coronary disease and therapy designed to modify these pathways is an important part of treating and preventing coronary syndromes.[10,11]

### TAPT

#### Cilostazol

Randomized controlled trials have been performed to assess the effectiveness of cilostazol, a phosphodiesterase III inhibitor that inhibits platelet aggregation,[12] in addition to DAPT, following PCI. The Drug-Eluting stenting followed by Cilostazol treatment REduces Adverse Serious cardiac Events (DECREASE) trial,[13] consisting of 3099 subjects, compared subjects who received aspirin and clopidogrel DAPT (n = 1656) with those who received cilostazol as part of TAPT (n = 1443). This study demonstrated that subjects who received TAPT were at lower risk of subsequent MI (hazard ratio [HR] 0.233, 95% CI 0.077–0.703, $P$ = .0097) and stent thrombosis (HR 0.136, 95% CI 0.035–0.521, $P$ = .0036) at the 12-month follow-up, with no increase in bleeding (HR 0.969, 95% CI 0.443–2.119, $P$ = .9372). No major difference was seen in the mortality rates between the two groups (HR 0.762, 95% CI 0.401–1.448, $P$ = .4062). Several meta-analyses using this strategy demonstrated similar results.[4,14,15]

Interestingly, a study by Yang and colleagues[16] demonstrated that DAPT containing the newer thienopyridine prasugrel was able to achieve superior platelet inhibition compared with a TAPT regime of aspirin, clopidogrel, and cilostazol. This study measured the level of platelet inhibition using the VerifyNow-P2Y12 rapid analyser,[17] and observed that the percentage platelet inhibition was higher among patients administered DAPT compared with the TAPT group (72.1% ± 12.2 vs 57.5% ± 23.5, P = .020).

### Glycoprotein IIb/IIIa inhibitors
Glycoprotein IIb/IIIa inhibitors have also been evaluated as part of TAPT following ACS. They can be administered orally or intravenously. However, oral use has declined owing to increased mortality rates observed in several trials.[18] Several trials have been performed to ascertain their effectiveness when given intravenously and their use has been found to be beneficial in treating patients presenting with STEMI (ST elevation MI), NSTEMI (non-ST elevation MI), and for elective PCI. Meta-analysis has demonstrated that patients with NSTEMI who receive a glycoprotein IIb/IIIa inhibitor in conjunction with DAPT are at a reduced risk of further MI (HR 0.70, 95% CI 0.56–0.88). They are at an equivalent risk of major bleeding (HR 1.15, 95% CI 0.69–1.91) and minor bleeding (HR 1.37, 95% CI 0.81–2.33) compared with those who received regular aspirin-based DAPT or aspirin alone. In patients with STEMI, the triple therapy was associated with significantly reduced rates of further MI (HR 0.26, 95% CI 0.17–0.38), similar rates of major bleeding (HR 1.86, 95% CI 0.43–8.17), and elevated rates of minor bleeding (HR 2.73, 95% CI 1.15–6.46). Among patients undergoing elective PCI, TAPT administration of glycoprotein IIb/IIIa inhibitors did not significantly reduce the rates of further MI (HR 0.77, 95% CI 0.54–1.11) but led to an increase in the rates of minor bleeding (HR 1.60, 95% CI 1.16–2.21). Rates of major bleeding were equivalent between the TAPT and control groups (HR 1.29, 95% CI 0.70–2.36).[5]

## OAT in the Management of Coronary Artery Disease

### Warfarin
There has been longstanding interest in the role of oral anticoagulants such as warfarin in preventing recurrent coronary events in at-risk patients. The beneficial effects on mortality and rates of reinfarction after MI from oral anticoagulants compared with placebo have been established in several trials that predate the era of mechanical reperfusion. However, two large meta-analyses demonstrated no mortality benefit from the addition of oral anticoagulants when added to aspirin, with a reduction in the incidence of stroke and reinfarction counterbalanced by an increase in major bleeding in the warfarin group. In the latter of these two analyses, reperfusion therapy was delivered to 25% of the subjects. All trials used aspirin monotherapy as a comparator.[19,20] With limited evidence of overall benefit and with the difficulties of maintaining reliable dosage with the existing anticoagulants, their use was largely abandoned in favor of a dual antiplatelet strategy. In a more recent trial, warfarin was demonstrated to be of potential prognostic benefit among subjects at risk of developing a left ventricular thrombus (LVT) after MI in combination with DAPT.[21]

## Novel Anticoagulants in the Management of ACS in Combination with DAPT

### Mechanisms of action
Unlike vitamin K antagonists, which reduce the synthesis of a range of vitamin K-dependent clotting factors by inhibition of the enzyme vitamin K epoxide reductase, the novel oral anticoagulants act on specific downstream enzymes in the clotting cascade. Factor Xa inhibitors (apixaban, rivaroxaban, and edoxaban) bind directly to factor Xa (as opposed to low molecular weight heparin and fondaparinux, which bind to factor Xa via antithrombin III). They are, therefore, able to affect both free and platelet-bound factor Xa. The direct thrombin inhibitor dabigatran acts on thrombin, preventing the conversion of fibrinogen to fibrin. Unlike heparin, which requires binding to antithrombin III to exert its effect on thrombin, dabigatran can act on both free and platelet-bound thrombin. In addition, it does not interact with platelet factor 4, the binding of which to heparin can induce formation of the antiplatelet antibodies underlying heparin-induced thrombocytopenia.[22]

### APIXABAN

Two studies, APPRAISE-1[23] (APixaban for the PRevention of Acute Ischemic and Safety Events) and APPRAISE-2[24] evaluated the use of apixaban, a factor Xa inhibitor,[25] in conjunction with DAPT among subjects with recent STEMI or NSTEMI (n = 1715). Subjects received either a placebo (n = 611) or the following apixaban regimes: 2.5 mg bid (n = 317), 10 mg OD (n = 318), 10 mg bid (n = 248), or 20 mg OD (n = 221). Apixaban 20 mg daily dose, consisting of 459 subjects, was discontinued after excessive rates of bleeding. Clinically significant bleeding (ie, bleeding that required medical attention) was seen in 7.8% of subjects taking 10 mg bid and 7.3% of subjects taking 20 mg OD. Among subjects on the placebo, 2.5 mg bid, and 10 mg OD apixaban regimes, 0.5%, 5%, and 5.6% risk of significant bleeds, respectively, were observed after 6-months follow-up. A decrease in the frequency of further cardiovascular events was observed, with a relative risk reduction of 27% observed among subjects administered 2.5 mg bid (HR 0.73, 95% CI 0.19–0.56, P = .21) and of 39% among those administered 10 mg OD (HR 0.61, 95% CI 0.04–0.65, $P$ = .07).

APPRAISE-1 was followed by the APPRAISE-2 study that evaluated 7392 subjects who were administered either placebo (n = 3687) or a 5 mg bid regimen of apixaban (n = 3705) in addition to aspirin and, for most, a further P2Y12 receptor antagonist, such as clopidogrel. There was a significant increase in major bleeding among subjects who received apixaban compared with those receiving placebo (HR 2.59, 95% CI 1.50–4.46, $P$ = .001). Of the bleeds occurring while on apixaban, a greater number were intracranial, or otherwise fatal, than in the placebo group. Rates of further MI, cardiovascular death, and stroke were 7.9% and 7.5% for the placebo and apixaban groups, respectively, after a mean 241 days of follow-up. These data suggest that the use of apixaban, even at the dose thought to be optimal based on the APPRAISE-1 study, increased the likelihood of major bleeding without significantly reducing the risk of further cardiovascular events or death.

One reason for the increased risk of adverse events seen in the APPRAISE-2 trial might be the inclusion of subjects with a range of other comorbidities such as age of at least 65 years, diabetes mellitus, MI within the previous 5 years, cerebrovascular disease, peripheral vascular disease, clinical heart failure or a left ventricular ejection fraction of less than 40% in association with the index event, impaired renal function (creatinine clearance <60 mL per minute), and/or no revascularization after the initial event. As a result, these subjects were more likely to be susceptible to adverse events.

## RIVAROXABAN

The ATLAS ACS-TIMI 46[26] (A Randomized, Double-Blind, Placebo-Controlled, Multicenter, Dose-Escalation and Dose-Confirmation Study to Evaluate the Safety and Efficacy of Rivaroxaban in Combination With Aspirin Alone or With Aspirin and a Thienopyridine in Subjects With Acute Coronary Syndromes) led into ATLAS ACS-2 TIMI 51.[27] The latter study evaluated the use of rivaroxaban (another factor Xa Inhibitor[28]) in addition to DAPT for the management of ACS. ATLAS ACS-TIMI 46 examined 3491 subjects who, after being stabilized following ACS, were treated with either aspirin alone (n = 761) or DAPT (n = 2730). Then they were given either a placebo or rivaroxaban 5 to 20 mg OD or 5 to 20 mg bid. This study demonstrated an increased risk of bleeding associated with increased doses of rivaroxaban used with DAPT within the once daily and twice daily regimes,

with the following doses: 5 mg OD (HR 3.28, 95% CI 1.57–6.84), 5 mg bid (HR 2.17, 95% CI 0.91–5.18), 10 mg OD (HR 3.21, 95% CI 2.06–5.00), 10 mg bid (HR 3.34, 95% CI 2.15–5.190), 15 mg OD (HR 3.69, CI 2.17–6.29), 15 mg bid (HR 3.41, CI 1.97–5.89), 20 mg OD (HR 5.12, CI 3.22–8.14), and 20 mg bid (HR 4.56, CI 2.83–7.33). There was a trend that rivaroxaban reduced risk of stroke, further MI, recurrent ischemia requiring revascularization, or death compared with the placebo (HR 0.79, 95% CI 0.60–1.05, $P$ = .10).

ATLAS ACS-2 TIMI 51 evaluated 15,526 subjects who were allocated to either placebo (n = 5176), or rivaroxaban 2.5 mg bid (n = 5174) or 5 mg bid (n = 5176) with a 13-month mean follow-up. In this study, rivaroxaban treatment (both doses combined) significantly reduced the risk of MI, stroke, or death (due to cardiovascular causes) by 16% (HR 0.84, 95% CI 0.74–0.96, $P$ = .008), with the absolute risk significantly lower among subjects receiving 5 mg bid compared with those receiving 2.5 mg bid (8.8% vs 9.1%). Rivaroxaban treatment (both doses) produced an increase in major bleeding (overall HR 3.96, 95% CI 2.46–6.38, $P$ = .001). However, rates of fatal bleeds were not increased significantly (HR 1.19, 95% CI 0.54–2.59, $P$ = .66). The rate of fatal bleeds in the group receiving the lower dose (2.5 mg bid) of rivaroxaban was reduced compared with the higher dose (5 mg bid) group (0.1% vs 0.4%). Death registries in different countries were used to ascertain the vital status of 1025 of 1295 subjects who withdrew from the ATLAS ACS 2 trial and the mortality benefit observed during the treatment phase of the study was maintained (C.M. Gibson, Transcatheter Cardiovascular Therapeutics 2012, FDA Redux).

## DABIGATRAN

The RE-DEEM trial[29] (RandomizEd Dabigatran Etexilate Dose Finding Study in Patients With Acute Coronary Syndromes Post Index Event With Additional Risk Factors for Cardiovascular Complications Also Receiving Aspirin and Clopidogrel) evaluated the use of dabigatran (a direct thrombin inhibitor) in combination with DAPT following treatment of ACS. The study included 1861 subjects who were given a placebo, 50 mg bid, 75 mg bid, 110 mg bid, or 150 mg bid of dabigatran. The trial demonstrated a 37% to 45% decrease in D-dimer concentrations among subjects who were administered dabigatran across all groups at 4-weeks follow-up. Over 6 months, subjects who were administered dabigatran were at an increased risk of bleeding compared with the placebo (DAPT only) group. Doses used were

50 mg bid (HR 1.77, 95% CI 0.70–4.50), 75 mg bid (HR 2.17, 95% CI 0.88–5.31), 110 mg bid (HR 3.92, 95% CI 1.72–8.95), and 150 mg bid (HR 4.27, 95% CI 1.86–9.81). Rates of cardiovascular death were comparable between the two lower doses of dabigatran and the placebo group (2.2% and 2.4% for 50 mg bid and 75 mg bid, respectively, vs 2.4%). Rates were lower in the higher dose group (1.2% for 110 mg and 150 mg). Rates of death were markedly lower in all dabigatran-receiving groups (3.8% for placebo vs 2.2% for 50 mg bid, 2.7% for 75 mg bid, 1.7% for 110 mg bid, and 2.0% for 50 mg bid).

## OAT to Prevent Thromboembolism

AF is the leading indication for OAT; lifetime risks are 25% for men and for women older than 40 years old. AF affects up to 8% of the population older than 65 years old at any one time.[30] Anticoagulation is indicated prophylactically in patients with prosthetic heart valves and in the treatment of deep vein thrombosis (DVT).[7] In these patients, the dose should be titrated up carefully with a target international normalized ratio (INR) of 2.0 to 3.0. In patients with further significant risk factors for thrombus formation, such as anterior-apical STEMI (**Fig. 1**), left atrial enlargement, a hypercoagulable state, or low ejection fraction, this should be increased to 2.5 to 3.5 (grade 1B).[31] Warfarin is the most widely used anticoagulant. It has been demonstrated by several studies to reduce stroke risk more effectively than an antiplatelet agent does, achieving a 64% relative risk reduction compared with 19% with antiplatelet agents such as aspirin and clopidogrel.[32] Warfarin is taken orally and, with recent developments in medical technology, self-monitoring

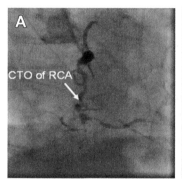
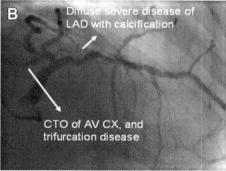
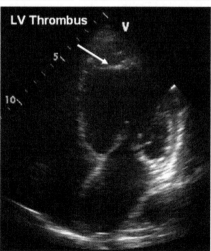

**Fig. 1.** Case example of 82-year-old man with multiple comorbidities who presented with troponin-positive ACS. Coronary angiography revealed severe three-vessel disease (*A* and *B*). Syntax score of 45. Cardiovascular risk calculated by EuroSCORE of 8%. HAS-BLED Score of 4. The lower panel is an echocardiogram showing severe left ventricular impairment with large apical thrombus. Given high risk for revascularization and high risk for bleeding, despite the need for triple therapy, patient was administered warfarin and was continued on medical therapy for coronary disease. AV CX, atrioventricular nodal circumflex artery; CTO, chronic total occlusion; LAD, left anterior descending artery; LV, left ventricular; RCA, right coronary artery.

and management is becoming an option that has the potential to significantly improve patients' quality of life[33] by reducing the inconvenience of patients having to attend specialist INR monitoring clinics and allowing them to monitor their INR more closely than these clinics are able to, resulting in a reduced risk of excessive bleeding or preventable thromboembolism.[34]

However, patients treated with warfarin are at a risk of significant adverse events, such as intracranial hemorrhage and gastrointestinal (GI) or other significant bleeds.[35] It can also be a challenging drug to prescribe; it has multiple interactions with other drugs and commonly ingested herbs or fruits that potentially alter its metabolism.[7] As a result, novel anticoagulants have been studied and demonstrated to achieve the same (if not superior) levels of protection against thrombus formation with more favorable side-effect profiles.[36]

ARISTOTLE (A Phase 3, Active [Warfarin] Controlled, Randomized, Double-Blind, Parallel Arm Study to Evaluate Efficacy and Safety of Apixaban in Preventing Stroke and Systemic Embolism in Subjects With Non-valvular Atrial Fibrillation) demonstrated that a 5 mg bid dose of apixaban was able to reduce the risk of stroke or embolism compared with warfarin among subjects with AF (HR 0.79, 95% CI 0.66–0.95, P<.001 for noninferiority, P = .01 for superiority) while also reducing the rates of significant bleeding (HR 0.69, 95% CI, 0.60–0.80, P<.001).[37]

ROCKET-AF (Rivaroxaban Once Daily Oral Direct Factor Xa Inhibition Compared with Vitamin K Antagonism for Prevention of Stroke and Embolism Trial in Atrial Fibrillation) observed that subjects administered rivaroxaban 20 mg OD in place of warfarin were at a reduced risk of thromboembolism (HR 0.79, 95% CI 0.66–0.96, P<.001) but at a similar risk of bleeding (HR 1.03, 95% CI 0.96–1.11, P = .44). Rivaroxaban treatment did, however, result in a lower risk of intracranial hemorrhage (HR 0.67, 95% CI, 0.47 to 0.93, P = .02).[38]

The RE-LY (Randomized Evaluation of Long-Term Anticoagulant Therapy) trial was able to demonstrate similar benefits associated with the use of dabigatran, with subjects administered either 110 mg bid or 150 mg bid of dabigatran and compared with subjects receiving warfarin. Subjects administered the 110 mg bid dose were at a similar risk of stroke to those who received warfarin (HR 0.91, 95% CI, 0.74–1.11, P = .34). Those who received 150 mg bid were at a reduced risk compared with warfarin (HR 0.66, 95% CI 0.53–0.82, P<.001). Subjects receiving 110 mg bid of dabigatran were at a reduced risk of major bleeding compared with those on warfarin (HR 0.80, 95% CI 0.69–0.93, P = .003) and those

receiving 150 mg bid were at an equivalent risk to the warfarin group (HR 0.93, 95% CI 0.81–1.07, P = .31). A further study, RE-LY ABLE (Long Term Multi-center Extension of Dabigatran Treatment in Patients With Atrial Fibrillation Who Completed the RE-LY Trial) evaluating the longer term outcomes of subjects in the initial study has recently been completed and the results are awaited.[39]

ENGAGE-AF TIMI 48 (Effective Anticoagulation With Factor Xa Next Generation in Atrial Fibrillation), a study to assess the effectiveness of edoxaban, another factor Xa inhibitor, is on-going.[40] Cost-effectiveness analysis has suggested that such drugs (dabigatran in particular) may be a cost-effective alternative to warfarin.[41]

### DAPT in Combination with Warfarin to Prevent Thromboembolism

When patients being treated for AF, or another condition requiring OAT, also require DAPT, the most common combination used is aspirin and clopidogrel (DAPT) with warfarin (OAT). This treatment may also be indicated to prevent formation of an LVT in patients with ventricular wall dysfunction following a (transmural) MI.[1] A study by Lamberts and colleagues[42] demonstrated that subjects treated with this combination are at an increased risk of spontaneous bleeding compared with subjects treated with DAPT alone (10.2% vs 3.2%, P = .01) and of fatal bleeding. This study compared bleeding risks of subjects treated with triple therapy to that for subjects treated with a vitamin K antagonist plus either aspirin or clopidogrel, DAPT only, or only a single antiplatelet drug. It suggested that there might not actually be a safe therapeutic window for the administration of OAT in combination with antiplatelet agents. The study evaluated 1495 subjects given OAT plus antiplatelet agents. It demonstrated that the risks of bleeding were greatest during the initial stages of treatment, with incidence of bleeds highest during the first 30 days of triple therapy (22.7 bleeds per 100 subject years). The incidence over the next 2 months reduced slightly (20.2 bleeds per 100 subject years) and approximately halved after 3 months (10.7 bleeds per 100 subject years). After 3 months, the rate of occurrences of bleeds in the DAPT plus OAT group was proportionately less elevated compared with groups of subjects receiving other therapies (OAT alone, DAPT alone, OAT and a single antiplatelet, or a single antiplatelet alone) than it was at the beginning of the treatment. However, it was still significantly raised (9.2 bleeds per 100 subject years vs 4.6 in the DAPT group). Similar observations were reported by Rogacka and colleagues,[44] who demonstrated that most bleeding in patients receiving DAPT plus OAT occurred within the first month.

This contrasts with Porter and colleagues,[45] who evaluated 180 subjects and demonstrated that triple therapy did not lead to rates of bleeding that should contraindicate its use. In this study, there were only 20 incidents of bleeding (18 minor and 2 major), with major bleeding only occurring during the time in which the subjects were receiving both warfarin and heparin while the dose of warfarin was titrated up. However, this study was performed at a single institution on a smaller sample size than Lambert and colleagues[42] and there was no control group.

More recently the WOEST (What is the Optimal antiplatElet & Anticoagulant Therapy in Subjects With Oral Anticoagulation and Coronary StenTing) study[46] randomized subjects undergoing PCI with an indication for anticoagulation to receive either triple therapy or the combination of clopidogrel and warfarin for 1 year. Most procedures were performed electively for stable angina. AF with a CHADS2 (congestive heart failure, hypertension, age, diabetes and stroke) score greater than 1 was the most common reason for anticoagulation. Drug-eluting stents (DESs) were used in about 65% of cases. The results demonstrated a lower risk of bleeding in subjects treated with dual, rather than triple, therapy (HR 0.36, 95% CI 0.26–0.50, $P$<.0001), with lower rates of both major and minor bleeding, though the difference in end points was driven mainly by minor bleeding. The rate of stent thrombosis in both groups was low, with no significant difference between the two treatments.

### DAPT in Combination with Novel Anticoagulants to Prevent Thromboembolism

Given the improved safety profiles of newer anticoagulants and noninferior clinical efficacy, it is hoped that it will be possible to coadminister these agents with DAPT to achieve this same benefit with similarly reduced risks among patients requiring DAPT plus OAT.

APPRAISE-2[24] evaluated apixaban use concurrently with DAPT. Although none of the subjects included had AF (it being an exclusion criteria for the study), it evaluated a group of subjects whose performance status and quality of life might have been impaired similarly to a patient with AF[47] with a dosage of apixaban that could be used clinically for AF.[37,48] It was associated with an unacceptably high risk of bleeding related complications.

The RE-LY trial[49] initially evaluated 18,113 subjects with AF who were then administered either warfarin according to INR or dabigatran 110 mg bid or 150 mg bid. Subsequent subgroup analysis[50] assessed subjects in the trial who were also taking antiplatelet therapy. Of 6952 subjects identified as having been administered antiplatelet therapy during the course of the trial, 5789 had received aspirin only, 351 had received clopidogrel only, and 812 had received DAPT. However, not all of these subjects were administered antiplatelet therapy throughout whole the trial. Therefore, this sample does not accurately represent subjects who were on a continuous course of antiplatelet therapy. Subjects on the lower (110 mg) dose of dabigatran with antiplatelets were at a lower risk of major bleeding than subjects taking warfarin with antiplatelets (HR 0.82, 95% CI 0.67–1.00) and at a similar risk of stroke or systemic emboli (SSE) (HR 0.93, 95% CI 0.70–1.25). Subjects taking the higher dose (150 mg) were at a similar risk of bleeds compared with those taking warfarin (HR 0.93, 95% CI 0.76–1.12), with the risk of SSE reduced by a similar degree to that observed amongst the group administered the lower dose (HR 0.80, 95% CI 0.59–1.08). This suggests that dabigatran may be an alternative anticoagulant that provides an equivocal benefit to warfarin with a significantly reduced risk of bleeds.

### Administering DAPT plus OAT in Clinical Practice

In either situation in which DAPT plus OAT may be indicated (following stent implantation when further anticoagulation is desirable, or when patients would otherwise need to be taking OAT as well as DAPT for comorbidities such as AF, DVT, or valve prosthesis), the decision to administer it must weigh the benefit that a patient may gain from the additional anticoagulant therapy against the risk of potentially life-threatening bleeding.[51]

Bleeding scores such as HAS-BLED (Hypertension, Abnormal renal/liver function, Stroke, Bleeding history or predisposition, Labile INR, Elderly, Drugs/alcohol concomitantly) and CRUSADE (Can Rapid risk stratification of Unstable angina patients Suppress ADverse outcomes with early implementation of the ACC/AHA [American College of Cardiology/American Heart Association] Guidelines) can be used to assess a patient's risk of bleeding to determine the optimal treatment. The former has been able to predict risk of bleeding with moderate accuracy among patients treated with DAPT in combination with

OAT[43] and the latter has been demonstrated to be an effective tool to assess a patient's baseline risk of bleeding.[52]

The CHADS2 score is an assessment tool in which a patient scores a point for having congestive heart failure, hypertension, age of or greater than 75 years, or diabetes mellitus, and two points for a previous history of stroke or TIA (to give a final score out of 6), and may be able to quantify risk of stroke in patients with AF and provide an indication of whether a patient may benefit from anticoagulation therapy.[53] More detailed tools such as the CHA2DS2-VASc (CHADS2, with two points for an age of 75 or greater, and additional points for other vascular disease, an age of 65–74, or being female [sex category]) may provide further indication in borderline cases.[54] Therefore, use of bleeding scores and stroke risk scores, when applicable, may be able to guide clinicians in the process of making the decision of whether to use OAT in combination with DAPT.

## Guidelines on DAPT in Combination with OAT in AF

### European Society of Cardiology

The European Society of Cardiology (ESC) Guidelines on STEMI advise that when anticoagulation therapy is used long-term in conjunction with DAPT, the target INR should be 2.0 to 2.5 (lower than the 2.0–3.0 usually used) and that patients at elevated risk of GI bleeds (elderly, previous history of GI bleeding, *Helicobacter pylori* infection, or nonsteroidal anti-inflammatory drug or steroid use) should be administered gastric protection in the form of a proton pump inhibitor (class IIA).[1]

The ESC also produced a consensus document specifically addressing the issue of managing patients with AF who require treatment of ACS.[55] The document provides detailed guidance on what is believed to be the optimal strategy for the management of the ACS based on the perceived risk of bleeding to the patient and the nature of the stent used during PCI (**Table 1**). In patients at low baseline risk of bleeding undergoing elective PCI who have a bare-metal stent (BMS) implanted, 1 month of warfarin, aspirin, and clopidogrel triple therapy is recommended, with a target INR of 2.0 to 2.5. If a DES is used, 3 to 6 months of triple therapy is recommended (depending on the nature of the DES) followed by up to 12 months of warfarin and a single antiplatelet agent (target INR 2.0–2.5 throughout). If a patient at low bleeding risk is treated for ACS, 6 months of DAPT plus OAT is recommended (irrespective of stent type), followed by up to 12 months of warfarin and either aspirin or clopidogrel (INR 2.0–2.5). Among patients at high risk of bleeding undergoing elective PCI, DAPT plus OAT should be used for just 2 to 4 weeks. When treating a patient at high risk of bleeding for ACS, up to 1 month of triple therapy is indicated,

**Table 1**
**ESC guidelines for the administration of DAPT in combination with OAT among patients with AF**

| Bleeding Risk[a] | Reason for PCI | Stent Used | Treatment Recommendation | Class of Recommendation |
|---|---|---|---|---|
| High | Elective | BMS | 2–4 wk DAPT + OAT<br>Lifelong OAT | IIA |
| | ACS | BMS | 2–4 wk DAPT + OAT<br>12 mo OAT + 1 antiplatelet<br>Lifelong OAT | IIA |
| Low (or intermediate) | Elective | BMS | 1 mo DAPT + OAT<br>Lifelong OAT | IIA |
| | Elective | DES | 3–6 mo DAPT + OAT<br>(depending on stent type)<br>12 mo OAT + 1 antiplatelet<br>Lifelong OAT | IIA |
| | ACS | BMS or DES | 6 mo DAPT + OAT<br>12 mo OAT + 1 antiplatelet<br>Lifelong OAT | IIA |

<sup>a</sup> Bleeding risk should be determined at the discretion of the physician.

*Adapted from* Lip GY, Huber K, Andreotti F, et al. Antithrombotic management of atrial fibrillation patients presenting with acute coronary syndrome and/or undergoing coronary stenting: executive summary—a Consensus Document of the European Society of Cardiology Working Group on Thrombosis, endorsed by the European Heart Rhythm Association (EHRA) and the European Association of Percutaneous Cardiovascular Interventions (EAPCI). Eur Heart J 2010;31:1311–8; with permission.

followed by up to 12 months of treatment with warfarin and a single antiplatelet agent. After these treatments (for both groups of patients), OAT should be continued as normal, with a target INR of 2.0 to 3.0 (Grade IIA).

### American College of Chest Physicians

Guidance from the American College of Chest Physicians (ACCP) on the management of AF[56] suggests that patients with AF receiving PCI to treat ACS who do not have a stent implanted should receive either DAPT alone or aspirin with warfarin, depending on whether their stroke risk according to CHADS2 score is low or high, respectively, with the warfarin and aspirin administered for 12 months before discontinuing aspirin (Grade 2C).

For patients undergoing stent implantation at high risk of stroke, the ACCP suggest triple therapy for either 1 or 3 to 6 months, depending on whether the stent is a BMS or DES. After this, they recommend discontinuation of one antiplatelet drug, continuing on a single antiplatelet drug and warfarin until 12 months after PCI. Following this, the antiplatelet should be stopped and OAT should be continued as required. If stroke risk is low, DAPT is recommended for 12 months before returning to regular treatment of AF. According ACCP guidelines, the target INR remains at 2.0 to 3.0 (Grade 2C) (**Table 2**).

Though the guidelines differ in how they stratify patients for treatment (ESC uses risk of bleeding, whereas the ACCP uses stroke risk) and their target INRs, both guidelines agree that there is a role for triple therapy in certain groups of patients. In addition, both agree that the optimal duration for continuation of DAPT plus OAT is no more than 6 months. No specific guidelines exist regarding the combination of DAPT with OAT for indications such as DVT or valve prosthesis; however, these guidelines should be applicable to these patients if risk of stroke, pulmonary embolism, or other SSE can be determined clinically.

### DAPT plus OAT and TAPT to Achieve Improved Outcome Following PCI

Currently, guidelines do not exist regarding the routine use of a third antithrombotic drug in managing a patient's risk of a MACE following PCI. OAT is clinically indicated following an MI in situations in which an MI causes ventricular dysfunction and, potentially, LVT, a case in which DAPT plus OAT is indicated to reduce MACEs and to prevent a stroke, which is addressed in the ESC guidelines[1]; and is advised for up to 6 months if echocardiography shows signs of recovery (class IIA). However, the use/utility of OAT purely as an adjunct to DAPT is still contentious, and ongoing research into the newer anticoagulants may find a role for it in the management of patients. However, in the meantime, its use should remain reserved for cases in which it is thought to be of particular necessity.

In some studies, Cilostazol as part of TAPT has been demonstrated to be associated with better outcomes than DAPT. Some studies have observed its benefits for groups of patients known

**Table 2**
**ACCP guidelines for the administration of DAPT plus OAT in patients with AF**

| Stoke Risk | Stent Used | Treatment Recommendation | Grade of Recommendation |
|---|---|---|---|
| High (CHADS2 score of 2 or greater) | BMS | 1 mo DAPT + OAT<br>12 mo OAT + 1 antiplatelet<br>Lifelong OAT | 2C |
| | DES | 3–6 mo DAPT + OAT (depending on stent type)<br>OAT + 1 antiplatelet until 12 mo post-PCI<br>Lifelong OAT | 2C |
| | None | 12 mo OAT + 1 antiplatelet<br>Lifelong OAT | 2C |
| Low (CHADS2 score of 0 or 1) | BMS or DES | 12 mo DAPT<br>Lifelong OAT or DAPT as needed. | 2C |
| | None | 12 mo DAPT<br>Lifelong OAT or DAPT as needed. | 2C |

*Adapted from* You JJ, Singer DE, Howard PA, et al. Antithrombotic therapy for atrial fibrillation: Antithrombotic Therapy and Prevention of Thrombosis, 9th ed: American College of Chest Physicians evidence-based clinical practice guidelines. Chest 2012;141:e531S–75S; with permission.

to be at elevated risk of ACS, such as patients who are obese[57] or have diabetes.[58] Guidelines on triple antiplatelet therapy from the ACCP[59] currently advise against the use of cilostazol to treat patients who have undergone elective PCI and stent implantation (Grade 1B) because of the high rates of skin rashes reported and limited evidence for its benefit on mortality rates. DAPT alone remains the mainstay of treatment following ACS.

The use of glycoprotein IIb/IIIa inhibitors was addressed in an update to the 2007 ACCP guidelines on the management of NSTEMI and unstable angina.[60] These guidelines advise against the use of abciximab in nonelective PCI (class III; level of evidence (LOE): A) and against the use of all glycoprotein IIb/IIIa in patients with unstable angina or NSTEMI who are at a low risk of ischemic events (Grade 3B). The drugs eptifibatide or tirofiban are recommended for use in patients suitable for glycoprotein IIb/IIIa inhibitor treatment before PCI (Grade 1A).

## SUMMARY

Although there is not yet complete consensus regarding the safety of DAPT in combination with oral anticoagulation, there are clearly a range of patients who stand to benefit from the intense antithrombotic treatment regime. Novel anticoagulants have shown promise as drugs that can provide added protection with superior safety profiles to that of the traditional warfarin. It is conceivable that they will be found suitable for use in patients considered for DAPT plus OAT combination in a variety of situations. If that is to be the case, the decision to administer DAPT plus OAT will have to involve carefully weighing the risk of bleeding against the risks of inadequate anticoagulation therapy, as it does now.

## REFERENCES

1. Hamm CW, Bassand JP, Agewall S, et al. ESC Guidelines for the management of acute myocardial infarction in patients presenting with ST-segment elevation. Eur Heart J 2012;33:2569–619.
2. Hamm CW, Bassand JP, Agewall S, et al. ESC Guidelines for the management of acute coronary syndromes in patients presenting without persistent ST-segment elevation: The Task Force for the management of acute coronary syndromes (ACS) in patients presenting without persistent ST-segment elevation of the European Society of Cardiology (ESC). Eur Heart J 2011;32:2999–3054.
3. Mulukutla SR, Marroquin OC, Vlachos HA, et al. Benefit of long-term dual anti-platelet therapy in patients treated with drug-eluting stents: from the NHLBI Dynamic Registry. Am J Cardiol 2013;111: 486–92.
4. Ding XL, Xie C, Jiang B, et al. Efficacy and safety of adjunctive cilostazol to dual antiplatelet therapy after stent implantation: an updated meta-analysis of randomized controlled trials. J Cardiovasc Pharmacol Ther 2013;18(3):222–8.
5. Geeganage C, Wilcox R, Bath PM. Triple antiplatelet therapy for preventing vascular events: a systematic review and meta-analysis. BMC Med 2010;8:36.
6. Costopoulos C, Niespialowska-Steuden M, Kukreja N, et al. Novel oral anticoagulants in acute coronary syndrome. Int J Cardiol 2012. [Epub ahead of print].
7. Tadros R, Shakib S. Warfarin—indications, risks and drug interactions. Aust Fam Physician 2010; 39:476–9.
8. Faxon DP, Eikelboom JW, Berger PB, et al. Consensus document: antithrombotic therapy in patients with atrial fibrillation undergoing coronary stenting. A North-American perspective. Thromb Haemost 2011;106:572–84.
9. Mega J, Carreras ET. Antithrombotic therapy: triple therapy or triple threat? Hematology Am Soc Hematol Educ Program 2012;2012:547–52.
10. Furie B, Furie BC. Mechanisms of thrombus formation. N Engl J Med 2008;359:938–49.
11. Furie B, Furie BC. Molecular and cellular biology of blood coagulation. N Engl J Med 1992;326:800–6.
12. Kim L, Charitakis K, Swaminathan RV, et al. Novel antiplatelet therapies. Curr Atheroscler Rep 2012; 14:78–84.
13. Lee SW, Park SW, Yun SC, et al. Triple antiplatelet therapy reduces ischemic events after drug-eluting stent implantation: Drug-Eluting stenting followed by Cilostazol treatment REduces Adverse Serious cardiac Events (DECREASE registry). Am Heart J 2010;159:284–91.e1.
14. Geng DF, Liu M, Jin DM, et al. Cilostazol-based triple antiplatelet therapy compared to dual antiplatelet therapy in patients with coronary stent implantation: a meta-analysis of 5,821 patients. Cardiology 2012;122:148–57.
15. Jang JS, Jin HY, Seo JS, et al. A meta-analysis of randomized controlled trials appraising the efficacy and safety of cilostazol after coronary artery stent implantation. Cardiology 2012;122:133–43.
16. Yang TH, Jin HY, Choi KN, et al. Randomized comparison of new dual-antiplatelet therapy (aspirin, prasugrel) and triple-antiplatelet therapy (aspirin, clopidogrel, cilostazol) using P2Y12 point-of-care assay in patients with STEMI undergoing primary PCI. Int J Cardiol 2012. [Epub ahead of print].
17. Malinin A, Pokov A, Spergling M, et al. Monitoring platelet inhibition after clopidogrel with the VerifyNow-P2Y12(R) rapid analyzer: the VERIfy

Thrombosis risk ASsessment (VERITAS) study. Thromb Res 2007;119:277–84.

18. Chew DP, Bhatt DL, Sapp S, et al. Increased mortality with oral platelet glycoprotein IIb/IIIa antagonists: a meta-analysis of phase III multicenter randomized trials. Circulation 2001;103:201–6.

19. Gao F, Zhou YJ, Wang ZJ, et al. Meta-analysis of the combination of warfarin and dual antiplatelet therapy after coronary stenting in patients with indications for chronic oral anticoagulation. Int J Cardiol 2011;148:96–101.

20. Zhao HJ, Zheng ZT, Wang ZH, et al. "Triple therapy" rather than "triple threat": a meta-analysis of the two antithrombotic regimens after stent implantation in patients receiving long-term oral anticoagulant treatment. Chest 2011;139:260–70.

21. Schwalm JD, Ahmad M, Salehian O, et al. Warfarin after anterior myocardial infarction in current era of dual antiplatelet therapy: a randomized feasibility trial. J Thromb Thrombolysis 2010;30:127–32.

22. Sikka P, Bindra VK. Newer antithrombotic drugs. Indian J Crit Care Med 2010;14:188–95.

23. Alexander JH, Becker RC, Bhatt DL, et al. Apixaban, an oral, direct, selective factor Xa inhibitor, in combination with antiplatelet therapy after acute coronary syndrome: results of the Apixaban for Prevention of Acute Ischemic and Safety Events (APPRAISE) trial. Circulation 2009;119:2877–85.

24. Alexander JH, Lopes RD, James S, et al. Apixaban with antiplatelet therapy after acute coronary syndrome. N Engl J Med 2011;365:699–708.

25. Roser-Jones C, Becker RC. Apixaban: an emerging oral factor Xa inhibitor. J Thromb Thrombolysis 2010; 29:141–6.

26. Mega JL, Braunwald E, Mohanavelu S, et al. Rivaroxaban versus placebo in patients with acute coronary syndromes (ATLAS ACS-TIMI 46): a randomised, double-blind, phase II trial. Lancet 2009;374:29–38.

27. Mega JL, Braunwald E, Wiviott SD, et al. Rivaroxaban in patients with a recent acute coronary syndrome. N Engl J Med 2012;366:9–19.

28. Turpie AG. Advances in oral anticoagulation treatment: the safety and efficacy of rivaroxaban in the prevention and treatment of thromboembolism. Ther Adv Hematol 2012;3:309–23.

29. Oldgren J, Budaj A, Granger CB, et al. Dabigatran vs. placebo in patients with acute coronary syndromes on dual antiplatelet therapy: a randomized, double-blind, phase II trial. Eur Heart J 2011;32: 2781–9.

30. Lloyd-Jones DM, Wang TJ, Leip EP, et al. Lifetime risk for development of atrial fibrillation: the Framingham Heart Study. Circulation 2004;110:1042–6.

31. Salem DN, O'Gara PT, Madias C, et al. Valvular and structural heart disease: American College of Chest Physicians Evidence-Based Clinical Practice Guidelines (8th edition). Chest 2008;133:593S–629S.

32. Hart RG, Pearce LA, Aguilar MI. Meta-analysis: antithrombotic therapy to prevent stroke in patients who have nonvalvular atrial fibrillation. Ann Intern Med 2007;146:857–67.

33. Verret L, Couturier J, Rozon A, et al. Impact of a pharmacist-led warfarin self-management program on quality of life and anticoagulation control: a randomized trial. Pharmacotherapy 2012;32(10):871–9.

34. Douketis JD. Patient self-monitoring of oral anticoagulant therapy: potential benefits and implications for clinical practice. Am J Cardiovasc Drugs 2001; 1:245–51.

35. Fang MC, Chang Y, Hylek EM, et al. Advanced age, anticoagulation intensity, and risk for intracranial hemorrhage among patients taking warfarin for atrial fibrillation. Ann Intern Med 2004;141:745–52.

36. Amin A. Oral anticoagulation to reduce risk of stroke in patients with atrial fibrillation: current and future therapies. Clin Interv Aging 2013;8:75–84.

37. Granger CB, Alexander JH, McMurray JJ, et al. Apixaban versus warfarin in patients with atrial fibrillation. N Engl J Med 2011;365:981–92.

38. Patel MR, Mahaffey KW, Garg J, et al. Rivaroxaban versus warfarin in nonvalvular atrial fibrillation. N Engl J Med 2011;365:883–91.

39. Boehringer Ingelheim Pharmaceuticals. RELY-ABLE long term multi-center extension of dabigatran treatment in patients with atrial fibrillation who completed RE-LY Trial. U.S. National Institutes of Health; 2008. Available at: http://clinicaltrials.gov/ct2/show/NCT00808067?term=re-ly+able&rank=1. Accessed February 28, 2013.

40. Daiichi Sankyo Inc. Global study to assess the safety and effectiveness of edoxaban (DU-176b) vs standard practice of dosing with warfarin in patients with atrial fibrillation (EngageAFTIMI48). U.S. National Institutes of Health; 2008. Available at: http://www.clinicaltrials.gov/ct2/show/NCT00781391?term=engage+AF&rank=1. Accessed February 27, 2013.

41. Kansal AR, Sorensen SV, Gani R, et al. Cost-effectiveness of dabigatran etexilate for the prevention of stroke and systemic embolism in UK patients with atrial fibrillation. Heart 2012;98:573–8.

42. Lamberts M, Olesen JB, Ruwald MH, et al. Bleeding after initiation of multiple antithrombotic drugs, including triple therapy, in atrial fibrillation patients following myocardial infarction and coronary intervention: a nationwide cohort study. Circulation 2012;126:1185–93.

43. Smith JG, Wieloch M, Koul S, et al. Triple antithrombotic therapy following an acute coronary syndrome: prevalence, outcomes and prognostic utility of the HAS-BLED score. EuroIntervention 2012;8:672–8.

44. Rogacka R, Chieffo A, Michev I, et al. Dual antiplatelet therapy after percutaneous coronary intervention with stent implantation in patients taking

chronic oral anticoagulation. JACC Cardiovasc Interv 2008;1:56–61.

45. Porter A, Konstantino Y, Iakobishvili Z, et al. Short-term triple therapy with aspirin, warfarin, and a thienopyridine among patients undergoing percutaneous coronary intervention. Catheter Cardiovasc Interv 2006;68:56–61.

46. Dewilde WJ, Oirbans T, Verheugt FW, et al. Use of clopidogrel with or without aspirin in patients taking oral anticoagulant therapy and undergoing percutaneous coronary intervention: an open-label, randomised, controlled trial. Lancet 2013;381(9872):1107–15.

47. Pepine CJ. Effects of pharmacologic therapy on health-related quality of life in elderly patients with atrial fibrillation: a systematic review of randomized and nonrandomized trials. Clin Med Insights Cardiol 2013;7:1–20.

48. Flaker GC, Eikelboom JW, Shestakovska O, et al. Bleeding during treatment with aspirin versus apixaban in patients with atrial fibrillation unsuitable for warfarin: the apixaban versus acetylsalicylic acid to prevent stroke in atrial fibrillation patients who have failed or are unsuitable for vitamin K antagonist treatment (AVERROES) trial. Stroke 2012;43:3291–7.

49. Connolly SJ, Ezekowitz MD, Yusuf S, et al. Dabigatran versus warfarin in patients with atrial fibrillation. N Engl J Med 2009;361:1139–51.

50. Dans AL, Connolly SJ, Wallentin L, et al. Concomitant use of antiplatelet therapy with dabigatran or warfarin in the randomized evaluation of long-term anticoagulation therapy (RE-LY) Trial. Circulation 2013;127:634–40.

51. Menozzi M, Rubboli A, Manari A, et al. Triple antithrombotic therapy in patients with atrial fibrillation undergoing coronary artery stenting: hovering among bleeding risk, thromboembolic events, and stent thrombosis. Thromb J 2012;10:22.

52. Subherwal S, Bach RG, Chen AY, et al. Baseline risk of major bleeding in non-ST-segment-elevation myocardial infarction: the CRUSADE (Can Rapid risk stratification of Unstable angina patients Suppress ADverse outcomes with Early implementation of the ACC/AHA Guidelines) Bleeding Score. Circulation 2009;119:1873–82.

53. Gage BF, Waterman AD, Shannon W, et al. Validation of clinical classification schemes for predicting stroke: results from the National Registry of Atrial Fibrillation. JAMA 2001;285:2864–70.

54. Coppens M, Eikelboom JW, Hart RG, et al. The CHA2DS2-VASc score identifies those patients with atrial fibrillation and a CHADS2 score of 1 who are unlikely to benefit from oral anticoagulant therapy. Eur Heart J 2013;34:170–6.

55. Lip GY, Huber K, Andreotti F, et al. Antithrombotic management of atrial fibrillation patients presenting with acute coronary syndrome and/or undergoing coronary stenting: executive summary–a Consensus Document of the European Society of Cardiology Working Group on Thrombosis, endorsed by the European Heart Rhythm Association (EHRA) and the European Association of Percutaneous Cardiovascular Interventions (EAPCI). Eur Heart J 2010;31:1311–8.

56. You JJ, Singer DE, Howard PA, et al. Antithrombotic therapy for atrial fibrillation: Antithrombotic Therapy and Prevention of Thrombosis, 9th edition. American College of Chest Physicians Evidence-Based Clinical Practice Guidelines. Chest 2012;141:e531S–75S.

57. Gao W, Zhang Q, Ge H, et al. Efficacy and safety of triple antiplatelet therapy in obese patients undergoing stent implantation. Angiology 2013. [Epub ahead of print].

58. Lee SW, Park SW, Kim YH, et al. Drug-eluting stenting followed by cilostazol treatment reduces late restenosis in patients with diabetes mellitus the DECLARE-DIABETES Trial (A Randomized Comparison of Triple Antiplatelet Therapy with Dual Antiplatelet Therapy After Drug-Eluting Stent Implantation in Diabetic Patients). J Am Coll Cardiol 2008;51:1181–7.

59. Vandvik PO, Lincoff AM, Gore JM, et al. Primary and secondary prevention of cardiovascular disease: Antithrombotic Therapy and Prevention of Thrombosis, 9th ed: American College of Chest Physicians Evidence-Based Clinical Practice Guidelines. Chest 2012;141:e637S–68S.

60. Wenger NK. 2011 ACCF/AHA focused update of the guidelines for the management of patients with Unstable Angina/Non-ST-Elevation Myocardial Infarction (updating the 2007 Guideline): highlights for the clinician. Clin Cardiol 2012;35:3–8.

# The Role of Platelet Function Testing in Risk Stratification and Clinical Decision-Making

Paul A. Gurbel, MD*, Udaya S. Tantry, PhD

## KEYWORDS

- P2Y$_{12}$ receptor • Platelet function testing • Clopidogrel • High on-treatment platelet reactivity
- Bleeding • Percutaneous coronary intervention

## KEY POINTS

- Clopidogrel (a widely used second-generation thienopyridine) therapy is associated with an unpredictable pharmacodynamic response whereby approximately 1 in 3 patients will have high on-treatment platelet reactivity to adenosine diphosphate (HPR).
- HPR is an established risk factor for ischemic event occurrence in patients undergoing percutaneous coronary intervention.
- Platelet function testing may have a role to monitor:
  - Therapeutic efficacy when clopidogrel is the chosen agent and
  - Safety when more potent drugs are used especially in patients with high bleeding risk.
- The concept of a "therapeutic window" of P2Y$_{12}$ receptor reactivity associated with both ischemic event occurrence (upper threshold, HPR) and bleeding risk (lower threshold, LPR) has been proposed.
- At this time it seems most reasonable to assess platelet function in high-risk clopidogrel-treated patients.

## INTRODUCTION

Platelets were first described as disclike structures in blood by Sir William Osler in 1873.[1] Seven years later, the anatomic structure and role of platelets in hemostasis and experimental thrombosis were described by Bizzozero.[2] Nearly a century later, Born[3] first described an in vitro method of quantifying platelet aggregation. In the 1962 *Nature* article, Born stated that, "If it can be shown that ADP (adenosine diphosphate) takes part in the aggregation of platelets in blood vessels, it is conceivable that AMP (adenosine monophosphate) or some other substance could be used to inhibit or reverse platelet aggregation in thrombosis." Moreover, subsequent studies by the same group indicated that there was an immediate decrease in the number of circulating platelets when ADP was injected into rabbits, cats, and even man. Furthermore, it was demonstrated that "thrombus-producing activity of the injured vessel wall" can be attenuated by the infusion of adenosine or 2-chloroadenosine. In 1965 Born

Disclosures: Dr Gurbel has received research funding from AstraZeneca, Daiichi Sankyo/Lilly, Sanofi-Aventis, CSL Pharmaceuticals, Nanosphere and Haemonetics; and honoraria and/or consultation fees from Merck, Daiichi Sankyo/Lilly, Boerhinger Ingleheim, Johnson and Johnson, AstraZeneca, Discovery Channel, and Bayer Healthcare. Dr Tantry reports receiving payment for lectures and receiving travel support from Accumetrics.
Cardiac Catheterization Laboratory, Sinai Center for Thrombosis Research, 2401 West Belvedere Avenue, Baltimore, MD 21215, USA
* Corresponding author.
*E-mail address:* pgurbel@lifebridgehealth.org

Intervent Cardiol Clin 2 (2013) 607–614
http://dx.doi.org/10.1016/j.iccl.2013.05.009

further stated that "these observations provide direct evidence that these inhibitors of platelet aggregation are able to inhibit thrombosis, and indirect evidence that the ADP mechanism is involved in thrombogenesis."[4] The observations by Born provided the fundamental basis for the development of $P2Y_{12}$ receptor blockers and also for the ex vivo measurement of platelet aggregation in patients with coronary artery disease (CAD). Since then, multiple in vitro and ex vivo studies, clinical trials, and translational research studies have supported the hypothesis that the ADP-induced platelet aggregation is central to occlusive thrombus generation and that an effective attenuation of ADP-induced platelet aggregation results in superior clinical outcomes with respect to thrombotic event occurrence in patients with high-risk CAD.

## ANTIPLATELET THERAPY STRATEGIES AND IMPORTANCE OF PLATELET FUNCTION TESTING

Dual antiplatelet therapy (DAPT) with aspirin and a $P2Y_{12}$ receptor blocker is the most important pharmacologic therapy administered to the high-risk percutaneous coronary intervention (PCI)/acute coronary syndromes (ACS) patient to block platelet reactivity and to prevent recurrent ischemic event occurrence. Although the clinical efficacy of DAPT has been demonstrated in a wide range of high-risk CAD patients, clopidogrel (a widely used second-generation thienopyridine) therapy is associated with an unpredictable pharmacodynamic response whereby approximately 1 in 3 patients will have high on-treatment platelet reactivity to ADP (HPR). Despite the fundamental importance of unblocked $P2Y_{12}$ receptors in the genesis of thrombosis and the clear demonstration of clopidogrel nonresponsiveness, cardiologists largely do not determine platelet function in their high-risk patients treated with clopidogrel to ensure that an antiplatelet effect is actually present. Indeed, this "nonselective" or "one-size-fits-all" approach to clopidogrel therapy to prevent catastrophic thrombotic event occurrence is paradoxic in comparison to the objective assessments and adjustments frequently made during treatment with most other cardiovascular drugs.[5]

There has been reluctance to accept platelet function testing (PFT) in routine practice because of the potential introduction of artifacts by laboratory methods, incomplete reflection of the actual in vivo thrombotic process, and failure to establish unequivocally a causal relation between the results of testing and thrombotic event occurrence.[6] In the last decade, improved understanding of

platelet receptor physiology has led to the development of more potent $P2Y_{12}$ receptor blockers. The introduction of more user-friendly platelet function assays that can reliably determine the antiplatelet effect of clopidogrel has somewhat changed the latter reluctant mindset and spurred great interest in antiplatelet therapy monitoring.[7]

## INITIAL EVIDENCE FOR HIGH PLATELET REACTIVITY TO ADP AS A RISK FACTOR

Barragan and colleagues[8] reported an association between posttreatment $P2Y_{12}$ reactivity and the occurrence of thrombotic events (clinical treatment failure) in a case-control study of PCI patients whereby platelet reactivity index greater than 50% measured by vasodilator-stimulated phosphoprotein phosphorylation (VASP-P) was associated with stent thrombosis. At the same time Matetzky and colleagues[9] observed that patients undergoing primary PCI for ST-segment elevation myocardial infarction (STEMI) who were in the lowest quartile of clopidogrel responsiveness (measured by aggregometry) had the highest rates of ischemic events during follow-up.

Given the interindividual variability in baseline ADP-induced platelet aggregation, the measurement of clopidogrel responsiveness (absolute or relative changes in platelet aggregation from baseline) may overestimate ischemic risk in nonresponders with low pretreatment reactivity as well as underestimate risk in responders who remain with high platelet reactivity after treatment.[10] Therefore, the absolute level of platelet reactivity during treatment (ie, on-treatment platelet reactivity) has been proposed as a better measure of thrombotic risk than responsiveness to clopidogrel.

Subsequent studies based on aggregometry demonstrated that a threshold of ~50% maximal periprocedural aggregation (20 μM ADP) was strongly associated with 6-month ischemic event occurrence; ~40% aggregation (20 μM ADP) was associated with stent thrombosis occurrence and ~40% preprocedural platelet aggregation (5 μM ADP) among patients before stenting was associated with 12-month ischemic event occurrence.[11–13] Using the VerifyNow $P2Y_{12}$ assay, it was demonstrated that patients with posttreatment reactivity greater than 235 PRU ($P2Y_{12}$ reaction units) (~upper quartile) had significantly higher rates of cardiovascular death (2.8 vs 0%, $P = .04$) and stent thrombosis (4.6 vs 0%, $P = .004$).[14] Low responders as indicated by upper quintile (~482 AU*min) using the Multiplate analyzer had a significantly higher risk of definite stent thrombosis and a higher mortality rate within

30 days compared with normal responders.[15–18] These initial studies stimulated a great interest in PFT in patients undergoing PCI during DAPT.

## HPR CUTOFF VALUES DEFINED BY RECEIVER OPERATING CHARACTERISTIC CURVE ANALYSIS

Receiver operating characteristic (ROC) curve analysis was used to define a threshold or cut point of on-treatment platelet reactivity associated with the optimal combination of sensitivity and specificity to identify thrombotic/ischemic risk. To date, cutoff values have been mainly investigated in patients undergoing PCI and a different cutoff value may be obtained in other settings depending on patient management or baseline risk profile. The observed cutoff values for platelet reactivity noted above had a very high negative predictive value for thrombotic/ischemic event occurrence, an observation of clinical importance. However, the positive predictive value is fairly low for all assays, which is consistent with the fact that although a major determinant of thrombotic events, high on-treatment platelet reactivity is not the sole factor responsible for these events and that overall event frequency is low.[19] A consensus statement was proposed with HPR cutoff values based on ROC curve analysis for various platelet function assays.[7]

In a time-dependent covariate Cox regression analysis of on-treatment platelet reactivity in the GRAVITAS (Gauging Responsiveness with A VerifyNow assay—Impact on Thrombosis And Safety) study (n = 2214, HPR defined as a PRU >208 was an independent predictor of event-free survival at 60 days (hazard ratio [HR] = 0.23, $P$ = .047) and strongly trended to be an independent predictor at 6 months (HR = 0.54, $P$ = .06).[20] In the ADAPT-DES (The Assessment of Dual Antiplatelet Therapy With Drug-Eluting Stents) trial (n = 8349) that included a higher risk population (~50% had ACS), patients with more than 208 PRU (42.5%) had a 3.9-fold adjusted hazard ratio for 30-day stent thrombosis ($P$ = .005) and a 2.49 adjusted hazard ratio for 1 year stent thrombosis ($P$ = .001).[21] The evidence from ADAPT drug-eluting stent suggests that short-term events are most closely related to HPR. Finally in a recent meta-analysis of 20 observational studies comprising a total of 9187 PCI patients, HPR (>208 PRU) was demonstrated to be a strong predictor of myocardial infarction, stent thrombosis, and the composite end point of reported ischemic events (HR = 3.0, 4.1, and 4.9, respectively; $P$<.00001 for all cases). Furthermore, the predicted risk for CV death, MI, or ST was not heterogeneous ($I^2$: 0%, 0%, and 12%, respectively; $P$ is not significant for all cases) despite large differences in the methodology and in the definition of HPR between studies.[22]

## PERSONALIZED ANTIPLATELET THERAPY TRIALS

In the GRAVITAS trial, primarily stable and low-risk PCI patients with HPR ($\geq$230 PRU) were randomized to 75 mg/d standard or 150 mg/d high clopidogrel dosing. High-dose clopidogrel treatment was ineffective in reducing 6-month composite ischemic event occurrence and there was an unexpectedly low event rate (2.3%) in both groups.[23] The pharmacodynamic effect of high-dose clopidogrel was relatively modest (~40% of the patients still had HPR) and unlikely to influence clinical outcomes in an overall low-risk population.[24] In support of this hypothesis, in the ELEVATE-TIMI 51 trial, up to a 225 mg daily clopidogrel dose was required to overcome HPR.[25] In the TRIGGER-PCI trial, the effects of a more potent active arm (prasugrel) compared with standard dose clopidogrel in low-risk patients with HPR (>208 PRU) undergoing nonurgent PCI was investigated.[26] This trial was prematurely terminated because of a very low incidence of cardiovascular events. Finally, in the ARCTIC study, 2440 patients scheduled for planned coronary stenting were randomly assigned to a strategy of platelet-function monitoring and drug adjustment or to a conventional strategy without monitoring. In the monitoring arm, one-third of patients had HPR (>235 PRU or <15% inhibition) before stent implantation and 80% of these patients received additional clopidogrel loading dose for PCI, whereas only 2.3% received prasugrel loading doses. The primary endpoint was not different in the monitoring arm compared with the conventional arm (34.6% vs 31.1%, HR = 1.13; $P$ = .10) and this may be because low-risk patients with HPR were mainly treated with high-dose clopidogrel. In this trial, the prevalence of ACS patients was low (27% Non ST-segment elevation-ACS vs 73% patients with stable CAD) and patients at very high risk for early atherothrombotic events (eg, STEMI patients) were excluded from the study.[27] In totality, these recent studies that included low-risk patients undergoing PCI with low event rates demonstrate that high-dose clopidogrel is not an optimal strategy to overcome HPR and suggest that future personalized antiplatelet therapy trials should focus on enrolling high-risk patients undergoing PCI and treating patients with HPR with prasugrel or ticagrelor. In addition, potent $P2Y_{12}$ receptor blocker should be administered as soon as possible and even before PCI to prevent early events. Finally, in a meta-analysis of personalized antiplatelet trials, tailored therapy was associated with significantly less cardiovascular death and stent thrombosis. However, intensification of antiplatelet therapy in patients with HPR was not associated with greater minor or major bleeding.[28]

## RELATION BETWEEN LOW ON-TREATMENT PLATELET REACTIVITY AND BLEEDING—THE THERAPEUTIC WINDOW CONCEPT

In addition to the upper threshold for ischemic risk (ie, HPR), small translational research studies have suggested a relation between low on-treatment platelet reactivity (LPR) with bleeding (**Table 1**).

**Table 1**
**Relation between platelet-function measurement and bleeding in patients treated with PCI**

| Study | Patients (n) and P2Y$_{12}$ Treatment | Platelet Function Test(s) | Bleeding Criteria | Outcome |
|---|---|---|---|---|
| Cuisset et al,[29] 2009 | NSTE-ACS (n = 597), Clopidogrel | LTA Preheparin ADP-induced aggregation and VASP-PRI | Non-CABG-related TIMI major and minor | <40% aggregation correlated with higher risk of 30 d postdischarge bleeding |
| Sibbing et al,[30] 2010 | PCI (n = 2533) Clopidogrel | Multiplatelet analyzer, ADP-induced aggregation | Procedure-related TIMI major bleeding | <188 AU*min associated with ×3.5 bleeding |
| Gurbel et al,[31] 2010 | PCI (n = 225) Clopidogrel | MA–ADP TEG platelet mapping assay | | ≤31 MA-ADP correlated with post-PCI bleeding |
| Bonello et al,[32] 2012 | ACS undergoing PCI (n = 301) Prasugrel | VASP assay | Major bleeding | VASP-PRI ≤16% associated with major bleedings |
| Mokhtar et al,[33] 2010 | Undergoing PCI (n = 346) Clopidogrel | VASP assay | Non-CABG TIMI minor and major | Low on treatment PRI independent predictor of bleedings |
| Patti et al,[34] 2011 | PCI (n = 310) CLP | VerifyNow P2Y12 assay | TIMI major bleeding | ROC analysis ≤189 PRU associated with bleeding |
| Parodi et al,[35] 2012 | Stenting (n = 298) Prasugrel | LTA | Entry site bleeding | LPR associated with bleeding |
| ARCITIC Study,[27] 2012 | Stenting (n = 2440) Clopidogrel, Prasugrel | VerifyNow P2Y12 assay | Major bleeding-STEEPLE trial | No correlation between bleeding and platelet reactivity |
| POPULAR study Breet et al,[36] 2010 | PCI (n = 1069) CLP | LTA, VerifyNowP2Y$_{12}$ assay; Plateletworks; IMPACT-R; PFA-100 with collagen–ADP; Innovance PFA P2Y | TIMI | No relation between bleeding and platelet reactivity measured by any assay |
| GRAVITAS Price et al,[23] 2011 | Undergoing PCI with DES implantation, treated with DAPT (n = 2214) | VerifyNow P2Y$_{12}$ assay | TIMI | No correlation between bleeding and platelet reactivity |

*Abbreviations:* CLP, clopidogrel; DES, drug-eluting stent; LTA, light transmittance aggregometry; NSTE-ACS, non-ST-segment elevation acute coronary syndrome; PFA-100, platelet function analyzer-100; PRI, platelet reactivity index; STEEPLE trial, Safety and Efficacy of Enoxaparin in Percutaneous Coronary Intervention Patients, an International Randomized Evaluation trial; TEG, thrombelastography.
*Data from* Refs.[30,32,34,37]

The first quartile of posttreatment ADP-induced platelet aggregation (<40%) was associated with postdischarge minor and major thrombolysis in myocardial infarction (TIMI) bleeding events in a cohort of patients undergoing PCI for NSTEMI and receiving clopidogrel (n = 597).[29] A 3.5-fold increased risk of procedure-related major bleeding in patients with less than 188 AU*min as assessed by the Multiplate analyzer was demonstrated in another prospective cohort of patients undergoing PCI (n = 2533).[30] Furthermore, a lower platelet reactivity index (VASP-PRI) was observed in patients with non-CABG-related major TIMI bleeding compared with patients without major bleeding (32.5 ± 22.4 vs 51.2 ± 21.9%; $P$ = .006) in a retrospective analysis of 346 patients undergoing PCI.[34] Similarly, in patients undergoing PCI who were treated with DAPT over 3 years, ADP-induced platelet fibrin clot strength (maximum amplitude [MA]) greater than 47 mm had the best predictive value of long-term ischemic events compared with light transmittance aggregometry ($P$<.0001). Moreover, ROC curve and quartile analysis suggested MA (ADP) ≤31 mm as a predictive value for post-PCI bleeding events.[31] Using VerifyNow P2Y12 assay, Campo and colleagues[37] demonstrated a therapeutic window (86–238 $P2Y_{12}$ reactivity units) with a lower incidence of both ischemic and bleeding complications in patients undergoing PCI.

Despite these observations from small studies, a large-scale single-center cohort study (POPULAR, n = 1069) and 3 personalized antiplatelet trials (GRAVITAS, TRIGGER-PCI, and ARCTIC) failed to show any meaningful relation between platelet reactivity and bleeding events, which may be attributed to a low incidence of major bleeding events in these trials.[23,26,27,36] However,

in the largest prospective registry, ADPAPT-DES, in a multivariable propensity score adjusted analysis, HPR (>208 PRU) was significantly associated with major bleeding (HR [95% confidence interval] = 0.73 [0.61, 0.89], $P$ = .002).[21]

The concept of a "therapeutic window" of $P2Y_{12}$ receptor reactivity associated with both ischemic event occurrence (upper threshold, HPR) and bleeding risk (lower threshold, LPR) has been proposed.[38] Based on observational studies, various cutoffs for HPR and LPR are presented in **Table 2**. These cutoffs could be used in future studies of personalized antiplatelet therapy.

## RELATION OF PLATELET REACTIVITY TO BLEEDING DURING SURGERY

In patients undergoing coronary artery bypass grafting (CABG), withdrawal of a $P2Y_{12}$ receptor blocker treatment for 5 to 7 days is recommended by the guidelines to avoid excessive perioperative bleeding by allowing platelet function recovery.[39,40] Because clopidogrel therapy is associated with response variability and nonresponsiveness, it was suggested that an objective measurement of the antiplatelet effect of clopidogrel before surgery may obviate the recommended waiting period in a substantial percentage of patients. In support of this hypothesis, in the prospective Time BAsed StRateGy to REduce Clopidogrel AssociaTed Bleeding During CABG (TARGET CABG) study, clopidogrel response was measured by thromboelastography with platelet mapping and surgery was scheduled with no delay in those with a maximum amplitude ($MA_{ADP}$) greater than 50 mm, within 3 to 5 days in those with a $MA_{ADP}$ = 35 to 50 mm, and after 5 days in those with an $MA_{ADP}$ less than 35 mm. This study demonstrated that stratifying clopidogrel-treated patients to specific waiting

**Table 2**
**Platelet reactivity cutoff associated with ischemic and bleeding events (therapeutic window)**

| | Cutoff Associated with Ischemic Event Occurrences | Cutoff Associated with Bleeding Event Occurrences |
|---|---|---|
| VerifyNow P2Y12 assay (PRU) | >208 | <85[37] |
| Multiplate analyzer | | |
|    ADP-induced aggregation (*AU) | >467 | <188[30] |
| Vasodilator stimulated phosphoprotein phosphorylation-platelet reactivity index (%) | >50% | 16%[32] |
| Thrombelastography platelet mapping assay | | |
|    ADP-induced platelet-fibrin clot strength (mm) | >47 | <29[31] |

*Data from* Refs.[30–32,37]

periods based on a preoperative assessment of clopidogrel response resulted in similar perioperative bleeding as compared with clopidogrel-naïve patients undergoing elective first-time on-pump CABG.[41] Despite the absence of evidence from a large-scale prospective trial, in the recent the Society of Thoracic Surgeons Guideline for cardiovascular surgeons, it was stated that "discontinuation of $P2Y_{12}$ inhibitors for a few days before cardiovascular operations is recommended to reduce bleeding and blood transfusion, especially in high-risk patients. Class I (Level of evidence B)."[42]

## SUMMARY

HPR is an established risk factor in patients undergoing PCI. Most of the studies linking HPR to thrombotic event occurrence have used a periprocedural platelet reactivity measurement. HPR may be most predictive of event occurrence in high-risk patients. Evidence also suggests that short-term events are more closely related to HPR than long-term events. It is uncertain that the "proof" of the clinical utility of PFT from an adequately powered randomized trial will ever be witnessed. Given the trend to lower event frequency in PCI trials, the required sample size to demonstrate the utility of PFT for guided therapy would be very large (n = ~7500–10,000). Thus, at this time the guidelines and the existing observational data must be relied on while considering the crucial role of platelet physiology in catastrophic event occurrence in the PCI patient. Recent American and European guidelines have included class IIb recommendations to measure platelet function in high-risk patients if the results of testing may alter management.[39,40]

Platelet function testing may have a role in monitoring (1) therapeutic efficacy when clopidogrel is the chosen agent and (2) safety when more potent drugs are used, especially in patients with high bleeding risk. Despite the lower overall on-treatment platelet reactivity during new $P2Y_{12}$ inhibitor therapy, there is evidence that selected patients have HPR and that these patients have increased MACE.[32]

Finally, platelet reactivity should not be regarded as an absolute and sole prognostic marker. Instead platelet reactivity should be evaluated in combination with demographic variables associated with risk, the time of platelet reactivity testing with respect to the time of PCI occurrence, and the presence of ACS.

Therefore, at this time it seems most reasonable to assess platelet function in high-risk clopidogrel-treated patients, for example, patients with current

or prior ACS, history of stent thrombosis and target vessel revascularization, poor left ventricular function, multivessel stenting, complex anatomy (eg, bifurcation, long, small stents), high body mass index, diabetes mellitus, and patients cotreated with proton-pump inhibitors. Treatment with more potent $P2Y_{12}$ receptor therapy would then be reserved for patients with HPR. Finally, it should be remembered that clopidogrel is pharmacodynamically effective in about two-thirds of the patients undergoing PCI; these patients do not have HPR. Therefore, selectively treating two-thirds of the patients with generic clopidogrel may provide significant cost savings. At the same time, unselected therapy with the new $P2Y_{12}$ receptor blockers is associated with increased bleeding. Based on the therapeutic window that defines optimal anti-ischemic efficacy and safety, the antiplatelet regimen is chosen, regardless of the cost.

## REFERENCES

1. Osler W. An account of certain organisms occurring in the liquor sanguinis. Proc R Soc Lond 1874;22: 391–8.
2. Bizzozero G. Su di un nuovo elemento morfologico del sangue dei mammiferi e della sua importanza nella trombosi e nella coagulazione. L'Osservatore 1881;17:785–7.
3. Born GV. Aggregation of blood platelets by adenosine diphosphate and its reversal. Nature 1962; 194:927–9.
4. Born GV. Platelets in thrombogenesis: mechanism and inhibition of platelet aggregation. Ann R Coll Surg Engl 1965;36:200–6.
5. Gurbel PA, Tantry US. Do platelet function testing and genotyping improve outcome in patients treated with antithrombotic agents?: platelet function testing and genotyping improve outcome in patients treated with antithrombotic agents. Circulation 2012;125: 1276–87.
6. Hirsh PD, Hillis LD, Campbell WB, et al. Release of prostaglandins and thromboxane into the coronary circulation in patients with ischemic heart disease. N Engl J Med 1981;304:685–91.
7. Bonello L, Tantry US, Marcucci R, et al, Working Group on High On-Treatment Platelet Reactivity. Consensus and future directions on the definition of high on-treatment platelet reactivity to adenosine diphosphate. J Am Coll Cardiol 2010;56:919–33.
8. Barragan P, Bouvier JL, Roquebert PO, et al. Resistance to thienopyridines: clinical detection of coronary stent thrombosis by monitoring of vasodilator-stimulated phosphoprotein phosphorylation. Catheter Cardiovasc Interv 2003;59:295–302.
9. Matetzky S, Shenkman B, Guetta V, et al. Clopidogrel resistance is associated with increased risk of

recurrent atherothrombotic events in patients with acute myocardial infarction. Circulation 2004;109: 3171–5.

10. Samara WM, Bliden KP, Tantry US, et al. The difference between clopidogrel responsiveness and posttreatment platelet reactivity. Thromb Res 2005; 115:89–94.

11. Gurbel PA, Bliden KP, Guyer K, et al. Platelet reactivity in patients and recurrent events post-stenting: results of the PREPARE POST-STENTING Study. J Am Coll Cardiol 2005;46:1820–6.

12. Gurbel PA, Bliden KP, Samara W, et al. The clopidogrel Resistance and Stent Thrombosis (CREST) study. J Am Coll Cardiol 2005;46:1827–32.

13. Bliden KP, DiChiara J, Tantry US, et al. Increased risk in patients with high platelet aggregation receiving chronic clopidogrel therapy undergoing percutaneous coronary intervention: is the current antiplatelet therapy adequate? J Am Coll Cardiol 2007;49:657–66.

14. Price MJ, Endemann S, Gollapudi RR, et al. Prognostic significance of post-clopidogrel platelet reactivity assessed by a point-of-care assay on thrombotic events after drug-eluting stent implantation. Eur Heart J 2008;29:992–1000.

15. Sibbing D, Morath T, Braun S, et al. Clopidogrel response status assessed with Multiplate point-of-care analysis and the incidence and timing of stent thrombosis over six months following coronary stenting. Thromb Haemost 2010;103:151–9.

16. Gurbel PA, Antonino MJ, Bliden KP, et al. Platelet reactivity to adenosine diphosphate and long-term ischemic event occurrence following percutaneous coronary intervention: a potential antiplatelet therapeutic target. Platelets 2008;19:595–604.

17. Bonello L, Paganelli F, Arpin-Bornet M, et al. Vasodilator-stimulated phosphoprotein phosphorylation analysis prior to percutaneous coronary intervention for exclusion of postprocedural major adverse cardiovascular events. J Thromb Haemost 2007;5:1630–6.

18. Sibbing D, Braun S, Morath T, et al. Platelet reactivity after clopidogrel treatment assessed with point-of-care analysis and early drug-eluting stent thrombosis. J Am Coll Cardiol 2009;53:849–56.

19. Dahlen JR, Price MJ, Parise H, et al. Evaluating the clinical usefulness of platelet function testing: considerations for the proper application and interpretation of performance measures. Thromb Haemost 2013;109(5):808–16.

20. Price MJ, Angiolillo DJ, Teirstein PS, et al. Platelet reactivity and cardiovascular outcomes after percutaneous coronary intervention: a time-dependent analysis of the Gauging Responsiveness with a Verify-Now P2Y12 assay: Impact on Thrombosis and Safety (GRAVITAS) trial. Circulation 2011;124:1132–7.

21. Stone GW. Assessment of dual antiplatelet therapy with drug-eluting stents a large-scale, prospective, multicenter registry examining the relationship between platelet responsiveness and stent thrombosis after DES implantation. Presented at TCT, San Francisco, October 27 - November 1, 2011 and Florida, October 22-26, 2012.

22. Aradi D, Komócsi A, Vorobcsuk A, et al. Prognostic significance of high on-clopidogrel platelet reactivity after percutaneous coronary intervention: systematic review and meta-analysis. Am Heart J 2010; 160:543–51.

23. Price MJ, Berger PB, Teirstein PS, et al, GRAVITAS Investigators. Standard- vs high-dose clopidogrel based on platelet function testing after percutaneous coronary intervention: the GRAVITAS randomized trial. JAMA 2011;305:1097–105.

24. Gurbel PA, Tantry US. An initial experiment with personalized antiplatelet therapy: the GRAVITAS trial. JAMA 2011;305:1136–7.

25. Mega JL, Hochholzer W, Frelinger AL 3rd, et al. Dosing clopidogrel based on CYP2C19 genotype and the effect on platelet reactivity in patients with stable cardiovascular disease. JAMA 2011;306:2221–8.

26. Trenk D, Stone GW, Gawaz M, et al. A randomized trial of prasugrel versus clopidogrel in patients with high platelet reactivity on clopidogrel after elective percutaneous coronary intervention with implantation of drug-eluting stents: results of the TRIGGER-PCI (Testing Platelet Reactivity In Patients Undergoing Elective Stent Placement on Clopidogrel to Guide Alternative Therapy With Prasugrel) study. J Am Coll Cardiol 2012;59:2159–64.

27. Collet JP, Cuisset T, Rangé G, et al, ARCTIC Investigators. Bedside monitoring to adjust antiplatelet therapy for coronary stenting. N Engl J Med 2012; 367:2100–9.

28. Aradi D, Komócsi A, Vorobcsuk A, et al. Impact of clopidogrel and potent P2Y 12-inhibitors on mortality and stroke in patients with acute coronary syndrome or undergoing percutaneous coronary intervention: a systematic review and meta-analysis. Thromb Haemost 2013;109:93–101.

29. Cuisset T, Cayla G, Frere C, et al. Predictive value of post-treatment platelet reactivity for occurrence of post-discharge bleeding after non-ST elevation acute coronary syndrome. Shifting from antiplatelet resistance to bleeding risk assessment? EuroIntervention 2009;5:325–9.

30. Sibbing D, Schulz S, Braun S, et al. Antiplatelet effects of clopidogrel and bleeding in patients undergoing coronary stent placement. J Thromb Haemost 2010;8:250–6.

31. Gurbel PA, Bliden KP, Navickas IA, et al. Adenosine diphosphate-induced platelet-fibrin clot strength: a new thrombelastographic indicator of long-term post-stenting ischemic events. Am Heart J 2010;160:346–54.

32. Bonello L, Mancini J, Pansieri M, et al. Relationship between post-treatment platelet reactivity and

ischemic and bleeding events at 1-year follow-up in patients receiving prasugrel. J Thromb Haemost 2012;10:1999–2005.

33. Mokhtar OA, Lemesle G, Armero S, et al. Relationship between platelet reactivity inhibition and non-CABG related major bleeding in patients undergoing percutaneous coronary intervention. Thromb Res 2010; 126:147–9.

34. Patti G, Pasceri V, Vizzi V, et al. Usefulness of platelet response to clopidogrel by point-of-care testing to predict bleeding outcomes in patients undergoing percutaneous coronary intervention (from the Antiplatelet Therapy for Reduction of Myocardial Damage During Angioplasty-Bleeding Study). Am J Cardiol 2011;107:995–1000.

35. Parodi G, Bellandi B, Venditti F, et al. Residual platelet reactivity, bleedings, and adherence to treatment in patients having coronary stent implantation treated with prasugrel. Am J Cardiol 2012;109:214–8.

36. Breet NJ, van Werkum JW, Bouman HJ, et al. Comparison of platelet function tests in predicting clinical outcome in patients undergoing coronary stent implantation. JAMA 2010;303:754–62.

37. Campo G, Parrinello G, Ferraresi P, et al. Prospective evaluation of on-clopidogrel platelet reactivity over time in patients treated with percutaneous coronary intervention relationship with gene polymorphisms and clinical outcome. J Am Coll Cardiol 2011;57:2474–83.

38. Gurbel PA, Becker RC, Mann KG, et al. Platelet function monitoring in patients with coronary artery disease. J Am Coll Cardiol 2007;50:1822–34.

39. Hamm CW, Bassand JP, Agewall S, et al. ESC Guidelines for the management of acute coronary syndromes in patients presenting without persistent ST-segment elevation: The Task Force for the management of acute coronary syndromes (ACS) in patients presenting without persistent ST-segment elevation of the European Society of Cardiology (ESC). Eur Heart J 2011;32:2999–3054.

40. Levine GN, Bates ER, Blankenship JC, et al, American College of Cardiology Foundation, American Heart Association Task Force on Practice Guidelines, Society for Cardiovascular Angiography and Interventions. 2011 ACCF/AHA/SCAI Guideline for Percutaneous Coronary Intervention. A report of the American College of Cardiology Foundation/American Heart Association Task Force on Practice Guidelines and the Society for Cardiovascular Angiography and Interventions. J Am Coll Cardiol 2011; 58:e44–122.

41. Mahla E, Suarez TA, Bliden KP, et al. Platelet function measurement-based strategy to reduce bleeding and waiting time in clopidogrel-treated patients undergoing coronary artery bypass graft surgery: the Timing Based on Platelet Function Strategy to Reduce Clopidogrel-Associated Bleeding Related to CABG (TARGET-CABG) Study. Circ Cardiovasc Interv 2012;5:261–9.

42. Ferraris VA, Saha SP, Oestreich JH, et al, Society of Thoracic Surgeons. 2012 update to the Society of Thoracic Surgeons guideline on use of antiplatelet drugs in patients having cardiac and noncardiac operations. Ann Thorac Surg 2012;94:1761–81.

# Pharmacogenomics in Interventional Pharmacology
## Present Status and Future Directions

Paddy M. Barrett, MD[a], Matthew J. Price, MD[a,b],*

## KEYWORDS

- Pharmacogenomics • Interventional pharmacology • Clopidogrel • P2Y12 inhibitors
- Cardiovascular medicine

## KEY POINTS

- Pharmacogenomics aims specifically to tailor drugs to an individual's unique genetic signature, thereby enhancing the likelihood that a patient experiences the greatest clinical efficacy with the least possibility of an adverse drug event.
- Candidate gene studies explore the influence of previously identified genes based on biologic plausibility. Simultaneously, genome-wide association studies test the associations between hundreds of thousands to several million single nucleotide polymorphisms and a phenotype of interest. Whole exome and whole genome sequencing are nonhypothesis-based techniques that can identify the specific causative variants associated with drug response, rather than relying on identifying common variants in linkage disequilibrium with potentially causative variants.
- CYP2C19 loss-of-function allele carriage is associated with lower levels of clopidogrel active metabolite, less platelet inhibition, lower bleeding risk, and a greater risk of myocardial infarction and stent thrombosis. The influence of CYP2C19 on outcomes is strongest in clopidogrel-treated patients undergoing percutaneous coronary intervention (PCI).
- CYP2C19 and other genes tested in candidate gene studies do not seem to influence the treatment effect of the other oral platelet P2Y12 inhibitors, prasugrel, and ticagrelor.
- Challenges to the broad adoption of pharmacogenomics in interventional cardiology include the lack of randomized trials, delays in result turnover, low event rates in elective PCI patients, and incomplete identification of the genomic determinants of clinical outcomes.

## INTRODUCTION

In the United States, more than 635,000 patients suffer a myocardial infarction (MI) annually and in approximately 280,000 of these cases it is a recurrent event.[1] Furthermore, nearly 2 million people undergo percutaneous coronary intervention (PCI) every year. These patients receive a multitude of pharmacologic agents, most of which have demonstrated clinical efficacy in large populations enrolled in randomized clinical trials.[2,3] However, many of these agents will be either partially or completely ineffective in a particular individual due to genetic factors and, thereby, expose patients to substantially higher risk of adverse events with limited clinical benefit.[4]

This work was supported in part by Clinical and Translational Science Award (CTSA) funding to the Scripps Translational Science Institute (NIH/NCATS UL1 TR000109).

[a] Scripps Translational Science Institute, 3344 North Torrey Pines Court, Suite 300, La Jolla, CA 92037, USA;
[b] Cardiac Catheterization Laboratory, Scripps Green Hospital, 10666 North Torrey Pines Road, Maildrop S1056, La Jolla, CA 92037, USA
* Corresponding author. Cardiac Catheterization Laboratory, Scripps Green Hospital, 10666 North Torrey Pines Road, Maildrop S1056, La Jolla, CA 92037.
E-mail address: price.matthew@scrippshealth.org

Intervent Cardiol Clin 2 (2013) 615–625
http://dx.doi.org/10.1016/j.iccl.2013.05.006
2211-7458/13/$ – see front matter © 2013 Elsevier Inc. All rights reserved.

Pharmacogenomics aims to specifically tailor drugs to an individual's unique genetic signature, thereby enhancing the likelihood that a patient experiences the greatest clinical efficacy with the least possibility of an adverse drug event. Although candidate gene studies and genome-wide association studies (GWASes) have demonstrated limited incremental value in the prediction of disease risk, their power is greatly amplified in the setting of pharmacogenomics because they provide exceptionally large improvements in the odds ratio for major side effects or drug responsiveness in the order of 300% to 2000%.[5] Additionally, the potential financial benefits of implementing pharmacogenomic approaches are considerable because lack of drug efficacy and adverse events costs the United States more than $100 billion annually.[5] Strategies are also needed to reduce the greater than $1 billion cost of taking a single drug to market.[6] Pharmacogenomics addresses such issues by improving the ability to select early stage compounds based on likelihood of efficacy and predicted adverse event profile, to reexamine previously failed compounds for select indications, and to reduce the likelihood of expensive postapproval drug recalls.

Although pharmacogenomics seems poised to enhance how the drugs of today and the future are designed, developed, and applied, the phenomenon of clopidogrel-response variability, combined with the importance of clopidogrel in interventional cardiology, has brought the potential benefit of genetic-guided therapy to current clinical practice. This article reviews the basic concepts of pharmacogenomics studies, delineates how the safety and efficacy of the oral platelet P2Y12 inhibitors are influencing genetics, and explores the future directions and limitations of pharmacogenomic approaches related to interventional cardiology.

## BASIC CONCEPTS OF PHARMACOGENETIC AND PHARMACOGENOMICS STUDIES

The tailoring of drug therapy to a patient metric is not a novel feature in cardiovascular medicine. As a daily part of clinical care, physicians adjust statin doses based on cholesterol levels, warfarin based on international normalized ratios, and antihypertensives based on blood pressure recordings. Furthermore, patient characteristics that influence circulating parent drug or active metabolite levels frequently dictate the appropriate dose or selection of a particular agent. An example is dose-adjustment for renal dysfunction for novel anticoagulants and intravenous direct antithrombins or contraindications in the presence of hepatic failure for cyclopentyl-triazolo-pyrimidine antiplatelet agents.[7–10] Pharmacogenomics takes this process to a greater depth of precision by choosing or adjusting a drug dependent on a variety of genomic factors.

There are several methodological approaches to determine the influence of genetic polymorphisms on drug effect or the risk of disease development (**Table 1**). Candidate gene studies explore the influence of previously identified genes based on biologic plausibility. This approach depends on the hypothesis that a particular gene may influence drug availability (eg, enzymes involved in

**Table 1**
**Methodological approaches for pharmacogenetic and pharmacogenomic studies**

| Sequencing Method | Concept | Cost | Advantages | Disadvantages |
|---|---|---|---|---|
| Candidate Gene Sequencing Studies | Study of previously defined biologically plausible genes | + | Inexpensive. Narrow gene focus. | Poor reproducibility |
| GWASes | Simultaneous comparison of multiple SNPs to a selected phenotype | ++ | Hundreds to thousands of data sets available for comparison | Excellent reproducibility |
| Exome Sequencing Studies | Sequencing of all protein coding regions of the genome | +++ | Efficient and cost-effective large-scale sequencing strategy | Does not explore noncoding regions of the genome |
| Whole Genome Sequencing Studies | Sequencing of all coding and non coding regions of the genome | ++++ | Complete nucleotide sequence assessment | Expensive and time consuming by comparison to other methods |

metabolism) or effect (eg, receptors involved in mechanism of action or a rare adverse effect). For example, Hulot and colleagues[11] tested the association between various genetic polymorphisms of CYP450 isoenzymes and clopidogrel effect based on previous knowledge of the biotransformation of the parent prodrug into active metabolite; this candidate gene approach first demonstrated that CYP2C19 loss-of-function (LOF) allele carriage significantly influenced clopidogrel pharmacodynamics. Despite these successes, the ability of a candidate gene approach to discover new genetic determinants is substantially restricted by such a narrowed, hypothesis-based focus. Moreover, false positive results can occur from repeated looks at different candidate genes within a cohort (often published separately) without statistical correction for multiple comparisons.

A GWAS simultaneously tests the associations between hundreds of thousands to several million single nucleotide polymorphisms (SNPs) and a phenotype of interest (eg, drug response or disease state). Although substantially more expensive than a candidate gene study, a GWAS can now be performed more easily due to decreased costs and exponential increases in computer processing power. Statistical significance requires associations with extremely small $P$-values to correct for the hundreds of thousands of simultaneous comparisons that are performed. A GWAS can be successful at delineating the influence of common sequence variants that occur with genome-wide significance ($P<10^{-8}$). For example, Shuldiner and colleagues[12] demonstrated through a GWAS approach that several polymorphisms within the CYP2C18-CYP2C19-CYP2C9-CYP2C8 cluster were associated with diminished clopidogrel response. Further candidate gene analysis showed that a significant SNP within this cluster was in high linkage disequilibrium with the CYP2C19*2 LOF allele, thereby confirming the earlier candidate gene studies in a more robust fashion at the level of genome-wide significance ($P = 4.3 \times 10^{-11}$). However, with regard to predicting disease risk, GWASes, in general, have identified loci with only modest odds ratios.[5] Because a GWAS is based on common sequence variants, it cannot identify rare functional variants, which often display much greater predictive ability. In addition, although most GWASs are not hypothesis-driven, the ability to identify novel variants is limited by the particular SNPs that are used in the analysis.

Whole exome sequencing, also known as hybridization oligonucleotide capture, enables the preferential enrichment and sequencing of protein-coding regions of the more than 21,000 genes within the genome. This approach has been used to identify novel genes associated with rare and common disorders.[13-16] Unlike candidate gene approaches, exome sequencing does not require a priori gene selection that may introduce biases in target selection. Exome sequencing offers better resolution, compared with a GWAS, which allows for identification of protein-based, potentially causative variants associated with disease rather than relying on identifying common variants in linkage disequilibrium with potentially causative variants. Whole genome sequencing is now available; however, cost has currently limited its application in large-scale pharmacogenomics studies. Complete knowledge of the sequence variants at a whole genome level (including the coding and noncoding regions of the genome) will provide much higher resolution genomic data. However, it still does not provide a complete picture because gene-gene interactions, epigenetic modifications, and proteomic and metabolomic features likely play a role in drug response, clinical efficacy, and safety.

### *Pharmacogenomics of Antiplatelet Therapy*

Platelet inhibitors are the cornerstone of adjunctive pharmacologic therapy in PCI because platelet activation and aggregation play a critical role in thrombosis. In randomized clinical trials of subjects with acute coronary syndrome (ACS), platelet P2Y12 antagonism combined with aspirin improves outcomes compared with aspirin alone. More intensive P2Y12 inhibition reduces thrombotic events, including stent thrombosis, in ACS patients treated with PCI.[17-22] Identifying patients who may not be receiving the intended effect of these antiplatelet agents can help determine the genomic variants that predict responsiveness to antiplatelet therapy. In addition, the downstream functional effects (measured by platelet reactivity assessment) could provide clinical value by adding to risk prediction and providing the clinician with the necessary information to tailor antiplatelet therapy dosing or selection.

## PHARMACOGENETICS OF CLOPIDOGREL

Platelet activation and aggregation are the proximate causes of thrombotic events after PCI. Activation of the platelet P2Y12 receptor by adenosine diphosphate (ADP) amplifies and sustains platelet activation during the extension phase of platelet plug formation after vascular injury.[23,24] Several randomized trials have demonstrated that treatment with the P2Y12 inhibitors ticlopidine, clopidogrel, prasugrel, and ticagrelor in combination with aspirin significantly reduces the likelihood of thrombotic cardiovascular events in patients with PCI or ACS.[18,20,25] The magnitude of clinical benefit afforded by these agents is primarily attributable to reduced platelet responsiveness to ADP. By extension, the patient with PCI who has enhanced responsiveness to ADP despite P2Y12 inhibitor therapy would be at higher risk of thrombosis, a supposition that has been borne out by observational studies and post hoc analysis of a randomized trial.[26–28] Therefore, platelet reactivity assessment and identification of the genomic variants that influence platelet reactivity could become critical components in the management of patients receiving such therapies. Clopidogrel has become a test case for the application of pharmacogenetics in interventional cardiology.

### Clopidogrel Metabolism

Although the clinical efficacy of clopidogrel has been demonstrated in patients presenting with ACS and in those undergoing PCI, its pharmacodynamic effect is variable.[18] This variability is associated with a variety of comorbidities, as well as genetic factors, that in large part influence the formation of clopidogrel active metabolite.[29] Clopidogrel, a thienopyridine, is an oral prodrug that first requires intestinal absorption. P-glycoprotein, an ATP-dependent efflux pump encoded by the ABCB1 gene that is expressed in intestinal epithelial cells, is thought to be involved in the absorption of clopidogrel prodrug. A substantial portion of prodrug is shunted into an inactive metabolite through hydrolysis by human carboxylesterase-1 in the liver. The remaining drug undergoes a two-step biotransformation into the active metabolite by the polymorphic cytochrome P450 enzymes (Fig. 1).[30,31] The thiophene ring of clopidogrel is first oxidized to 2-oxo-clopidogrel, which is then hydrolyzed to a highly labile active metabolite that forms a disulfide bond with the P2Y$_{12}$ receptor as platelets pass through the liver, irreversibly binding and antagonizing the receptor for the platelet's lifespan (7–10 days). In vitro experiments using enzyme kinetic analysis have demonstrated that the first reaction is catalyzed by CYP2C19, CYP1A2, and CYP2B6, with each enzyme contributing approximately 45%, 36%, and 19%, respectively. In the second step, CYP3A4, CYP2B6, CYP2C19, and CYP2C9 are involved with a relative contribution of 40%, 33%, 21%, and 7%, respectively.[32,33] An alternative pathway for the oxidative biotransformation of clopidogrel that does not involve CYP2C19 has been suggested.[34]

### CYP2C19 and Clopidogrel Effect

Several candidate gene studies based on the mechanism of clopidogrel effect have identified the genetic variants of CYP2C19, CYP2C9, CYP2B6, CYP3A4, ABCB1, and PON1 as playing a potential role in the antiplatelet effect of clopidogrel.[2,35] Whereas the data supporting a strong influence of CYP2C9, CYP3A4, ABCB1, and PON1 on clopidogrel effect have been mixed,[33,36–40] the evidence base for CYP2C19 is more robust, supported by pharmacokinetic, pharmacodynamics, and clinical outcomes studies.[35,36] The CYP2C19 LOF variant accounts for approximately 12% of the drug's variable antiplatelet effect.[41] Carriage of one or more CYP2C19 LOF allele is associated with reduced clopidogrel active metabolite levels, diminished platelet inhibition, and higher rates of adverse cardiovascular events after PCI.[12,35,41–43]

Single-center, observational studies have demonstrated that carriers of the CYP2C19*2 allele undergoing PCI[12,44,45] have a 2.4-fold to 3.6-fold higher risk of a major adverse cardiovascular event compared with noncarriers. The genetic substudy of the large, randomized, multicenter Assess Improvement in Therapeutic Outcomes by Optimizing Platelet Inhibition with Prasugrel-Thrombolysis in Myocardial Infarction (TRITON-TIMI) 38 trial demonstrated that, among ACS subjects treated with PCI, clopidogrel-treated carriers of the CYP2C19*2 allele displayed a significantly greater risk of cardiovascular death, MI, or stroke and a threefold increased risk of stent thrombosis.

Two meta-analyses of populations predominantly consisting of ACS patients undergoing PCI found significant associations between CYP2C19 genotype and poor clinical outcomes, particularly stent thrombosis. Carriage of at least one CYP2C19 risk allele was associated with increased cardiovascular risk.[46,47] There seemed to be a gradient of risk with increasing allele carriage. Mega and colleagues[47] observed that subjects with a single LOF allele have a 2.7-fold increased risk for stent thrombosis, which rises to a 4-times increased risk for those carrying both LOF alleles when compared with noncarriers.[44] The population significance of this is substantial, with approximately 25% to 40% of the population carrying a single LOF allele and approximately 2% to 5% carrying both LOF alleles.[47–49]

Holmes and colleagues[50] recently performed the largest meta-analysis to date using both treatment-only (ie, assessing the influence of CYP2C19 LOF allele carriage on outcomes among clopidogrel-treated subjects) and effect-modification analysis

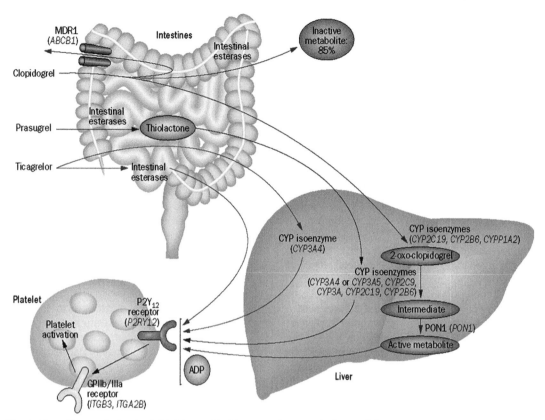

**Fig. 1.** The efficacy of platelet inhibition with thienopyridines might be modified by genetic variation in proteins involved in the absorption, metabolism, and response to these drugs. Bioavailability of the prodrug clopidogrel is determined by intestinal absorption, which might be limited by the efflux pump MDR1 (encoded by *ABCB1*). Subsequently, most of the prodrug is inactivated by ubiquitous esterases, but the remainder is activated in a two-step process by CYP isoenzymes in the liver. Genetic variation in the activity of *CYP2C19* is particularly important in determining clopidogrel response. Hydrolytic cleavage by the hepatic esterase PON1 yields the bioactive metabolite, which irreversibly binds to P2Y$_{12}$ receptors (encoded by *P2RY12*) on platelets, and subsequently prevents ADP-induced stimulation of the GPIIb/IIIa receptor (encoded by *ITGB3* and *ITGA2B*) and thus platelet activation. The prodrug prasugrel is hydrolyzed to a thiolactone derivative in the intestine and is then oxidized to its active metabolite by CYP isoenzymes in the liver, but seems to be unaffected by genetic variation in *CYP2C19*. Ticagrelor is a direct-acting, reversible, P2Y$_{12}$-receptor inhibitor, and seems to be unaffected by genetic variation in the CYP isoenzymes. Abbreviations: CYP, cytochrome P450; GP, glycoprotein; MDR1, multidrug resistance protein 1; PON1, serum paraoxonase/arylesterase 1. (*From* Ahmad T, Voora D, Becker RC. The pharmacogenetics of antiplatelet agents: toward personalized therapy? Nat Rev Cardiol 2011;8(10):560–71; with permission.)

(ie, assessing the influence of allele carriage on the treatment effect of clopidogrel vs placebo). According to treatment-only analysis of 26 studies involving 26,251 individuals, *CYP2C19* LOF allele carriage was associated with lower levels of active metabolite, less platelet inhibition, lower bleeding risk, and greater risks of MI (hazard ratio [HR] 1.37; 95% CI: 1.13–1.65) and stent thrombosis (HR 1.75; 95% CI: 1.50–2.03). However, in larger studies, there was a trend toward the null for the risk of the composite cardiovascular outcome, including target vessel revascularization (which has never proven to be influenced by clopidogrel). According to effect-modification analysis of four placebo-controlled randomized

trials, *CYP2C19* genotype did not influence clopidogrel efficacy relative to placebo. With the exception of a small fraction of the subjects in CURE (Clopidogrel in Unstable Angina to Prevent Recurrent Events) trial, these randomized trials did not include PCI subjects, in whom the treatment effect of clopidogrel and the influence of *CYP2C19* genotype on outcomes seem to be strongest (see previous discussion).[47] Synthesizing the data, it seems that the primary role for genotyping patients treated with clopidogrel is in those undergoing PCI, but not in clinical scenarios in which the absolute benefit of clopidogrel is marginal (eg, atrial fibrillation[51] or primary and secondary prevention[52]).[53]

## Clopidogrel dosing, platelet function, and CYP2C19 genotype

In 2010, the Federal Drug Administration (FDA) included a black box warning on all clopidogrel labeling with the recommendation that physicians should be aware of the genetic variants that may influence the drug's metabolism and a suggestion that alternative treatment approaches or strategies may be necessary.[54] **Box 1** shows the current American College of Cardiology Foundation/American Heart Association (ACCF/AHA) guidelines for PCI. On-treatment platelet reactivity (OTR) while receiving clopidogrel has been associated with clinical outcomes after PCI in several observational studies and a post hoc study of a randomized clinical trial.[26–28,55] Several studies have evaluated the relationship between CYP2C19 genotype and the antiplatelet effect of higher clopidogrel dosing regimens.

The Genotype Information and Functional Testing (GIFT) study explored the influence of a panel of genetic polymorphisms related to platelet reactivity in more than 1000 subjects undergoing PCI who were randomly assigned to clopidogrel either 75 mg or 150 mg daily maintenance dose (MD) as part of the Gauging Responsiveness with a VerifyNow P2Y12 assay: Impact on Thrombosis and Safety (GRAVITAS) trial.[36,56] Carriage of the CYP2C19*2 allele was significantly associated with high OTR at 12 to 24 hours ($P = 2.2 \times 10^{-15}$), 30 days ($P = 1.3 \times 10^{-7}$), and 6 months ($P = 1.9 \times 10^{-11}$) after PCI, thereby providing definitive evidence supporting a pharmacodynamic basis for the reported association between CYP2C19 and cardiovascular outcomes. Carriers of one or two reduced-function CYP2C19 alleles were significantly more likely to display persistently high OTR at 30 days and 6 months than noncarriers were, irrespective of treatment assignment. A clopidogrel 150 mg MD had only a marginal pharmacodynamic effect in carriers of two CYP2C19 LOF alleles.

The Escalating Clopidogrel by Involving a Genetic Strategy—Thrombolysis in Myocardial Infarction (ELEVATE-TIMI)-56 trial was a dose-ranging, randomized, pharmacodynamic study that evaluated the antiplatelet effect of increasing daily dose of clopidogrel in carriers of the CYP2C19*2 LOF allele.[48] In carriers of one CYP2C19*2 allele, a tripling the MD of clopidogrel to 225 mg daily achieved the same level of platelet inhibition as the standard 75 mg MD in subjects who were noncarriers. However, among carriers of two CYP2C19*2 alleles, a clopidogrel 300 mg MD failed to demonstrated comparable platelet inhibition as clopidogrel 75 mg MD did in noncarriers. Therefore, the use of higher doses of clopidogrel in poor metabolizers is a suboptimal strategy to improve platelet reactivity. In addition, the marginal effect of clopidogrel 150 mg MD may in part explain the negative results of randomized clinical trials of high-dose clopidogrel in patients with high OTR to standard dosing.[56,57] Pharmacodynamic studies have demonstrated that prasugrel is more effective compared with high-dose clopidogrel in reducing platelet reactivity, particularly in CYP2C19*2 carriers.[58]

## AHA/ACCF/Society for Cardiovascular Angiography and Interventions Guidelines

The 2011 AHA/ACCF/SCAI (Society for Cardiovascular Angiography and Interventions) guidelines for PCI recommend that genetic testing might be considered to identify whether a patient at high risk for poor clinical outcomes is predisposed to inadequate platelet inhibition with clopidogrel (Class IIB, level of evidence C), and that alternative P2Y12 inhibitors (eg, prasugrel or ticagrelor) might be considered when a patient at risk is identified by genetic testing (Class IIB, level of Evidence C).[59]

## GENETIC DETERMINANTS OF PRASUGREL EFFICACY

Prasugrel, a next-generation thienopyridine has more rapid and greater platelet inhibition compared with clopidogrel[60] and is superior to clopidogrel in reducing recurrent cardiovascular events in ACS patients undergoing PCI.[20] Prasugrel undergoes a more efficient generation of the active metabolite by the CYP450 system[61] (see **Fig. 1**) and small pharmacodynamic studies showed no influence of polymorphisms of CYP450 isoenzymes on prasugrel's

---

**Box 1**
**Warning for clopidogrel**

1. The effectiveness of clopidogrel depends on activation to an active metabolite by the cytochrome P450 (CYP) system, principally CYP2C19.

2. Poor metabolizers treated with clopidogrel at recommended doses exhibit higher cardiovascular event rates following ACS or PCI than patients with normal CYP2C19 function.

3. Tests are available to identify a patient's CYP2C19 genotype and can be used as an aid in determining therapeutic strategy.

4. Consider alternative treatment or treatment strategies in patients identified as CYP2C19 poor metabolizers.

active metabolite formation or its antiplatelet effect.[42,62] The genetic substudy of the TRITON TIMI-38 trial demonstrated that subjects randomly assigned to prasugrel had similar pharmacodynamic outcomes and similar rates of cardiovascular death, MI, and stroke at 15 months in all groups irrespective of CYP2C19 or ABCB1 genotype, unlike that observed with clopidogrel.[40,43,63] However, a small observational, single-center study detected significantly greater rates of high OTR in CYP2C19*2 carriers treated with prasugrel 10 mg daily MD compared to noncarriers as measured by vasodilator-stimulated phosphoprotein phosphorylation (VASP) analysis. This effect was not detected by ADP-induced light transmittance aggregometry, which may be a less specific test for P2Y12 receptor activity compared with VASP.

## GENETIC DETERMINANTS OF TICAGRELOR EFFICACY

Ticagrelor, a cyclopentyl-triazolo-pyrimidine, is a direct-acting agent that is metabolized by the CYP3A4/5 isoenzyme but does not require biotransformation to exert an antiplatelet effect.[64] Its onset of action is rapid and it provides a greater magnitude of platelet inhibition compared with clopidogrel.[65] CYP2C19 and ABCB1 polymorphisms do not influence the antiplatelet effect of the drug in pharmacodynamic studies.[37] The Platelet Inhibition and Patient Outcomes (PLATO) trial compared the safety and efficacy of ticagrelor with clopidogrel in ACS subjects treated with both conservative and early invasive strategies and demonstrated a significant reduction in the primary endpoint of cardiovascular death, MI, and stroke (HR, 0.84; 95% CI, 0.77 to 0.92; $P<.001$) with ticagrelor.[25] A genetic substudy demonstrated that there was no significant interaction between the treatment effect of ticagrelor and CYP2C19 genotype.[39] However, within the clopidogrel group there was a significantly higher rate of ischemic outcomes during the first 30 days in subjects with any LOF allele compared with clopidogrel-treated subjects with no LOF allele; the absolute risk reduction with ticagrelor in noncarriers was approximately half that of carriers. Of note, only 64% of subjects randomized underwent PCI, thus likely underestimating the effect of CYP2C19 in that cohort.[39]

## FUTURE DIRECTIONS

Several hurdles challenge the broad adoption of genomics into routine interventional cardiology practice. Although the weight of the data supports a strong association between CYP2C19 LOF allele

carriage and poor outcomes in PCI patients treated with clopidogrel, large randomized clinical trials of genotype-guided care are lacking and are likely never to be performed. The low absolute event rates among elective PCI patients with second-generation drug-eluting stents, even in patients with high OTR, may result in little absolute benefit and increased harm for intensive antiplatelet therapy in CYP2C19 LOF allele carriers undergoing PCI for stable coronary artery disease.[56,66] A strategy of selective intensification of $P2Y_{12}$ inhibition only in patients identified to be at high risk for cardiovascular events while receiving clopidogrel therapy (eg, those with ACS undergoing PCI) could maximize ischemic risk reduction while minimizing bleeding risk. Currently, sequencing is performed primarily by central laboratories, resulting in a lag period of several days to get actionable clinical data to the physician. The application of genotyping in ACS and other areas of interventional cardiology will require the development and adoption of inexpensive, point-of-care genotyping platforms that do not require batching[67] because clinical decisions are made within minutes to hours of patient presentation.

The panel of variants used today to determine platelet response and clinical efficacy include candidate gene discovery techniques and GWASs, which are limited in their exploratory power. Future variants that influence the safety and efficacy of interventional pharmaceuticals and devices could be discovered by means of higher resolution analyses such as whole exome and whole genome sequencing, which can identify rare variants of much greater functional significance not previously identified. Even with complete disclosure of the entire nucleotide sequence of the genome, the functional impact of genomics is still likely to be underrealized as further elucidation of gene-gene interactions, epigenomic factors, and other findings are factored into the algorithms used to determine risk.

Genomics may also influence the size and design of future trials in interventional cardiology. Smaller, shorter, and less costly genomically guided trials have been successful in other disease states. A phase 3 trial of ivacaftor, a drug used to treat a genetically distinct subset of cystic fibrosis patients, was completed in 48 weeks and with only 167 subjects.[68] Such strategies could provide more targeted therapies with greater clinical efficacy, less potential for adverse events, and substantially reduced costs. For example, costly ventures such as Merck's recent decision no longer to pursue approval of the combination therapy niacin/laropiprant in the United States based on of its lack of clinical efficacy and the increase in adverse events could be far less likely.[69]

## SUMMARY

Although randomized controlled trials of genotype-guided therapy in interventional cardiology are lacking, there is a strong body of evidence that supports the prognostic value for pharmacodynamic and clinical outcomes with clopidogrel. The current knowledge of genetic determinants of the safety and efficacy of interventional therapies is limited by candidate gene approaches, which are dependent on prior knowledge of mechanisms of action. *CYP2C19* LOF alleles and clinical characteristics only explain a fraction of clopidogrel response variability, despite its strong heritability. With the development of exploratory pharmacogenomics through cheaper, high throughput techniques, such as whole exome and whole genome sequencing, combined with the evolution of rapid bedside genotyping, the prospective determination of the complete panel of genomic and other variants will allow more optimal strategies to be selected at an individual level. Only with the complete accounting of all factors involved will the potential of enhanced patient outcomes predicted by precision medicine be fully realized.

## REFERENCES

1. Go AS, Mozaffarian D, Roger VL, et al. Executive summary: heart disease and stroke statistics–2013 update: a report from the American Heart Association. Circulation 2013;127(1):143–52.
2. Topol EJ, Schork NJ. Catapulting clopidogrel pharmacogenomics forward. Nat Med 2011;17(1):40–1.
3. O'Gara PT, Kushner FG, Ascheim DD, et al. 2013 ACCF/AHA Guideline for the management of ST-elevation myocardial infarction: a report of the American College of Cardiology Foundation/American Heart Association Task Force on Practice Guidelines. Circulation 2013;127(4):e362–425.
4. Voora D, Ginsburg GS. Clinical application of cardiovascular pharmacogenetics. J Am Coll Cardiol 2012;60(1):9–20.
5. Harper AR, Topol EJ. Pharmacogenomics in clinical practice and drug development. Nat Biotechnol 2012;30(11):1117–24.
6. Herper M. The truly staggering cost of inventing new drugs. 2012 [cited 2013 02/19/2013]. Available at: http://www.forbes.com/sites/matthewherper/2012/02/10/the-truly-staggering-cost-of-inventing-new-drugs/.
7. Boehringer-ingelheim. PRADAXA Highlights of prescribing information. 2012 [cited 2013 03/19/2013]. Available at: http://bidocs.boehringer-ingelheim.com/BIWebAccess/ViewServlet.ser?docBase=renetnt&folderPath=/PrescribingInformation/PIs/Pradaxa/Pradaxa.pdf. Accessed March 21, 2013.
8. Bristol-Myers-Squibb/Pfizer. ELIQUIS Highlights of prescribing information. 2012 [cited 2013 03/19/2013]; ELIQUIS package insert]. Available at: http://packageinserts.bms.com/pi/pi_eliquis.pdf. Accessed March 21, 2013.
9. Pharmaceuticals J. XARELTO Highlights of prescribing information. 2013 [cited 2013 03/19/2013]; XARELTO Package Insert]. Available at: http://www.janssenmedicalinformation.com/assets/pdf/products/files/Xarelto/pi/ENC-010330-11.pdf. Accessed March 21, 2013.
10. Pharmaceuticals, A.Z. BRILINTA Highlights of prescribing information. 2013 [cited 2013 03/19/2013]; Brilinta Package Insert]. Available at: http://www1.astrazeneca-us.com/pi/brilinta.pdf. Accessed March 21, 2013.
11. Hulot JS, Bura A, Villard E, et al. Cytochrome P450 2C19 loss-of-function polymorphism is a major determinant of clopidogrel responsiveness in healthy subjects. Blood 2006;108(7):2244–7.
12. Shuldiner AR, O'Connell JR, Bliden KP, et al. Association of cytochrome P450 2C19 genotype with the antiplatelet effect and clinical efficacy of clopidogrel therapy. JAMA 2009;302(8):849–57.
13. Ng SB, Turner EH, Robertson PD, et al. Targeted capture and massively parallel sequencing of 12 human exomes. Nature 2009;461(7261):272–6.
14. Choi M, Scholl UI, Ji W, et al. Genetic diagnosis by whole exome capture and massively parallel DNA sequencing. Proc Natl Acad Sci U S A 2009;106(45):19096–101.
15. Ng SB, Buckingham KJ, Lee C, et al. Exome sequencing identifies the cause of a mendelian disorder. Nat Genet 2010;42(1):30–5.
16. Biesecker LG. Exome sequencing makes medical genomics a reality. Nat Genet 2010;42(1):13–4.
17. Leon MB, Baim DS, Popma JJ, et al. A clinical trial comparing three antithrombotic-drug regimens after coronary-artery stenting. Stent Anticoagulation Restenosis Study Investigators. N Engl J Med 1998;339(23):1665–71.
18. Yusuf S, Zhao F, Mehta SR, et al. Effects of clopidogrel in addition to aspirin in patients with acute coronary syndromes without ST-segment elevation. N Engl J Med 2001;345(7):494–502.
19. Mehta SR, Yusuf S, Peters RJ, et al. Effects of pretreatment with clopidogrel and aspirin followed by long-term therapy in patients undergoing percutaneous coronary intervention: the PCI-CURE study. Lancet 2001;358(9281):527–33.
20. Wiviott SD, Braunwald E, McCabe CH, et al. Prasugrel versus clopidogrel in patients with acute coronary syndromes. N Engl J Med 2007;357(20):2001–15.
21. Cannon CP, Harrington RA, James S, et al. Comparison of ticagrelor with clopidogrel in patients with a planned invasive strategy for acute coronary

syndromes (PLATO): a randomised double-blind study. Lancet 2010;375(9711):283–93.

22. De Luca G, Suryapranata H, Stone GW, et al. Abciximab as adjunctive therapy to reperfusion in acute ST-segment elevation myocardial infarction: a meta-analysis of randomized trials. JAMA 2005; 293(14):1759–65.

23. Gurbel PA, Bliden KP, Hayes KM, et al. Platelet activation in myocardial ischemic syndromes. Expert Rev Cardiovasc Ther 2004;2(4):535–45.

24. Becker RC, Gurbel PA. Platelet P2Y12 receptor antagonist pharmacokinetics and pharmacodynamics: a foundation for distinguishing mechanisms of bleeding and anticipated risk for platelet-directed therapies. Thromb Haemost 2010;103(3):535–44.

25. Wallentin L, Becker RC, Budaj A, et al. Ticagrelor versus clopidogrel in patients with acute coronary syndromes. N Engl J Med 2009;361(11):1045–57.

26. Bonello L, Tantry US, Marcucci R, et al. Consensus and future directions on the definition of high on-treatment platelet reactivity to adenosine diphosphate. J Am Coll Cardiol 2010;56(12):919–33.

27. Price MJ, Angiolillo DJ, Teirstein PS, et al. Platelet reactivity and cardiovascular outcomes after percutaneous coronary intervention: a time-dependent analysis of the Gauging Responsiveness with a VerifyNow P2Y12 assay: Impact on Thrombosis and Safety (GRAVITAS) trial. Circulation 2011;124:1132–7.

28. Brar SS, ten Berg J, Marcucci R, et al. Impact of platelet reactivity on clinical outcomes after percutaneous coronary intervention: a collaborative meta-analysis of individual participant data. J Am Coll Cardiol 2011;58(19):1945–54.

29. Musunuru K, Roden DM, Boineau R, et al. Cardiovascular pharmacogenomics: current status and future directions-report of a national heart, lung, and blood institute working group. J Am Heart Assoc 2012;1(2):e000554.

30. Verschuren JJ, Trompet S, Wessels JA, et al. A systematic review on pharmacogenetics in cardiovascular disease: is it ready for clinical application? Eur Heart J 2012;33(2):165–75.

31. Ahmad T, Voora D, Becker RC. The pharmacogenetics of antiplatelet agents: towards personalized therapy? Nat Rev Cardiol 2011;8(10):560–71.

32. Kazui M, Nishiya Y, Ishizuka T, et al. Identification of the human cytochrome P450 enzymes involved in the two oxidative steps in the bioactivation of clopidogrel to its pharmacologically active metabolite. Drug Metab Dispos 2010;38(1):92–9.

33. Price MJ. Genetic considerations. Adv Cardiol 2012;47:100–13.

34. Bouman HJ, Schomig E, van Werkum JW, et al. Paraoxonase-1 is a major determinant of clopidogrel efficacy. Nat Med 2011;17(1):110–6.

35. Price MJ, Tantry US, Gurbel PA. The influence of CYP2C19 polymorphisms on the pharmacokinetics, pharmacodynamics, and clinical effectiveness of P2Y(12) inhibitors. Rev Cardiovasc Med 2011;12(1):1–12.

36. Price MJ, Murray SS, Angiolillo DJ, et al. Influence of genetic polymorphisms on the effect of high- and standard-dose clopidogrel after percutaneous coronary intervention: the GIFT (Genotype Information and Functional Testing) study. J Am Coll Cardiol 2012;59(22):1928–37.

37. Tantry US, Bliden KP, Wei C, et al. First analysis of the relation between CYP2C19 genotype and pharmacodynamics in patients treated with ticagrelor versus clopidogrel: the ONSET/OFFSET and RESPOND genotype studies. Circ Cardiovasc Genet 2010;3(6):556–66.

38. Sibbing D, Koch W, Massberg S, et al. No association of paraoxonase-1 Q192R genotypes with platelet response to clopidogrel and risk of stent thrombosis after coronary stenting. Eur Heart J 2011;32(13):1605–13.

39. Wallentin L, James S, Storey RF, et al. Effect of CYP2C19 and ABCB1 single nucleotide polymorphisms on outcomes of treatment with ticagrelor versus clopidogrel for acute coronary syndromes: a genetic substudy of the PLATO trial. Lancet 2010;376(9749):1320–8.

40. Mega JL, Close SL, Wiviott SD, et al. Genetic variants in ABCB1 and CYP2C19 and cardiovascular outcomes after treatment with clopidogrel and prasugrel in the TRITON-TIMI 38 trial: a pharmacogenetic analysis. Lancet 2010;376(9749):1312–9.

41. Steinhubl SR. Genotyping, clopidogrel metabolism, and the search for the therapeutic window of thienopyridines. Circulation 2010;121(4):481–3.

42. Brandt JT, Close SL, Iturria SJ, et al. Common polymorphisms of CYP2C19 and CYP2C9 affect the pharmacokinetic and pharmacodynamic response to clopidogrel but not prasugrel. J Thromb Haemost 2007;5(12):2428–36.

43. Mega JL, Close SL, Wiviott SD, et al. Cytochrome p-450 polymorphisms and response to clopidogrel. N Engl J Med 2009;360(4):354–62.

44. Gurbel PA, Tantry US. Do platelet function testing and genotyping improve outcome in patients treated with antithrombotic agents?: platelet function testing and genotyping improve outcome in patients treated with antithrombotic agents. Circulation 2012;125(10):1276–87 [discussion: 1287].

45. Simon T, Verstuyft C, Mary-Krause M, et al. Genetic determinants of response to clopidogrel and cardiovascular events. N Engl J Med 2009;360(4):363–75.

46. Hulot JS, Collet JP, Silvain J, et al. Cardiovascular risk in clopidogrel-treated patients according to cytochrome P450 2C19*2 loss-of-function allele or

proton pump inhibitor coadministration: a systematic meta-analysis. J Am Coll Cardiol 2010;56(2):134–43.

47. Mega JL, Simon T, Collet JP, et al. Reduced-function CYP2C19 genotype and risk of adverse clinical outcomes among patients treated with clopidogrel predominantly for PCI: a meta-analysis. JAMA 2010;304(16):1821–30.

48. Mega JL, Hochholzer W, Frelinger AL 3rd, et al. Dosing clopidogrel based on CYP2C19 genotype and the effect on platelet reactivity in patients with stable cardiovascular disease. JAMA 2011;306(20):2221–8.

49. Scott SA, Sangkuhl K, Gardner EE, et al. Clinical Pharmacogenetics Implementation Consortium guidelines for cytochrome P450-2C19 (CYP2C19) genotype and clopidogrel therapy. Clin Pharmacol Ther 2011;90(2):328–32.

50. Holmes MV, Perel P, Shah T, et al. CYP2C19 genotype, clopidogrel metabolism, platelet function, and cardiovascular events: a systematic review and meta-analysis. JAMA 2011;306(24):2704–14.

51. Connolly SJ, Pogue J, Hart RG, et al. Effect of clopidogrel added to aspirin in patients with atrial fibrillation. N Engl J Med 2009;360(20):2066–78.

52. Bhatt DL, Fox KA, Hacke W, et al. Clopidogrel and aspirin versus aspirin alone for the prevention of atherothrombotic events. N Engl J Med 2006;354(16):1706–17.

53. Pare G, Mehta SR, Yusuf S, et al. Effects of CYP2C19 genotype on outcomes of clopidogrel treatment. N Engl J Med 2010;363(18):1704–14.

54. Holmes DR Jr, Dehmer GJ, Kaul S, et al. ACCF/AHA clopidogrel clinical alert: approaches to the FDA "boxed warning": a report of the American College of Cardiology Foundation Task Force on clinical expert consensus documents and the American Heart Association endorsed by the Society for Cardiovascular Angiography and Interventions and the Society of Thoracic Surgeons. J Am Coll Cardiol 2010;56(4):321–41.

55. Stone G. ADAPT-DES: a Large-Scale, Multicenter, Prospective, Observational Study of the Impact of Clopidogrel Hyporesponsiveness on Patient Outcomes—One Year Results. 2012 [cited 2013 02/21/2013]. Available at: http://www.clinicaltrialresults.org/Files/Homepages for disease states/clopidogrel.htm. Accessed March 26, 2013.

56. Price MJ, Berger PB, Teirstein PS, et al. Standard-vs high-dose clopidogrel based on platelet function testing after percutaneous coronary intervention: the GRAVITAS randomized trial. JAMA 2011;305(11):1097–105.

57. Collet JP, Cuisset T, Range G, et al. Bedside monitoring to adjust antiplatelet therapy for coronary stenting. N Engl J Med 2012;367(22):2100–9.

58. Alexopoulos D, Dimitropoulos G, Davlouros P, et al. Prasugrel overcomes high on-clopidogrel platelet reactivity post-stenting more effectively than high-dose (150-mg) clopidogrel: the importance of CYP2C19*2 genotyping. JACC Cardiovasc Interv 2011;4(4):403–10.

59. Levine GN, Bates ER, Blankenship JC, et al. 2011 ACCF/AHA/SCAI Guideline for Percutaneous Coronary Intervention: a Report of the American College of Cardiology Foundation/American Heart Association Task Force on Practice Guidelines and the Society for Cardiovascular Angiography and Interventions. Circulation 2011;124(23):e574–651.

60. Jernberg T, Payne CD, Winters KJ, et al. Prasugrel achieves greater inhibition of platelet aggregation and a lower rate of non-responders compared with clopidogrel in aspirin-treated patients with stable coronary artery disease. Eur Heart J 2006;27(10):1166–73.

61. Sugidachi A, Ogawa T, Kurihara A, et al. The greater in vivo antiplatelet effects of prasugrel as compared to clopidogrel reflect more efficient generation of its active metabolite with similar antiplatelet activity to that of clopidogrel's active metabolite. J Thromb Haemost 2007;5(7):1545–51.

62. Varenhorst C, James S, Erlinge D, et al. Genetic variation of CYP2C19 affects both pharmacokinetic and pharmacodynamic responses to clopidogrel but not prasugrel in aspirin-treated patients with coronary artery disease. Eur Heart J 2009;30(14):1744–52.

63. Mega JL, Close SL, Wiviott SD, et al. Cytochrome P450 genetic polymorphisms and the response to prasugrel: relationship to pharmacokinetic, pharmacodynamic, and clinical outcomes. Circulation 2009;119(19):2553–60.

64. Teng R, Oliver S, Hayes MA, et al. Absorption, distribution, metabolism, and excretion of ticagrelor in healthy subjects. Drug Metab Dispos 2010;38(9):1514–21.

65. Gurbel PA, Bliden KP, Butler K, et al. Randomized double-blind assessment of the ONSET and OFFSET of the antiplatelet effects of ticagrelor versus clopidogrel in patients with stable coronary artery disease: the ONSET/OFFSET study. Circulation 2009;120(25):2577–85.

66. Trenk D, Stone GW, Gawaz M, et al. A randomized trial of prasugrel versus clopidogrel in patients with high platelet reactivity on clopidogrel after elective percutaneous coronary intervention with implantation of drug-eluting stents: results of the TRIGGER-PCI (Testing Platelet Reactivity In Patients

Undergoing Elective Stent Placement on Clopidogrel to Guide Alternative Therapy With Prasugrel) study. J Am Coll Cardiol 2012;59(24):2159–64.

67. Roberts JD, Wells GA, Le May MR, et al. Point-of-care genetic testing for personalisation of antiplatelet treatment (RAPID GENE): a prospective, randomised, proof-of-concept trial. Lancet 2012;379(9827):1705–11.

68. Ramsey BW, Davies J, McElvaney NG, et al. A CFTR potentiator in patients with cystic fibrosis and the G551D mutation. N Engl J Med 2011; 365(18):1663–72.

69. Nainggolan L. Niacin/laropiprant products to be withdrawn in EU next week. 2013 [cited 2013 02/21/2013]. Available at: http://www.theheart.org/article/1497081.do. Accessed March 26, 2013.

# Antithrombotic Strategies in Endovascular Interventions
## Current Status and Future Directions

Mehdi H. Shishehbor, DO, MPH, PhD[a],*, Barry T. Katzen, MD[b]

KEYWORDS

- Antithrombotic therapy • Endovascular intervention • Peripheral artery disease • Antiplatelet agents
- EUCLID trial

KEY POINTS

- Antithrombotic therapy is an important part of endovascular intervention.
- Despite many studies, the role of antithrombotic and antiplatelet therapy remains undefined.
- Newer agents such as prasugrel and ticagrelor may provide additional benefit in patients undergoing endovascular intervention but need to be tested in randomized clinical trials.
- The Examining Use of tiCagreLor In paD (EUCLID) trial will provide important data regarding efficacy and safety of ticagrelor for treating peripheral artery disease.

## INTRODUCTION

Peripheral vascular disease (PVD) affects the cerebral circulation and extracranial vessels, the aorta, great vessels, mesenteric and renal arteries, and the lower extremity arteries. It has significant morbidity and mortality beyond the known risk factors such as diabetes mellitus, hypertension, and hyperlipidemia. However, despite its clinical significance and prevalence, little level 1 evidence is available regarding the role of antithrombotic therapy in patients undergoing endovascular intervention. The current practice in this regard is heterogeneous and has mainly been driven by data from coronary artery disease and percutaneous coronary intervention (PCI). This article discusses the role of antithrombotic agents for endovascular intervention.

## PATHOPHYSIOLOGY

Arterial thrombosis is the underpinning of most morbidity and mortality associated with cardiovascular, cerebrovascular, and peripheral artery disease (PAD). In addition to inflammation and atherosclerosis it seems that hemostatic factors may also play significant role in the pathogenesis of PVD. Both plasma fibrinogen and cross-linked fibrin degradation products have been shown to be increased in patients with claudication.[1–4] Furthermore, individuals with PVD have increased levels of thrombin-antithrombin III complex, D-dimer, von Willebrand factor, tissue plasminogen activator antigen, plasminogen activator inhibitor-1 levels, C-reactive protein, and prothrombin fragments 1 and 2.[1–4] These hemostatic factors have collectively been shown to be associated with increased clinical events or higher incidence of restenosis.

Endovascular intervention can activate platelets and the hemostatic system resulting in restenosis. Thrombin has been linked to restenosis by activation of thrombin receptors on the smooth muscle cells, macrophages, fibroblasts, and endothelial cells.[5–9] A recent study compared thrombelastometry-derived value coagulation time (CT) among patients with severe in-stent

Disclosures: The authors have nothing to disclose.
[a] Endovascular Services, Heart & Vascular Institute, Cleveland Clinic, 9500 Euclid Avenue, J3-05, Cleveland, OH 44195, USA; [b] Baptist Cardiac & Vascular Institute, 8900 North Kendall Drive, Miami, FL 33176, USA
* Corresponding author.
E-mail address: shishem@ccf.org

interventional.theclinics.com

restenosis and those without. The thrombelas-tometry-derived CT was significantly shorter in the severe in-stent restenosis group compared with that of patients without restenosis.[10] Furthermore, high levels of plasma heparin factor II, an inhibitor of thrombin, has been associated with reduced incidence of in-stent restenosis.[11]

Platelets are also important mediators of atherosclerosis and thrombosis.[12] In the setting of endovascular intervention vascular injury occurs, resulting in activation of platelets by exposure to collagen and von Willebrand factor.[13] Through activation of integrin receptors an array of inflammatory and prothrombotic mediators such as ADP, thromboxane $A_2$ ($TxA_2$), and thrombin are released.[13] These mediators then result in further platelet activation.[14] Rapid recruitment and activation of platelets leads to further thrombus formation.

## ASPIRIN

Aspirin is the most widely studied thromboxane inhibitor. It acts indirectly through irreversible inhibition of prostaglandin H-synthase, and inhibits the actions of thromboxane.[15] It is a cyclooxygenase-1 selective inhibitor, resulting in impaired synthesis of $TxA_2$. The role of aspirin in cardiovascular disease has been well established; however, controversy exists as to whether aspirin could have a net clinical benefit in patients with PVD. A recent meta-analysis of 18 trials with 5269 patients with PAD revealed a reduction in cardiovascular events (adjusted hazard ratio, 0.88; 95% confidence interval [CI], 0.76–1.04); however, this was not statistically significant.[16] No significant reduction in all-cause or cardiovascular mortality was identified.[16] The current American College of Cardiology (ACC)/American Heart Association (AHA) guidelines give a class I indication for the use of aspirin in patients with PAD.[17] Limited data are available on the impact of aspirin after endovascular intervention; however, the combination of aspirin and dipyridamole have been shown to reduce recurrent obstruction after endovascular angioplasty for up to 12 months.[18–20] High-dose aspirin had no advantage compared with low-dose therapy in these trials and was associated with significant gastrointestinal symptoms.[18–20]

Although the current guidelines and many experts continue to support the use of aspirin for prevention of cardiovascular endpoints in patients with PAD, few studies have shown benefit with low-dose aspirin for prevention of limb associated adverse events. As noted earlier, the combination of aspirin and dipyridamole failed to show a significant reduction in reocclusion after lower extremity

angioplasty.[18–20] Early epidemiologic studies such as the Physicians' Health Study revealed a significant reduction in the rate of lower extremity revascularization with the use of low-dose aspirin in men.[21] However, in the current era of stents and other advanced therapies, there is no level 1 evidence that chronic aspirin therapy results in better patency, lower rate of in-stent restenosis, or better limb-associated outcomes.

## TICLOPIDINE

A first generation ADP receptor antagonist, ticlopidine is no longer available in the United States. This ADP receptor antagonist inhibits the $P2Y_{12}$ subtype. The two main drugs in this class are ticlopidine and clopidogrel. Early data in patients undergoing PCI showed encouraging results with ticlopidine; however, the Clopidogrel Aspirin Stent International Cooperative (CLASSIC) trial compared ticlopidine with clopidogrel and showed better safety and efficacy profiles with clopidogrel.[22]

There are no randomized data with ticlopidine in patients undergoing endovascular intervention. However, ticlopidine has been shown to be superior to aspirin for maintaining vein graft patency.[23] However, the combination of aspirin plus ticlopidine was not superior to aspirin alone in maintaining graft patency in the Clopidogrel and Acetylsalicylic Acid in Bypass Surgery for Peripheral Arterial Disease (CASPAR) trial.[24]

## CLOPIDOGREL

An ADP receptor antagonist, clopidogrel has the most clinical data for prevention of thrombosis after aspirin. There is a significant body of evidence supporting the use of clopidogrel in patients undergoing PCI and in those presenting with acute coronary syndrome.[25–28] However, the data for the use of clopidogrel in patients with PAD to prevent cardiovascular endpoints remain controversial. The first signal showing potential benefit with clopidogrel in patients with PAD was derived from the Clopidogrel versus Aspirin in Patients at Risk of Ischemic Events (CAPRIE) study (**Fig. 1**).[29,30] In this study, an 8.7% relative risk reduction was seen with clopidogrel compared with aspirin alone and the benefit was mostly seen in those with symptomatic PAD (**Fig. 2**). However, the Clopidogrel and Aspirin in the Management of Peripheral Endovascular Revascularization (CAMPER) trial was withdrawn because of lack of enrollment. Another trial that evaluated the role of clopidogrel for primary and secondary prevention was Clopidogrel for High Atherothrombotic Risk and Ischemic Stabilization Management

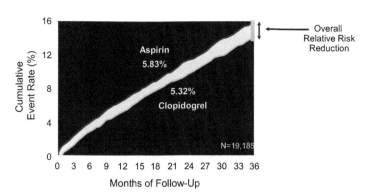

**Fig. 1.** Efficacy of clopidogrel versus aspirin in reducing myocardial infarction, ischemic stroke, or vascular death in the CAPRIE trial. (*Adapted from* CAPRIE Steering Committee. A randomised blinded, trial of clopidogrel versus aspirin in patients at risk of ischaemic events (CAPRIE). Lancet 1996;348:1333; with permission.)

and Avoidance (CHARISMA).[31] A total of 15,063 patients were randomized to clopidogrel plus aspirin versus aspirin alone. In the overall population, dual antiplatelet therapy was not superior to aspirin alone for preventing cardiovascular death, stroke, and myocardial infarction (**Fig. 3**).[31] However, in a subgroup analysis, in those with established cardiovascular disease, dual antiplatelet therapy resulted in 12.5% significant relative risk reduction. Dual antiplatelet therapy was associated with a higher risk of bleeding compared with aspirin alone (**Table 1**). Despite the overwhelming data in support of dual antiplatelet therapy for acute coronary syndrome and PCI, currently there are few data to support its use for endovascular intervention. The current ACC/AHA guidelines recommend clopidogrel as monotherapy for those individuals who cannot tolerate aspirin; however, dual antiplatelet therapy is not recommended.[17]

Despite these recommendations there is a variable treatment approach for patients undergoing endovascular intervention. Recent survey revealed variable treatment duration and a mixture of approaches.[32] Most operators treat with dual antiplatelet therapy after most endovascular interventions; however, the duration of dual antiplatelet therapy remains undefined.[32]

## OTHER ADP RECEPTOR ANTAGONISTS

Because of issues related to clopidogrel resistance, onset of action, and degree of platelet inhibition, new antiplatelet therapies have recently been developed.[12] Of these, prasugrel and ticagrelor have received US Food and Drug Administration approved for coronary indications. Prasugrel is a prodrug whose active metabolite irreversibly binds to $P2Y_{12}$ receptor. Ticagrelor is a cyclopentyl triazolopyrimidine that directly and reversibly inhibits the $P2Y_{12}$ receptor. However, few data are available for their use in patients with PAD or in patients undergoing endovascular intervention. The Examining Use of tiCagreLor In paD (EUCLID) trial will examine the role of ticagrelor versus clopidogrel monotherapy for patients with PAD. This trial allows enrollment of patients 30 days post endovascular or surgical revascularization; therefore, data from this trial should help guide antiplatelet therapy for patients with PAD with or without revascularization.

## DIPYRIDAMOLE

Dipyridamole is an inhibitor of the cyclic AMP (cAMP) phosphodiesterase and cyclic GMP phosphodiesterase type V enzyme. It is also a potent inhibitor of adenosine deaminase, resulting in increased concentrations of adenosine. In a recent Cochrane meta-analysis of 6 randomized trials with a total of 356 patients, aspirin and dipyridamole combination failed to prevent reocclusion at 6 months (fixed-effect odds ratio [OR], 0.69; 95% CI, 0.44–1.10; $P = .12$).[33]

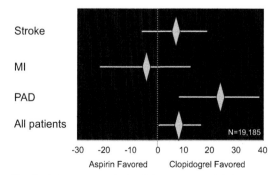

**Fig. 2.** Subgroup analysis of the CAPRIE trial showing a significant benefit in patients with PAD. (*Adapted from* CAPRIE Steering Committee. A randomised blinded, trial of clopidogrel versus aspirin in patients at risk of ischaemic events (CAPRIE). Lancet 1996;348:1333; with permission.)

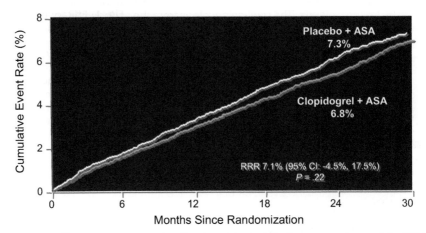

**Fig. 3.** No significant differences were noted in the CHARISMA trial when comparing aspirin (ASA) alone with aspirin plus clopidogrel. (*Data from* Bhatt DL, Fox KA, Hacke W, et al. Clopidogrel and aspirin versus aspirin alone for the prevention of atherothrombotic events. N Engl J Med 2006;354:1713.)

## LOW-MOLECULAR-WEIGHT HEPARINS

Peri-interventional treatment with low-molecular-weight heparin (LMWH) has been shown to be superior to unfractionated heparin in femoropopliteal obstructions.[34] However, long-term therapy (for 3 months) with dalteparin failed to reduce femoropopliteal occlusions after angioplasty.[35]

## GLYCOPROTEIN IIB/IIIA RECEPTOR ANTAGONIST

These agents prevent binding of fibrinogen to the platelet and hence prevent fibrinogen cross-linking. Their role in the setting of PCI has been well established. However, they have had a more limited role for endovascular intervention.

Three clinical trials compared the effects of abciximab versus placebo and 1 trial compared abciximab plus urokinase with urokinase alone.[36–39] The results from these trials were mixed. Duda and colleagues[39] showed no significant advantage

with abciximab at 24 hours and 3 months. However, another trial found better patency at 24 hours and 3 months.[38] Overall, there seemed to be higher rates of bleeding with abciximab. Because of limited efficacy, potential cost, and risk of bleeding, abciximab is rarely used as an adjunct to endovascular intervention.

## VITAMIN K ANTAGONIST

Vitamin K antagonist (VKA) has been compared with aspirin plus dipyridamole. A pooled comparison of 2 trials showed no benefit with VKA at 1, 3, 6, and 12 months.[40,41] Tan and colleagues[42] conducted another randomized trial comparing clopidogrel plus aspirin versus low-molecular-weight heparin (LMWH) and Coumadin. No statistically significant difference was noted between the two groups at 1, 6, and 12 months. As expected, patients treated with LMWH followed by warfarin had higher bleeding complications.[42] The combination of VKA and suloctidil also was not superior

**Table 1**
**Risk of bleeding among the two treatment arms in the CHARISMA trial**

| Safety Outcome[a] | Clopidogrel + ASA (n = 7802) | Placebo + ASA (n = 7801) | RR (95% CI) |
|---|---|---|---|
| GUSTO severe bleeding, N (%) | 130 (1.7) | 104 (1.3) | 1.25 (0.97, 1.61) |
| Fatal bleeding, N (%) | 26 (0.3) | 17 (0.2) | 1.53 (0.83, 2.82) |
| Primary ICH, N (%) | 26 (0.3) | 27 (0.3) | 0.96 (0.56, 1.65) |
| GUSTO moderate bleeding, N (%) | 164 (2.1) | 101 (1.3) | 1.62 (1.27, 2.08) |

*Abbreviations:* ASA, aspirin; ICH, intracranial hemorrhage; RR, relative risk.
   [a] Adjudicated outcomes by intention-to-treat analysis.
   *Data from* Bhatt DL, Fox KA, Hacke W, et al. Clopidogrel and aspirin versus aspirin alone for the prevention of atherothrombotic events. N Engl J Med 2006;354:1706–17.

to VKA alone.[43] VKA was compared with ticlopidine in 197 patients. VKA was not superior to ticlopidine in preventing primary occlusion; however, it was associated with more side effects.

## CILOSTAZOL

Cilostazol is a phosphodiesterase inhibitor with therapeutic focus on cAMP. It is a potent inhibitor of platelet aggregation and is a direct arterial vasodilator. There is strong evidence to support its use for prevention of restenosis in patients undergoing coronary stenting.[44–46] Iida and colleagues[47] conducted a randomized clinical trial of 127 patients with de novo femoropopliteal lesions, and cilostazol plus aspirin showed a high rate of patency at 12, 24, and 36 months compared with ticlopidine plus aspirin. In a retrospective analysis, cilostazol similarly showed better primary patency rates than ticlopidine.[48]

## BIVALIRUDIN

A direct thrombin-specific anticoagulant now used widely in the setting of PCI, bivalirudin has also been considered for endovascular interventions.[49] Because of its short half life, it has potential advantages compared with unfractionated heparin by offering decreased vascular complications (both access and non–access site related), earlier sheath removal, and potentially earlier ambulation. Furthermore, it eliminates the need for frequent activated coagulation time checks and offers a steady level of anticoagulation during the procedure. In a registry from 4 institutions no adverse events were reported, with 100% procedural success rate. Bivalirudin has also been evaluated in the setting of endovascular abdominal aneurysm repair (EVAR). Overall, bivalirudin was a safe and feasible alternative to unfractionated heparin in patients undergoing EVAR.[50] In retrospective studies bivalirudin has also been shown to be safe and effective compared with heparin alone in patients undergoing carotid artery stenting.[51] Several other registries have evaluated the role of bivalirudin in different endovascular settings. These reports have been presented at various national and international meetings but they have yet to be published in peer-reviewed journals. A large international randomized trial of bivalirudin versus heparin in percutaneous endovascular interventions is currently underway (Endovascular Interventions with Angiomax [ENDOMAX] trial).

## SUMMARY

Despite technical advances and higher prevalence of endovascular procedures, little progress has

been made with regard to antithrombotic therapy for these procedures. Although most investigator use some form of anticoagulation during the procedure and continue antiplatelet therapy afterwards, little evidence exist to support this approach. In the meantime, antiplatelet and anticoagulant therapies are evolving rapidly with new antiplatelet agents like ticagrelor and prasugrel and antithrombotic agents like rivaroxaban, Eliquis, and dabigatran. Future trials with these agents will invariably impact the field of endovascular interventions.

## REFERENCES

1. Lassila R, Peltonen S, Lepantalo M, et al. Severity of peripheral atherosclerosis is associated with fibrinogen and degradation of cross-linked fibrin. Arterioscler Thromb 1993;13(12):1738–42.
2. Lee AJ, Fowkes FG, Rattray A, et al. Haemostatic and rheological factors in intermittent claudication: the influence of smoking and extent of arterial disease. Br J Haematol 1996;92(1):226–30.
3. Lowe GD, Fowkes FG, Dawes J, et al. Blood viscosity, fibrinogen, and activation of coagulation and leukocytes in peripheral arterial disease and the normal population in the Edinburgh Artery Study. Circulation 1993;87(6):1915–20.
4. Smith FB, Lowe GD, Fowkes FG, et al. Smoking, haemostatic factors and lipid peroxides in a population case control study of peripheral arterial disease. Atherosclerosis 1993;102(2):155–62.
5. Aihara K, Azuma H, Akaike M, et al. Heparin cofactor II is an independent protective factor against peripheral arterial disease in elderly subjects with cardiovascular risk factors. J Atheroscler Thromb 2009;16(2):127–34.
6. Hasenstab D, Lea H, Hart CE, et al. Tissue factor overexpression in rat arterial neointima models thrombosis and progression of advanced atherosclerosis. Circulation 2000;101(22):2651–7.
7. Hering J, Amann B, Angelkort B, et al. Thrombin-antithrombin complex and the prothrombin fragment in arterial and venous blood of patients with peripheral arterial disease. Vasa 2003;32(4):193–7.
8. Patterson C, Stouffer GA, Madamanchi N, et al. New tricks for old dogs: nonthrombotic effects of thrombin in vessel wall biology. Circ Res 2001; 88(10):987–97.
9. Wilensky RL, Pyles JM, Fineberg N. Increased thrombin activity correlates with increased ischemic event rate after percutaneous transluminal coronary angioplasty: lack of efficacy of locally delivered urokinase. Am Heart J 1999;138(2 Pt 1):319–25.
10. Cvirn G, Hoerl G, Schlagenhauf A, et al. Stent implantation in the superficial femoral artery: short thrombelastometry-derived coagulation times

identify patients with late in-stent restenosis. Thromb Res 2012;130(3):485–90.

11. Takamori N, Azuma H, Kato M, et al. High plasma heparin cofactor II activity is associated with reduced incidence of in-stent restenosis after percutaneous coronary intervention. Circulation 2004;109(4):481–6.

12. Meadows TA, Bhatt DL. Clinical aspects of platelet inhibitors and thrombus formation. Circ Res 2007; 100(9):1261–75.

13. Ruggeri ZM. Platelets in atherothrombosis. Nat Med 2002;8(11):1227–34.

14. Offermanns S. Activation of platelet function through G protein-coupled receptors. Circ Res 2006;99(12):1293–304.

15. Weiss HJ, Aledort LM. Impaired platelet-connective-tissue reaction in man after aspirin ingestion. Lancet 1967;2(7514):495–7.

16. Berger JS, Krantz MJ, Kittelson JM, et al. Aspirin for the prevention of cardiovascular events in patients with peripheral artery disease: a meta-analysis of randomized trials. JAMA 2009; 301(18):1909–19.

17. Hirsch AT, Haskal ZJ, Hertzer NR, et al. ACC/AHA 2005 practice guidelines for the management of patients with peripheral arterial disease (lower extremity, renal, mesenteric, and abdominal aortic): a collaborative report from the American Association for Vascular Surgery/Society for Vascular Surgery, Society for Cardiovascular Angiography and Interventions, Society for Vascular Medicine and Biology, Society of Interventional Radiology, and the ACC/AHA Task Force on Practice Guidelines (Writing Committee to Develop Guidelines for the Management of Patients With Peripheral Arterial Disease): endorsed by the American Association of Cardiovascular and Pulmonary Rehabilitation; National Heart, Lung, and Blood Institute; Society for Vascular Nursing; TransAtlantic Inter-Society Consensus; and Vascular Disease Foundation. Circulation 2006;113(11):e463–654.

18. Weichert W, Meents H, Abt K, et al. Acetylsalicylic acid–reocclusion–prophylaxis after angioplasty (ARPA-study). A randomized double-blind trial of two different dosages of ASA in patients with peripheral occlusive arterial disease. Vasa 1994; 23(1):57–65.

19. Minar E, Ahmadi A, Koppensteiner R, et al. Comparison of effects of high-dose and low-dose aspirin on restenosis after femoropopliteal percutaneous transluminal angioplasty. Circulation 1995; 91(8):2167–73.

20. Ranke C, Creutzig A, Luska G, et al. Controlled trial of high- versus low-dose aspirin treatment after percutaneous transluminal angioplasty in patients with peripheral vascular disease. Clin Investig 1994;72(9):673–80.

21. Goldhaber SZ, Manson JE, Stampfer MJ, et al. Low-dose aspirin and subsequent peripheral arterial surgery in the Physicians' Health Study. Lancet 1992;340(8812):143–5.

22. Theroux P, Ouimet H, McCans J, et al. Aspirin, heparin, or both to treat acute unstable angina. N Engl J Med 1988;319(17):1105–11.

23. Becquemin JP. Effect of ticlopidine on the long-term patency of saphenous-vein bypass grafts in the legs. Etude de la Ticlopidine apres Pontage Femoro-Poplite and the Association Universitaire de Recherche en Chirurgie. N Engl J Med 1997; 337(24):1726–31.

24. Belch JJ, Dormandy J, Biasi GM, et al. Results of the randomized, placebo-controlled Clopidogrel and Acetylsalicylic Acid in Bypass Surgery for Peripheral Arterial Disease (CASPAR) trial. J Vasc Surg 2010;52(4):825–33, 833.e1–2.

25. Thompson PD, Zimet R, Forbes WP, et al. Meta-analysis of results from eight randomized, placebo-controlled trials on the effect of cilostazol on patients with intermittent claudication. Am J Cardiol 2002;90(12):1314–9.

26. Randomised trial of intravenous streptokinase, oral aspirin, both, or neither among 17,187 cases of suspected acute myocardial infarction: ISIS-2. ISIS-2 (Second International Study of Infarct Survival) Collaborative Group. Lancet 1988;2(8607): 349–60.

27. Baigent C, Collins R, Appleby P, et al. ISIS-2: 10 year survival among patients with suspected acute myocardial infarction in randomised comparison of intravenous streptokinase, oral aspirin, both, or neither. The ISIS-2 (Second International Study of Infarct Survival) Collaborative Group. BMJ 1998; 316(7141):1337–43.

28. Roux S, Christeller S, Ludin E. Effects of aspirin on coronary reocclusion and recurrent ischemia after thrombolysis: a meta-analysis. J Am Coll Cardiol 1992;19(3):671–7.

29. Collaborative overview of randomised trials of antiplatelet therapy–I: prevention of death, myocardial infarction, and stroke by prolonged antiplatelet therapy in various categories of patients. Antiplatelet Trialists' Collaboration. BMJ 1994;308(6921): 81–106.

30. CAPRIE Steering Committee. A randomised, blinded, trial of clopidogrel versus aspirin in patients at risk of ischaemic events (CAPRIE). CAPRIE Steering Committee. Lancet 1996;348(9038): 1329–39.

31. Bhatt DL, Fox KA, Hacke W, et al. Clopidogrel and aspirin versus aspirin alone for the prevention of atherothrombotic events. N Engl J Med 2006; 354(16):1706–17.

32. Allemang MT, Rajani RR, Nelson PR, et al. Prescribing patterns of antiplatelet agents are highly

variable after lower extremity endovascular procedures. Ann Vasc Surg 2013;27(1):62–7.

33. Robertson L, Ghouri MA, Kovacs F. Antiplatelet and anticoagulant drugs for prevention of restenosis/ reocclusion following peripheral endovascular treatment. Cochrane Database Syst Rev 2012;(8): CD002071.

34. Schweizer J, Muller A, Forkmann L, et al. Potential use of a low-molecular-weight heparin to prevent restenosis in patients with extensive wall damage following peripheral angioplasty. Angiology 2001; 52(10):659–69.

35. Koppensteiner R, Spring S, Amann-Vesti BR, et al. Low-molecular-weight heparin for prevention of restenosis after femoropopliteal percutaneous transluminal angioplasty: a randomized controlled trial. J Vasc Surg 2006;44(6):1247–53.

36. Ansel GM, Silver MJ, Botti CF Jr, et al. Functional and clinical outcomes of nitinol stenting with and without abciximab for complex superficial femoral artery disease: a randomized trial. Catheter Cardiovasc Interv 2006;67(2):288–97.

37. Baumgartner DA Jr. A time to say no. Ohio Med 1988;84(10):783–4.

38. Dorffler-Melly J, Mahler F, Do DD, et al. Adjunctive abciximab improves patency and functional outcome in endovascular treatment of femoropopliteal occlusions: initial experience. Radiology 2005; 237(3):1103–9.

39. Duda SH, Tepe G, Luz O, et al. Peripheral artery occlusion: treatment with abciximab plus urokinase versus with urokinase alone–a randomized pilot trial (the PROMPT Study). Platelet Receptor Antibodies in Order to Manage Peripheral Artery Thrombosis. Radiology 2001;221(3):689–96.

40. Do DD, Mahler F. Low-dose aspirin combined with dipyridamole versus anticoagulants after femoropopliteal percutaneous transluminal angioplasty. Radiology 1994;193(2):567–71.

41. Pilger E, Lammer J, Bertuch H, et al. Nd:YAG laser with sapphire tip combined with balloon angioplasty in peripheral arterial occlusions. Long-term results. Circulation 1991;83(1):141–7.

42. Tan JY, Shi WH, He J, et al. A clinical trial of using antiplatelet therapy to prevent restenosis following peripheral artery angioplasty and stenting. Zhonghua Yi Xue Za Zhi 2008;88(12):812–5 [in Chinese].

43. Mahler F, Schneider E, Gallino A, et al. Combination of suloctidil and anticoagulation in the prevention of reocclusion after femoro-popliteal PTA. Vasa 1987; 16(4):381–5.

44. Ge J, Han Y, Jiang H, et al. RACTS: a prospective randomized antiplatelet trial of cilostazol versus ticlopidine in patients undergoing coronary stenting: long-term clinical and angiographic outcome. J Cardiovasc Pharmacol 2005;46(2):162–6.

45. Kozuma K, Hara K, Yamasaki M, et al. Effects of cilostazol on late lumen loss and repeat revascularization after Palmaz-Schatz coronary stent implantation. Am Heart J 2001;141(1):124–30.

46. Park SW, Lee CW, Kim HS, et al. Effects of cilostazol on angiographic restenosis after coronary stent placement. Am J Cardiol 2000;86(5):499–503.

47. Iida O, Nanto S, Uematsu M, et al. Cilostazol reduces restenosis after endovascular therapy in patients with femoropopliteal lesions. J Vasc Surg 2008;48(1):144–9.

48. Ikushima I, Yonenaga K, Iwakiri H, et al. A better effect of cilostazol for reducing in-stent restenosis after femoropopliteal artery stent placement in comparison with ticlopidine. Med Devices (Auckl) 2011;4:83–9.

49. Bittl JA, Chaitman BR, Feit F, et al. Bivalirudin versus heparin during coronary angioplasty for unstable or postinfarction angina: final report reanalysis of the Bivalirudin Angioplasty Study. Am Heart J 2001;142(6):952–9.

50. Stamler S, Katzen BT, Tsoukas AI, et al. Clinical experience with the use of bivalirudin in a large population undergoing endovascular abdominal aortic aneurysm repair. J Vasc Interv Radiol 2009;20(1):17–21.

51. Stabile E, Sorropago G, Tesorio T, et al. Heparin versus bivalirudin for carotid artery stenting using proximal endovascular clamping for neuroprotection: results from a prospective randomized study. J Vasc Surg 2010;52(6):1505–10.

# Antithrombotic Strategies in Valvular and Structural Heart Disease Interventions
## Current Status and Future Directions

Davide Capodanno, MD, PhD[a,b,*], Corrado Tamburino, MD, PhD[a,b]

## KEYWORDS

- TAVI • Dual antiplatelet therapy • Bivalirudin • Heparin

## KEY POINTS

- Transcatheter therapies for valvular and structural heart disease require the introduction of large and potentially thrombogenic materials through the venous or arterial system to the site of the intervention, as well as the release or implantation of devices that require some time for full endothelization.
- Stroke is one of the most feared complications of interventional catheter procedures, being associated not only with increased acute mortality but also with increased morbidity and physical disability.
- The approach to antithrombotic prophylaxis in valvular and structural transcatheter intervention is currently empiric. Research questions include type, doses, timing, and duration of antiplatelet and antithrombotic therapies.
- A careful, patient-centered risk-benefit assessment is needed for any antithrombotic combination.

Valvular and structural heart disease intervention is an exponentially growing field within interventional cardiology. Transcatheter therapies for both valvular and congenital heart disease disorders imply the introduction of large and potentially thrombogenic materials through the venous or arterial system to the site of the intervention, as well as the release or implantation of devices that require some time for full endothelization. In addition, a proportion of these patients have a greater propensity for hemodynamic compromise, which may increase the risk of ischemic stroke. For these reasons, the use of antithrombotic drugs for reducing the risk of stroke, systemic embolism, or valve/device thrombosis in the early-term and mid-term period is key to achieve successful procedural results and improve the overall outcomes of transcatheter procedures. However, drugs and doses for antiplatelet and anticoagulant therapy for valvular and structural interventions are mostly empiric in daily practice and typically administered at the operator's discretion. The objectives of this article are (1) to review the evidence supporting the rationale for antithrombotic management of patients undergoing transcatheter aortic valve implantation (TAVI), percutaneous mitral valve repair

Financial Disclosure: None.
[a] Cardiovascular Department, Ferrarotto Hospital, University of Catania, Via Citelli 6, Catania 95124, Italy;
[b] Excellence Through Newest Advances (ETNA) Foundation, Via Citelli 6, Catania 95124, Italy
* Corresponding author. Cardiovascular Department, Ferrarotto Hospital, University of Catania, Via Citelli 6, Catania 95124, Italy.
E-mail address: dcapodanno@gmail.com

Intervent Cardiol Clin 2 (2013) 635–642
http://dx.doi.org/10.1016/j.iccl.2013.05.005
2211-7458/13/$ – see front matter

interventional.theclinics.com

with the Mitraclip system, patent foramen ovale (PFO), and atrial septal defect (ASD) closure; (2) to describe common strategies for managing antiplatelet and anticoagulant therapy in valvular and structural heart disease patients undergoing transcatheter procedures; (3) to provide insights on future directions and research lines in this field.

## EMBOLISM AND THROMBOSIS IN VALVULAR AND STRUCTURAL TRANSCATHETER INTERVENTIONS

Embolic stroke is one of the most feared complications of interventional catheter procedures, being associated not only with increased acute mortality but also with increased morbidity and physical disability.

### TAVI

Cerebral silent embolic events have been reported post-TAVI by magnetic resonance in 68% to 84% of cases (**Fig. 1**).[1–5] On a more clinical level, a weighted meta-analysis of 53 studies including a total of 10,037 patients estimated the incidence of periprocedural stroke and subsequent outcomes in patients undergoing transfemoral, transapical, or transsubclavian TAVI. Pooled rates of stroke within 24 hours and 30 days were 1.5 ± 1.4% and 3.3 ± 1.8%, and 6 of every 7 stroke events were classified as major strokes. The route chosen for TAVI significantly affected the stroke rate, with the transapical access associated with the lowest risk. Not surprisingly, patients who experienced a stroke also experienced a 3.5-fold increased risk of mortality at 30 days (25.5 ± 21.9% vs 6.9 ± 4.2%).[6] Similarly, another weighted meta-analysis using Valve Academic Research Consortium definitions reported a 3.2% (95% confidence interval [95% CI] 2.1%–4.8%) risk of major stroke at 30 days.[7] Of note, the incidence of stroke peaks within 2 days, but slightly continues

afterward, reflecting the high baseline risk of patients who are currently referred to TAVI.[8] Valve thrombosis is estimated at a nonnegligible weighted rate of 1.2% (95% confidence interval 0.3–2.2).[7]

### MitraClip

In the EVEREST II (Endovascular Valve Edge-to-Edge Repair Study), the only randomized trial to date reporting data of MitraClip versus surgical mitral repair or replacement, 2 strokes occurred within 30 days in the interventional arm (1.1% vs 2.1% in the surgical arm, $P = .89$).[9] Observational series with different baseline case-mix reported major strokes in 0% to 2.6% of cases.[10–15] A weighted meta-analysis could meaningfully increase the precision of this risk estimate, given the small number of patients enrolled in the above mentioned studies, mostly reflecting the early experience of single institutions with percutaneous mitral valve repair. In the EVEREST II trial, clip thrombosis was uncommon, being detected in 1 of 184 cases (0.5%).

### PFO/ASD

Data on periprocedural stroke as the consequence of percutaneous closure of a PFO or an ASD cannot be easily disconnected from the underlying risk of recurrent stroke owing to suboptimal sealing of the shunt area or cerebrovascular embolism from alternative sources. In addition, closure devices may differ in terms of thrombogenicity and the incidence of new-onset conditions at high embolic potential, including atrial fibrillation.[16–20] In 499 patients from the Amplatzer PFO closure device arm of the RESPECT (Randomized Evaluation of Recurrent Stroke Comparing PFO Closure to Established Current Standard of Care Treatment) trial, one ischemic stroke (0.2%) occurred 1 week after implant and another one 5 months

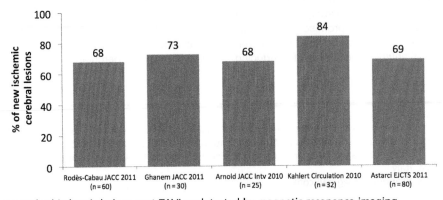

**Fig. 1.** New cerebral ischemic lesions post-TAVI as detected by magnetic resonance imaging.

after implant with findings of severe shunting related to previously undiagnosed sinus venosus defect, requiring surgical closure.[20] No thrombus was detected on any implanted device. In observational series, thromboembolic events while on antiplatelet treatment have been reported in 1.6% to 8.2% of patients within the year after PFO closure.[21-27] Also, many cases of device thrombosis have been reported within the first months after ASD device implantation, with an incidence of up to 7%, depending on the device.[17,28]

## PATHOPHYSIOLOGY OF STROKE AND SYSTEMIC EMBOLISM IN VALVULAR AND STRUCTURAL TRANSCATHETER INTERVENTIONS

Not surprisingly, embolism of thrombotic material is more commonly detected in left heart catheterization procedures, which require advancing the catheter through the aorta, thus increasing the risk of embolization by scraping of aortic plaques with subsequent direct embolization of debris to the brain. Indeed, scraping of aortic plaques occurs more commonly with large catheters, such as those used for TAVI. Embolic stroke may also theoretically occur in the setting of right heart catheterization in patients with PFO or ASD, or following transseptal puncture in patients undergoing Mitraclip implantation.

### TAVI

The aortic arch is recognized as a source of embolic material. In fact, retrograde progression of atheroma from the descending aorta to the arch has been shown to correlate significantly with the presence of cardiovascular risk factors and advanced age, conditions that are frequently encountered in patients referred to TAVI.[29] In addition, elderly patients present with a higher prevalence of comorbidities at embolic potential, including atrial fibrillation (pre-existing or new onset) and carotid artery disease. Given these anatomic considerations, the choice of the arterial access may play a pivotal role in the determination of embolic risk with the potential advantage of nontransfemoral approaches. However, no differences in the rates of in-hospital stroke were noted in a propensity-matched comparison between the subclavian and transfemoral access from the Italian registry of the self-expanding Medtronic CoreValve (Medtronic Inc., Minneapolis, MN) (2.1% vs 2.1%; $P = .99$).[30] It should be noted that the process of propensity matching typically excludes several patients who are not suitable for both TAVI approaches, mimicking the selection

process of a randomized clinical trial. Indeed, despite propensity matching, peripheral artery disease, a marker of more advanced and extended atherosclerosis, was still more prevalent in patients from the Italian CoreValve registry treated via the subclavian approach than those treated transfemorally (85% vs 21%, $P<.0001$) and therefore the advantages of nontransfemoral accesses in this kind of comparisons are likely underestimated. Variables that are more specifically linked with the TAVI procedure include device manipulation in the arch, the possibility of dislocating plaque or calcium particles while crossing the native valve and the act of deploying/postdilating the prosthesis. A transcranial Doppler study during TAVI showed that the most procedural embolic events occurred during balloon valvuloplasty, manipulation of catheters across the aortic valve, and valve implantation.[31] Differences in the risk of stroke could be theoretically attributable to different mechanisms of valve deployment (self-expanding vs balloon-expandable) and characteristics of the available systems. Ideally, this hypothesis should be investigated in the setting of a large head-to-head randomized comparison. In a propensity-matched comparison of the self-expanding Medtronic CoreValve and the balloon-expandable Edwards SAPIEN/SAPIEN XT (Edwards Lifesciences, Irvine, CA) transcatheter heart valves from the PRAGMATIC Plus (Pooled-RotterdAm-MilAno-Toulouse In Collaboration) initiative, the rates of stroke were numerically higher with the CoreValve system but did not significantly differ at 30 days, likely as the reflection of the small sample size (2.9% vs 1.0%, odds ratio [OR] 3.06, 95% CI 0.61–15.35; $P = .17$).[32]

There is a range of other explanations for periprocedural stroke in TAVI patients. First, thromboemboli may arise from the bioprosthesis before endothelialization completes. Aggregation of platelet and fibrin has been known to occur on valve leaflets within a few hours after implantation.[8] Second, hypotension associated with rapid ventricular pacing or hemodynamic instability during the procedure may impact the risk of ischemic stroke. Finally, the operator's experience plays a major role, including a meticulous technique and proper management of antiplatelet and anticoagulant therapy. A list of potential explanations for the risk of stroke in TAVI patients is shown in **Table 1**.

### Mitraclip

Embolic stroke is uncommon in the setting of right heart catheterization. However, blood clots can form in and around catheters inside the venous system in patients who are not adequately

**Table 1**
**Stroke determinants in patients undergoing transcatheter aortic valve implantation**

| | |
|---|---|
| Patient-related | • Aortic atherosclerosis<br>• Atrial fibrillation<br>• Carotid artery disease |
| Procedure-related | • Device manipulation<br>• Crossing of the native valve<br>• Prosthesis deployment<br>• Postdilation<br>• Access-related<br>• Operator's experience |
| Device-related | • Valve<br>• Frame |
| Postprocedure-related | • Antiplatelet therapy<br>• Anticoagulation therapy |

anticoagulated. The execution of a transseptal puncture during the procedure determines a transient direct communication between the venous and the arterial circulation, thereby creating the premise of paradoxic embolism. Reasons for clot formation vary according to host factors, catheter characteristics, cannulation site, and antithrombotic prophylaxis. Right and left heart thromboemboli in the setting of Mitraclip procedures rarely include thrombi that may develop within the cardiac chambers on injured endothelium and implanted devices.

## PFO/ASD

Adding to thrombotic mechanisms described above for the Mitraclip procedure, transcatheter closure of PFO has been shown to induce significant activation of the coagulation system, which reaches maximal levels 7 days after the device deployment, gradually returning to baseline by day 90.[33] On the other hand, implantation of the device does not seem to be associated with any increase in platelet activation in aspirin-treated patients. These findings are similar to those obtained after transcatheter closure of ASD.[34]

## ANTITHROMBOTIC STRATEGIES IN PATIENTS UNDERGOING VALVULAR AND STRUCTURAL PERCUTANEOUS INTERVENTIONS

The approach to antithrombotic prophylaxis against valve/device-related thromboembolic complications in valvular and structural transcatheter intervention is currently empiric. Downsides of antithrombotic management include the risk of bleeding, especially in elderly patients, like those undergoing valvular procedures.[35]

## TAVI

There is no consensus on the optimal duration of dual antiplatelet therapy after TAVI. For example, in the PARTNER (Placement of Aortic Transcatheter Valves) trial, antiplatelet therapy included aspirin and clopidogrel for 6 months after the procedure.[36] Differently, in the large FRANCE-2 (French Aortic National CoreValve and Edwards) registry, patients were on aspirin (≤160 mg daily) and clopidogrel (300-mg loading dose, then 75 mg daily) before the procedure and aspirin alone after 1 month of dual therapy.[37] In general, it seems that most centers adopt a strategy of low-dose aspirin and a short to intermediate period with a thienopyridine. The American College of Chest Physicians practice guidelines for antithrombotic and thrombolytic therapy in valvular heart disease support this strategy, but with a low grade of recommendation and level of evidence.[38]

The underlying rationale for adding clopidogrel to aspirin derives from the initial TAVI experience, when extracorporeal bypass for hemodynamic support was used during the procedure. Grube and colleagues[39] observed 2 cases of prolonged and severe postprocedural thrombocytopenia in patients who were not treated with clopidogrel, likely as the reflection of platelet activation processes and consumption. TAVI is now performed mostly under local anesthesia and/or light sedation with no need for extracorporeal circulatory support, and very infrequent cases of mild and transient thrombocytopenia have been reported.[40] As noted above, the need for a course of dual antiplatelet therapy is theoretically supported by the delay of time needed for incorporation of the prosthesis within the aortic wall for neointimal tissue growth and endothelialization. This process begins with early fibrin deposition, linked to inflammatory response and foreign body reactions. Three months later, smooth muscle cells and endothelial cells replace fibrin.[41] Although these findings derive from histopathologic studies of CoreValve explants, clinical evidence for the benefit of dual antiplatelet therapy after TAVI remains elusive. In a small study from a single center, 79 patients were randomized to dual antiplatelet therapy with a 300-mg loading dose of clopidogrel on the day before TAVI followed by a 3-month maintenance daily dose of 75 mg on a background of aspirin

100 mg versus aspirin alone. The primary efficacy endpoint, a composite of major cardiac and cerebrovascular events, including overall mortality, myocardial infarction, major stroke, urgent or emergency conversion to surgery, or life-threatening bleeding, occurred with a similar frequency between the 2 groups both at 30 days (13% vs 15%; $P = .71$) and 6 months (18% vs 15%; $P = .85$). There were no differences in Valve Academic Research Consortium –defined major and minor bleeding between the 2 strategies. Although limited by the small sample size, this study does not seem to support a strategy of short-term adjunctive use of clopidogrel added to aspirin after TAVI, but more investigations are needed.[42]

Intraprocedural anticoagulation with weight-adjusted unfractionated heparin (UFH) has been a well-established standard of care in all major published registries of TAVI. Using UFH and protamine sulfate to reverse the anticoagulant effect at the end of the procedure has the advantage of being intuitive, relatively economic, and broadly familiar in the interventional and surgical setting. On the downside, this approach may suffer from ample variability in pharmacokinetics and pharmacodynamics of heparin, resulting in wide interindividual response. In addition, late anticoagulant effects of heparin, which dissociates from cells and proteins, and protamine, with rebound bleeding, have been described. Finally, rapid reversal of anticoagulation may lead to prothrombotic rebound with detrimental clinical consequences. Interestingly, oral anticoagulation proved to be effective in 3 reported cases of late valve thrombosis.[43]

### MitraClip

The manufacturer leaves antithrombotic management of Mitraclip to the discretion of the operator, because of a lack of specific investigations aimed at comparing different treatment strategies after percutaneous mitral valve repair. Indicatively, in the EVEREST II, patients were treated with heparin during the procedure, and a combination of aspirin (at a dose of 325 mg daily) for 6 months and clopidogrel (at a dose of 75 mg daily) for 30 days after the procedure. A case of large thrombus formation in the posterolateral wall of the left atrium and on the right atrial side of the septum has been reported on day 5 after Mitraclip implantation, and the authors reported a note of caution on the need for a course of anticoagulation in patients undergoing percutaneous mitral valve repair.[44]

### PFO/ASD

There are no studies on the most appropriate antithrombotic therapy after transcatheter closure of PFO/ASD, and the choice of antithrombotic drugs after these procedures has been empirically determined, with aspirin as the agent most frequently used. In the CLOSURE-1 (A Prospective, Multicenter, Randomized Controlled Trial to Evaluate the Safety and Efficacy of the STARFlex Septal Closure System vs Best Medical Therapy in Patients With a Stroke and/or Transient Ischemic Attack Due to Presumed Paradoxic Embolism Through a Patent Foramen Ovale) trial, after PFO closure with the StarFlex device, all patients were given a standard antiplatelet regimen including clopidogrel (75 mg daily) for 6 months, and aspirin (81–325 mg daily) for 2 years. Experimental studies have demonstrated that the Amplatzer PFO occluder is partially endothelialized 1 month after implantation and completely covered by neoendothelial cells at 3 months.[45] Thus, the first weeks after PFO closure may constitute a vulnerable window with newer devices, in which the closure system is potentially more thrombogenic.[46,47] Remarkably, most of the patients who experience device thrombosis are receiving antiplatelet treatment, and most of them are successfully treated with heparin or warfarin. Therefore, some operators advocate short-term anticoagulation (1–3 months) after PFO/ASD closure. Once device endothelialization is completed and no residual shunt is observed, anticoagulant treatment is then switched to antiplatelet therapy or no antithrombotic treatment.

## FUTURE DIRECTIONS AND CONCLUSIONS

Bivalirudin is a direct selective inhibitor of the activated coagulation factor II (thrombin).

Direct thrombin inhibitors have some advantages over the heparins, such as lack of dependence on plasma protein, which results in a more predictable response and makes them very attractive for use in populations at high risk of bleeding (**Table 2**). The BRAVO 2/3 (Effect of Bivalirudin on Aortic Valve Intervention Outcomes 2/3) is an ongoing international, multicenter, open-label, randomized controlled trial of bivalirudin in patients undergoing transfemoral TAVI (NCT01651780). Approximately 550 patients will be randomly assigned to either standard dosing of bivalirudin (bolus 0.75 mg/kg plus infusion) or UFH (targeting an activated coagulation time $\geq$250 seconds) as control. Use of antiplatelet agents before, during, and post procedure, and possibly oral anticoagulants post procedure, will be according to the sites' standard practice. The primary endpoint will be major bleeding defined as Bleeding Academic Research Consortium type $\geq$3 at 48 hours or hospital discharge, whichever occurs first.[48]

**Table 2**
**Pharmacologic properties of heparins and bivalirudin**

|  | UFH | Bivalirudin |
|---|---|---|
| Bioavailability | 35% | 100% |
| Action independent of antithrombin III | No | Yes |
| Nonspecific protease binding | Yes | No |
| Predictable PK-PD | No | Yes |
| Inhibits fibrin-bound thrombin | No | Yes |
| Activates/aggregates platelet | Yes | No |
| Half-life in minutes | 60' to 90' | 25' |

Several relatively novel antiplatelet (ie, prasugrel, ticagrelor) and anticoagulant (dabigatran, rivaroxaban, apixaban) agents have recently entered the cardiologist's armamentarium in Europe and the United States. None of these drugs is currently approved from European or US regulatory agencies for antithrombotic management of patients undergoing valvular or structural percutaneous intervention. Randomized clinical trials remain the most appropriate setting to establish the safety and efficacy of a drug for any novel indication. The safety and efficacy of the current approach for either TAVI, Mitraclip implantation, or PFO/ASD closure, mostly using a short- to intermediate-term combination of aspirin and clopidogrel after the procedure, and unfractionated heparin during the procedure, have never been prospectively investigated in a randomized clinical trial. Therefore, at present, the apparent superiority of any antithrombotic approach over another remains speculative. Research questions include which antiplatelet anticoagulant agents to use after valvular and structural interventions, when they should be administered, at which doses, and for how long. Careful and tailored risk-benefit assessment is needed for any antithrombotic combination in patients undergoing valvular or structural transcatheter interventions.

## REFERENCES

1. Rodés-Cabau J, Dumont E, Boone RH, et al. Cerebral embolism following transcatheter aortic valve implantation: comparison of transfemoral and transapical approaches. J Am Coll Cardiol 2011; 57:18–28.
2. Ghanem A, Müller A, Nähle CP, et al. Risk and fate of cerebral embolism after transfemoral aortic valve implantation: a prospective pilot study with diffusion-weighted magnetic resonance imaging. J Am Coll Cardiol 2010;55:1427–32.
3. Arnold M, Schulz-Heise S, Achenbach S, et al. Embolic cerebral insults after transapical aortic valve implantation detected by magnetic resonance imaging. JACC Cardiovasc Interv 2010;3:1126–32.
4. Kahlert P, Al-Rashid F, Döttger P, et al. Cerebral embolization during transcatheter aortic valve implantation: a transcranial Doppler study. Circulation 2012;126:1245–55.
5. Astarci P, Glineur D, Kefer J, et al. Magnetic resonance imaging evaluation of cerebral embolization during percutaneous aortic valve implantation: comparison of transfemoral and trans-apical approaches using Edwards Sapiens valve. Eur J Cardiothorac Surg 2011;40:475–9.
6. Eggebrecht H, Schmermund A, Voigtländer T, et al. Risk of stroke after transcatheter aortic valve implantation (TAVI): a meta-analysis of 10,037 published patients. EuroIntervention 2012;8:129–38.
7. Généreux P, Head SJ, Van Mieghem NM, et al. Clinical outcomes after transcatheter aortic valve replacement using valve academic research consortium definitions: a weighted meta-analysis of 3,519 patients from 16 studies. J Am Coll Cardiol 2012;59:2317–26.
8. Tay EL, Gurvitch R, Wijesinghe N, et al. A high-risk period for cerebrovascular events exists after transcatheter aortic valve implantation. JACC Cardiovasc Interv 2011;4:1290–7.
9. Feldman T, Foster E, Glower DD, et al, EVEREST II Investigators. Percutaneous repair or surgery for mitral regurgitation. N Engl J Med 2011;364: 1395–406.
10. Franzen O, Baldus S, Rudolph V, et al. Acute outcomes of MitraClip therapy for mitral regurgitation in high-surgical-risk patients: emphasis on adverse valve morphology and severe left ventricular dysfunction. Eur Heart J 2010;31:1373–81.
11. Tamburino C, Ussia GP, Maisano F, et al. Percutaneous mitral valve repair with the MitraClip system: acute results from a real world setting. Eur Heart J 2010;31:1382–9.
12. Rudolph V, Knap M, Franzen O, et al. Echocardiographic and clinical outcomes of MitraClip therapy in patients not amenable to surgery. J Am Coll Cardiol 2011;58:2190–5.
13. Baldus S, Schillinger W, Franzen O, et al. Mitra-Clip therapy in daily clinical practice: initial results from the German transcatheter mitral valve interventions (TRAMI) registry. Eur J Heart Fail 2012; 14:1050–5.
14. Grasso C, Capodanno D, Scandura S, et al. One- and twelve-month safety and efficacy outcomes of patients undergoing edge-to-edge percutaneous mitral valve repair (from the GRASP Registry). Am J Cardiol 2013;111(10):1482–7.

15. Whitlow PL, Feldman T, Pedersen WR, et al, EVEREST II Investigators. Acute and 12-month results with catheter-based mitral valve leaflet repair: the EVEREST II (Endovascular Valve Edge-to-Edge Repair) High Risk Study. J Am Coll Cardiol 2012;59:130–9.

16. Taaffe M, Fischer E, Baranowski A, et al. Comparison of three patent foramen ovale closure devices in a randomized trial (Amplatzer versus CardioSEAL-STARflex versus Helex occluder). Am J Cardiol 2008;101:1353–8.

17. Krumsdorf U, Ostermayer S, Billinger K, et al. Incidence and clinical course of thrombus formation on atrial septal defect and patient foramen ovale closure devices in 1,000 consecutive patients. J Am Coll Cardiol 2004;43:302–9.

18. Furlan AJ, Reisman M, Massaro J, et al. Closure or medical therapy for cryptogenic stroke with patent foramen ovale. N Engl J Med 2012;366:991–9.

19. Windecker S. The PC trial: percutaneous closure of patent foramen ovale versus medical treatment in patients with cryptogenic embolism. Paper presented at Transcatheter Therapeutics. Miami, October 25, 2012.

20. Carroll JD. The RESPECT trial: a randomized evaluation of recurrent stroke comparing PFO closure to established current standard of care treatment. Paper presented at Transcatheter Therapeutics. Miami, October 25, 2012.

21. Martín F, Sánchez PL, Doherty E, et al. Percutaneous transcatheter closure of patent foramen ovale in patients with paradoxical embolism. Circulation 2002;106:1121–6.

22. Windecker S, Wahl A, Chatterjee T, et al. Percutaneous closure of patent foramen ovale in patients with paradoxical embolism: long-term risk of recurrent thromboembolic events. Circulation 2000;101:893–8.

23. Braun M, Fassbender D, Schoen SP, et al. Transcatheter closure of patent foramen ovale in patients with cerebral ischemia. J Am Coll Cardiol 2002;39:2019–25.

24. Braun M, Gliech V, Boscheri A, et al. Transcatheter closure of patent foramen ovale (PFO) in patients with paradoxical embolism: periprocedural safety and mid-term follow-up results of three different device occluder systems. Eur Heart J 2004;25:424–30.

25. Windecker S, Wahl A, Nedeltchev K, et al. Comparison of medical treatment with percutaneous closure of patent foramen ovale in patients with cryptogenic stroke. J Am Coll Cardiol 2004;44:750–8.

26. Beitzke A, Schuchlenz H, Gamillscheg A, et al. Catheter closure of the persistent foramen ovale: mid-term results in 162 patients. J Interv Cardiol 2001;14:223–30.

27. Wahl A, Meier B, Haxel B, et al. Prognosis after percutaneous closure of patent foramen ovale for paradoxical embolism. Neurology 2001;57:1330–2.

28. Sherman JM, Hagler DJ, Cetta F. Thrombosis after septal closure device placement: a review of the current literature. Catheter Cardiovasc Interv 2004;63:486–9.

29. Di Tullio MR, Sacco RL, Savoia MT, et al. Aortic atheroma morphology and the risk of ischemic stroke in a multiethnic population. Am Heart J 2000;139:329–36.

30. Petronio AS, De Carlo M, Bedogni F, et al. 2-year results of CoreValve implantation through the subclavian access: a propensity-matched comparison with the femoral access. J Am Coll Cardiol 2012;60:502–7.

31. Drews T, Pasic M, Buz S, et al. Transcranial Doppler sound detection of cerebral microembolism during transapical aortic valve implantation. Thorac Cardiovasc Surg 2011;59:237–42.

32. Chieffo A, Buchanan GL, Van Mieghem NM, et al. Transcatheter aortic valve implantation with the Edwards SAPIEN versus the Medtronic CoreValve Revalving system devices: a multicenter collaborative study: the PRAGMATIC Plus Initiative (Pooled-RotterdAm-Milano-Toulouse In Collaboration). J Am Coll Cardiol 2013;61:830–6.

33. Bédard E, Rodés-Cabau J, Houde C, et al. Enhanced thrombogenesis but not platelet activation is associated with transcatheter closure of patent foramen ovale in patients with cryptogenic stroke. Stroke 2007;38:100–4.

34. Rodés-Cabau J, Palacios A, Palacio C, et al. Assessment of the markers of platelet and coagulation activation following transcatheter closure of atrial septal defects. Int J Cardiol 2005;98:107–12.

35. Capodanno D, Angiolillo DJ. Antithrombotic therapy in the elderly. J Am Coll Cardiol 2010;56:1683–92.

36. Smith CR, Leon MB, Mack MJ, et al. Transcatheter versus surgical aortic-valve replacement in high-risk patients. N Engl J Med 2011;364:2187–98.

37. Gilard M, Eltchaninoff H, Iung B, et al. Registry of transcatheter aortic-valve implantation in high-risk patients. N Engl J Med 2012;366:1705–15.

38. Whitlock RP, Sun JC, Fremes SE, et al. Antithrombotic and thrombolytic therapy for valvular disease: Antithrombotic Therapy and Prevention of Thrombosis, 9th ed: American College of Chest Physicians Evidence-Based Clinical Practice Guidelines. Chest 2012;141:e576S–600S.

39. Grube E, Laborde JC, Gerckens U, et al. Percutaneous implantation of the CoreValve self-expanding valve prosthesis in high-risk patients with aortic valve disease: the Siegburg first-in-man study. Circulation 2006;114:1616–24.

40. Ussia GP, Scarabelli M, Mulè M, et al. Postprocedural management of patients after transcatheter aortic valve implantation procedure with self-expanding bioprosthesis. Catheter Cardiovasc Interv 2010;76:757–66.

41. Noble S, Asgar A, Cartier R, et al. Anatomo-pathological analysis after CoreValve Revalving system implantation. EuroIntervention 2009;5:78–85.

42. Ussia GP, Scarabelli M, Mulè M, et al. Dual antiplatelet therapy versus aspirin alone in patients undergoing transcatheter aortic valve implantation. Am J Cardiol 2011;108:1772–6.

43. Cota L, Stabile E, Agrusta M, et al. Bioprostheses "thrombosis" after transcatheter aortic valve replacement. J Am Coll Cardiol 2013;61:789–91.

44. Bekeredjian R, Mereles D, Pleger S, et al. Large atrial thrombus formation after MitraClip implantation: is anticoagulation mandatory? J Heart Valve Dis 2011;20:146–8.

45. Han YM, Gu X, Titus JL, et al. New self-expanding patent foramen ovale occlusion device. Catheter Cardiovasc Interv 1999;47:370–6.

46. Cenni E, Ciapetti G, Cervellati M, et al. Activation of the plasma coagulation system induced by some biomaterials. J Biomed Mater Res 1996;31:145–8.

47. Hong J, Azens A, Ekdahl KN, et al. Material-specific thrombin generation following contact between metal surfaces and whole blood. Biomaterials 2005;26:1397–403.

48. Sergie Z, Lefèvre T, Van Belle E, et al. Current peri-procedural anticoagulation in transcatheter aortic valve replacement: could bivalirudin be an option? Rationale and design of the BRAVO 2/3. studies. J Thromb Thrombolysis 2013;35(4):483–93.

# Monitoring and Reversal of Anticoagulation and Antiplatelets

Gregory W. Yost, DO*, Steven R. Steinhubl, MD

## KEYWORDS

- Anticoagulation • Antiplatelets • Antithrombotics • PCI • Monitoring • Reversal • Bleeding

## KEY POINTS

- Combination therapy with anticoagulants and antiplatelets during percutaneous coronary intervention reduces incidence of stent thrombosis.
- The role of monitoring during percutaneous coronary intervention is variable depending on the type of antithrombotic used.
- Clinical benefit of tailored antiplatelet therapy based on point-of-care tests has yet to be proved.
- Reversal agents (if available) for the various antithrombotics may be necessary when major bleeding occurs or emergent surgery is needed.

## INTRODUCTION

Since the beginnings of percutaneous transluminal coronary angioplasty (PTCA), the biggest concern with performing the intervention has been abrupt closure of the vessel. Even despite advances in the technical aspects of percutaneous coronary intervention (PCI), especially with stenting, the possibility of thrombosis remains a prominent issue. Thrombogenic potential exists in a newly placed stent until there is complete endothelialization[1] (approximately after 28 days for bare metal stent; longer for drug-eluting stents, because of delayed neointimal proliferation).[2,3] There is overwhelming clinical evidence that the use of anticoagulants and antiplatelets lowers the risk of vessel closure during and after PCI. Anticoagulation and dual antiplatelet therapy with stent placement is a standard of treatment and class I indication according to current practice guidelines.[4] Anticoagulation has been used since before the stent era and continues to be used during PCI for 2 major reasons: preventing arterial thrombus formation and reducing thrombogenicity of catheters and guidewires used during the invasive procedures.[5]

Since PTCA was first described[6,7] and the breakthrough studies of the role of stents,[8,9] the evolution in anticoagulation and antiplatelet therapy used during PCI has led to reductions in periprocedural ischemic events and stent thrombosis.[10] Although greater combinations and doses of anticoagulation with antiplatelets in general seem to provide the best protection against thrombogenic and embolic events, there is a significant trade-off with a higher risk of major and minor bleeding episodes.[11] The goal of this review article is to expand on each of the commonly used antiplatelet and anticoagulants used at time of PCI, with specific focus on drug monitoring and reversal, if applicable.

Disclosure: The authors have nothing to disclose.
Department of Cardiology, Geisinger Medical Center, 100 North Academy Avenue, Danville, PA 17822, USA
* Corresponding author.
E-mail address: gwyost@geisinger.edu

## ANTICOAGULANTS

Predisposition to thrombosis during catheterization exists because of exposure of clotting factors to disrupted endothelium, catheters, and guidewires. The goals of anticoagulation therapy are to minimize thrombus propagation on the endovascular surface and formation of new thrombi from PCI equipment use.[5,12] Ideal anticoagulation would effectively prevent thrombus formation, have low risk of bleeding, have safe monitoring profile, have short duration of effect (half-life), and could be reversed if needed. The options available for anticoagulation during PCI include unfractionated heparin (UFH), low-molecular-weight heparin (LMWH), direct thrombin inhibitors, and indirect factor Xa inhibitors (**Table 1**).[12,13]

### UFH

Thrombus propagation occurs when thrombin is produced on the surface of activated platelets, converting fibrinogen to fibrin. Fibrin gets cross-linked with factor XIIIa, reinforcing platelet aggregation and culminating in clot formation. Heparin combines with antithrombin to indirectly inactivate thrombin, factors Xa, and intrinsic pathway factors (XIIa, XIa, and IXa).[14,15] UFH has been proved beneficial in the treatment of unstable angina or and non-ST segment increase in myocardial infarction (MI).[16–18] Although anticoagulants have been shown to inactivate von Willebrand factor, there may be differences between anticoagulants in curbing its release: enoxaparin may lessen the release more so than UFH. This situation is important in unstable angina, when there may be an early increase of von Willebrand factor. This early release of von Willebrand factor may be associated with worse outcomes.[19,20]

Use of intravenous (IV) UFH given before PCI to prevent intracoronary thrombosis was started at the time of the first percutaneous intervention by Andreas Gruntzig and has remained the gold standard through the current age of routine stenting and use of dual antiplatelets.[5] In early phases of PTCA, the vessel closure rate during or after dilatation was 2% to 11%.[21] Use of UFH decreased these rates, but there remained a risk for closure, because there was no clear consensus for proper dosing. The dosing recommendations for heparin have changed over time with the advancements in PCI.[12] UFH remains the most commonly used anticoagulant, despite availability of newer medications.

Despite UFH being the most widely used anticoagulant, there are several limitations to its use beyond the risk of bleeding seen in all

### Table 1
### Anticoagulants

| | Mechanism of Action | Onset of Action (Half-Life) | Method of Monitoring | Recommended Point-of-Care Test | Reversal for Bleeding |
|---|---|---|---|---|---|
| UFH | Inactivates thrombin, factors IXa, Xa, XIa, XIIa | Immediate, IV (dose dependent, 30–90 min) | aPTT | ACT | Protamine sulfate (1 mg per 100 units of UFH) |
| LMWH | Inactivates thrombin (less affinity) and factor Xa (higher affinity) | Immediate, IV 3–5 h, SQ (3–6 h) | Anti–factor Xa level | None | Partial with protamine sulfate (1 mg per 100 anti-Xa units) |
| Bivalirudin | Transiently inhibits thrombin | <5 min, IV (25 min, longer with renal failure) | ACT | ACT | None[a] |
| Argatroban | Reversibly inhibits thrombin | Immediate, IV (30–60 min) | aPTT | ACT | None[a] |
| Fondaparinux | Inactivates factor Xa | 2 h, SQ (17–21 h) | Anti–factor Xa | None | None[a] |

*Abbreviations:* ACT, activated clotting time; aPTT, activated partial thromboplastin time; SQ, subcutaneous.
[a] Recombinant factor VIIa can be used to help reduce bleeding.

anticoagulants. UFH has a pharmacologic profile that is less predictable. Several of the heparin-binding proteins are acute-phase reactants, which typically increase in the setting of unstable angina or MIs. Studies have confirmed that thrombin bound to fibrin is protected from inactivation by heparin.[22] In addition, there is decreased affinity of antithrombin III when factor Xa is bound to phospholipid surfaces within a prothrombinase complex, which may account for the variable effect with UFH.[23,24] There may even be a pro-thrombotic risk (outside heparin-induced thrombocytopenia [HIT]) because of its weaker control of von Willebrand factor, possibility of rebound thrombin generation after its discontinuation, and platelet activation and enhanced aggregation with therapeutic concentrations of UFH.[19,20,25] Because of its unpredictability, UFH needs to be closely and continually monitored, especially while being used during PCI.

### Monitoring

UFH is typically monitored with activated partial thromboplastin time (aPTT). There are variations in response to heparin between different commercial aPTT reagents.[26] Another problem is that aPTT becomes prolonged beyond measure when heparin concentrations exceed 1 U/mL.[24] This is typically the case during coronary artery bypass surgery and PCI, when high concentrations of heparin are required to prevent clotting. Monitoring is performed in these cases by using activated clotting time (ACT). Earlier studies identified a narrow therapeutic window for UFH and that lower ACT levels may be associated with higher incidence of ischemia.[27–29] One meta-analysis identified an optimal ACT range of 350 to 375 in patients undergoing PCI. This finding was associated with a 6.6% ischemic event rate defined by the composite end point of death, MI, or urgent revascularization at 7 days. The relative risk reduction in ischemic events at 7 days was 34% with these higher levels of ACT relative to lower. The lowest level of bleeding (8.6%) was observed in the range of 325 to 350 seconds, and it progressively increased to 12.4% at 350 to 375 seconds. There was a substantial increase in bleeding events when ACT values exceeded 400 seconds.[30] In contrast, a subanalysis from the more modern STEEPLE (The Safety and Efficacy of Enoxaparin in PCI Patients, an International Randomized Evaluation) trial suggested that an ACT of 325 seconds may be the optimal target when balancing risk versus benefits. This finding paralleled similar findings from a meta-analysis performed by Brener and colleagues[31] showing no further protection against ischemic events but still a greater bleeding

risk with higher ACT levels. This finding holds especially true in the modern era of PCI, when P2Y12 and glycoprotein (GP) IIb/IIIa inhibitors are frequently used. Based on these results, lower ACT levels in the low 200s are not associated with higher incidences of ischemia, but higher ACT levels and weight-indexed dosing of UFH may cause more bleeding.[32]

Different models for measuring ACT levels may have different results.[33] The 2011 PCI guidelines recommend an ACT level of 200 to 250 seconds after an initial UFH bolus of 50 to 70 units/kg when GP IIb/IIIa inhibitors are used. ACT levels of 250 to 300 seconds (for HemoTec device [HemoTec Inc, Englewood, CO]) or 300 to 350 seconds (for Hemochron device [International Technidyne Corporation, Edison, NJ]) after an initial bolus of 70 to 100 units/kg of UFH are the goals when not using GP IIb/IIIa inhibitors.[34]

### Reversal

Heparin has a short half-life; however, it has a nonlinear response when used at therapeutic doses: half-life of heparin increases from $\approx$30 minutes after an IV bolus of 25 U/kg to 60 minutes with an IV bolus of 100 U/kg and 150 minutes with a bolus of 400 U/kg.[15] IV protamine sulfate can be used when immediate reversal of heparin is needed. One milligram of protamine sulfate neutralizes 100 units of heparin (eg, 50 mg protamine sulfate should be given for heparin IV bolus of 5000 units). When a patient is on continuous heparin infusion, only the preceding 1 to 2 hours of heparin needs considered for dosing of protamine sulfate because of the short half-life of heparin (eg, 25 mg of protamine sulfate given to neutralize heparin at 1200 units/h for the past 2 hours). Slow infusion of protamine may reduce chances of bradycardia, hypotension (no faster than 20 mg/min and no more than 50 mg in any 10-minute period). The aPTT should normalize after administration of protamine. Because protamine is derived from fish sperm, patients with allergic reactions to fish can be pretreated with corticosteroids or antihistamines.[35–37]

### LMWH (Enoxaparin)

LMWH (3000–5000 Da) is produced by chemical or enzymatic depolymerization of UFH (weight ranges 3000–30,000 Da).[38] This change in molecular weight and size creates several important differences between UFH and LMWH. Heparin has a unique pentasaccharide sequence allowing it to bind to antithrombin. This interaction causes a conformational change inactivating factor Xa. A ternary complex must be formed to inactivate thrombin-heparin binding to antithrombin and thrombin. This complex can be formed only by pentasaccharide chains consisting of 18 saccharide units. UFH is composed of at least 18 saccharide units; however, LMWH typically have shorter chain units. This creates an important difference, in that LMWH has a higher affinity for factor Xa as opposed to UFH, which has equal activity against factor Xa and thrombin.[12,24,37,39–41]

LMWH has a more predictable anticoagulant profile and can be given IV or subcutaneously. It can typically be given in fixed or weight-adjusted doses without routine monitoring (renal insufficiency, obesity, and children may be exceptions).[35] Less binding of LMWH to plasma proteins is a major reason for this situation, which establishes better bioavailability, longer half-life, and dose-independent clearance.[22,37,42] LMWH may reduce risk of bleeding because it causes less vessel wall permeability, less platelet activation, less susceptibility to inactivation by platelet factor 4, and less risk of HIT than seen with UFH,[42,43] although the clinical data supporting this are mixed.

Further exploration of using LMWH over UFH during acute coronary syndrome (ACS) and PCI was undertaken because of its potentially better predictability and less harm. Gurfunkel and colleagues[44] first noted a decrease in rates of silent ischemia, recurrent angina, revascularization, and minor bleeding in the group who received LMWH and aspirin (ASA) versus UFH and ASA when used for treatment of unstable angina. The FRIC (Fragmin in Unstable Coronary Artery Disease Study) trial[45] found no significant differences between LMWH and UFH when used for treatment of unstable angina or non-Q wave MIs. Since then, several more studies have offered more support for benefits of LMWH over UFH. TIMI 11B (The Thrombolysis in Myocardial Infarction B Trial Investigators) and ESSENCE (Efficacy and Safety of Subcutaneous Enoxaparin in Non-Q wave Coronary Events) separately showed superiority of enoxaparin over UFH in reducing end points of death, nonfatal MI, and urgent revascularization when used for treatment of unstable angina and non–ST elevation MI (NSTEMI). A meta-analysis of the 2 studies showed persistence of lower end points over 43 days. There was a significant increase in minor bleeding but not for major bleeding rates.[46–48] The SYNERGY (The Superior Yield of the New Strategy of Enoxaparin, Revascularization and Glycoprotein IIb/IIIa Inhibitors) trial showed that enoxaparin was not inferior to UFH but may have a slightly increased risk of bleeding. However, there were a nonnegligible number of patients who crossed over to the other antithrombotic agent. The study concluded that despite an increase in bleeding, enoxaparin is likely superior when used as initial first-line therapy without changing to UFH.[49] Crossing over or giving additional UFH after initially treating with enoxaparin should be avoided, as supported by the STACKENOX (STACK-on to ENOXaparin) trial.[50]

The STEEPLE trial compared use of enoxaparin with UFH with GP IIb/IIIa inhibitors in patients undergoing elective PCI. The results showed that enoxaparin (compared with UFH) had a significantly higher rate of achieving target anticoagulation levels, and bleeding rates were similar to or lower than those with UFH (depending on dose used at time of elective PCI).[51] This finding provides stronger support for better bioavailability and predictability of LMWH over UFH without the need for close monitoring.[19] Use of IV enoxaparin in combination with GP inhibitors was shown to be a safe alternative to UFH when used during PCI in the NICE 1 and NICE 4 (National Investigators Collaborating on Enoxaparin) studies (dosed at 1 mg/kg and 0.75 mg/kg, respectively). NICE 3 showed that the combination can also be used safely as initial anticoagulation for ACSs and continued during the transition to the catheterization laboratory for PCI.[43,52] Further, Bhatt and colleagues[53] performed a randomized study comparing enoxaparin with GP IIb/IIIa inhibitors versus UFH with GP IIb/IIIa inhibitors. The results showed that there was no significant difference in bleeding and that enoxaparin was no less efficacious than UFH when used during urgent or elective PCI. A meta-analysis of 13 studies performed by Dumaine and colleagues[54] showed that use of LMWH was associated with less major bleeding and no differences in end point of death and MI when compared with UFH. There may also be less incidence of bleeding associated with sheath removal.[53,55]

### Monitoring

Despite the safe findings shown in previous trials using LMWH and GP IIb/IIIa inhibitors, there remains concern over monitoring therapeutic levels of anticoagulation especially in select populations (ie, elderly, obesity, renal failure). Because LMWH has minimal effect on thrombin, it has only a modest effect on aPTT levels. Unlike UFH, with which ACT is the standard for monitoring, LWMH does not significantly prolong ACT levels and cannot be reliably used during PCI.[56,57] Measuring anti–factor Xa levels most accurately reflects LMWH levels because of its predominant anti–factor Xa activity.[58] Peak anti–factor Xa levels occur 3 to 5 hours after a subcutaneous dose of LMWH and are longer in patients with renal insufficiency.[37] An optimal anti–factor Xa level has not been clearly defined; however, a therapeutic range of 0.5 to 1.8 IU/mL has been suggested based on several different studies.[52,59–62] The standard anti–factor Xa activity laboratory study is not a method that can be readily used at the time of a catheterization procedure. In this scenario, a point-of-care test (POCT) may be useful in determining if a patient is therapeutically anticoagulated at time of PCI.[63]

Several POCT methods have been developed. The ELECT (Evaluating Enoxaparin Clotting Times) study used the Rapidpoint ENOX (PharmaNetics, Morrisville, NC) test, which was specific to enoxaparin. This study aimed to determine appropriate therapeutic ranges of anticoagulation, but this POCT method is no longer available.[64,65] The Heptest (Heptest Laboratories, St. Louis, MO) is a clotting assay that is sensitive to both low molecular compounds with exclusive anti–factor Xa activity as well as agents affecting anti–factor IIa. Its correlation with both assays makes it useful when it is necessary to monitor LMWH as well as UFH.[58]

HEMONOX assay (International Technidyne Corporation, Edison, NJ) is another POCT used to monitor the anticoagulation effects of LMWH. Rouby and colleagues[63] found good correlation between HEMONOX and anti-Xa activity levels. This observational study investigated the correlation between HEMONOX clotting times (CTs) and anti-Xa levels in 2 treatment groups: enoxaparin plus GP IIb/IIIa inhibitor and enoxaparin alone. There was a significant increase in HEMONOX CT and anti-Xa levels from baseline (HEMONOX CT <100 seconds correlated with undetectable anti-Xa levels) in all patients. There was less of an increase in both HEMONOX CT as well as anti-Xa levels in the enoxaparin plus GP IIb/IIIa group versus the enoxaparin alone group. The HEMONOX CT for patients receiving enoxaparin alone was $257 \pm 95$ (130–431) seconds versus $207 \pm 74$ (104–386) seconds in the patients receiving enoxaparin plus GP IIb/IIIa inhibitors. This finding corresponded with peak anti-Xa levels of $0.86 \pm 0.11$ (0.69–1.14) U/mL for the enoxaparin alone group and $0.78 \pm 0.12$ (0.61–1.10) U/mL for the enoxaparin plus GP IIb/IIIa group. The changes in HEMONOX CT were proportional the anti-Xa activity levels during PCI. The study also pointed out that regardless of the decline in HEMONOX in the presence of GP IIb/IIIa inhibitors, the anti-Xa levels remained within therapeutic ranges.

Although monitoring is not indicated in all situations, certain populations may be at higher risk of bleeding. The clearance of the anti-Xa effect of LMWH is largely correlated with creatinine clearance ($Cl_{cr}$). Decreased clearance of anti-Xa effects correlates with greater risk for major bleeding events.[66] Monitoring and dosing of different LMWH agents in obese patients has been studied. Anti–factor Xa activity levels increased to appropriate levels when administered based on body weight up to 144 kg for enoxaparin, 190 kg for dalteparin, and 165 kg for tinazaparin.[37] Increased age and history of gastrointestinal bleeding are other groups that have higher risk of major bleeding and may warrant clinical monitoring while using LMWH.[58]

Until there is a universally accepted recommendation for monitoring, the guidelines advocate that additional dosing of LMWH before PCI is dependent on timing of the most recent dose. If the last dose of enoxaparin was less than 8 hours before PCI, then no additional anticoagulation therapy is needed. If the last dose of enoxaparin was between 8 and 12 hours before PCI, it is recommended to give a 0.3 mg/kg bolus of IV enoxaparin at time of PCI. If the last dose of enoxaparin was greater than 12 hours before PCI, then conventional anticoagulation therapy is suggested.[67]

### Reversal

The half-life of LMWH is 3 to 6 hours after subcutaneous administration and, as mentioned before, is longer in patients with kidney disease. A major concern for most clinicians in using LMWH is that there is no proven reversal. Protamine sulfate only partially reverses the effects of LMWH.[68] The reason for its partial effect is that it only neutralizes the anti–factor IIa activity and has little to no effect on the anti-Xa activity. When immediate reversal is needed, it is generally recommended to give 1 mg of protamine sulfate per 100 anti-Xa units of LMWH given in the last 8 hours (where 1 mg of enoxaparin equals 100 anti-Xa units). A second dose of 0.5 mg protamine sulfate per 100 anti-Xa units can be given if bleeding continues. The maximum single dose of protamine sulfate is 50 mg.[69]

### Pentasaccharides (Fondaparinux)

Fondaparinux is a synthetic derivative of the natural pentasaccharide sequence found in heparin. This derivative works through antithrombin to indirectly inhibit factor Xa with greater specificity than UFH and LMWH. Fondaparinux is a short molecule and unable to bridge antithrombin to thrombin; it does not increase rate of thrombin inhibition by antithrombin. Fondaparinux is subcutaneously injected, reaches peak levels in 2 hours, and is excreted in urine, with a half-life of 17 hours in the younger population and ~21 hours in the elderly. Like LMWH, fondaparinux has less binding to other plasma proteins as seen with UFH. Because of its long half-life, bioavailability, and predictable anticoagulant response, it is typically administered once daily without monitoring. Renal insufficiency is a contraindication to its use ($Cl_{cr}$ <30 mL/min).[13,35,37]

A pilot study by Vuillemenot and colleagues[70] suggested that use of fondaparinux during PCI may be considered without significantly worse complication rates compared with historical studies. Since then, subsequent studies have further expanded on its potential. The PENTALYSE (Synthetic Pentasaccharide as an Adjunct to fibrinolysis in ST-elevation Acute Myocardial Infarction) study[71] showed that administration of pentasaccharide inhibiting factor Xa with alteplase may be as safe and effective at revascularizing as UFH. The PENTUA (Pentasaccharide in Unstable Angina) study[72] suggested that fondaparinux may have similar safety and efficacy as enoxaparin when used for treatment of ACS. This study also showed no significant dose responses between different doses of fondaparinux (2.5, 4, 8, and 12 mg once daily). OASIS 5 (Organization to Assess Strategies in Ischemic Syndromes 5)[73] held up the notion that fondaparinux was noninferior to enoxaparin in the subsequent 9-day end point outcomes of death, MI, and refractory ischemia. Also, fondaparinux was superior to enoxaparin in respect to significant reductions in major bleeding at 9 days, deaths at 30 days, and deaths at 180 days. The results from the ASPIRE (Arixtra Study in Percutaneous Coronary Intervention: a Randomized Evaluation) study showed that fondaparinux was just as efficacious and safe as using UFH for patients undergoing elective or urgent PCI, regardless whether or not a GP IIb/IIIa inhibitor was being used. In this trial, fondaparinux was given in 2.5-mg and 5-mg doses. There were no significant differences in bleeding complications between the 2 doses, but there was a trend for lower incidences with the 2.5-mg dose. The procedural success rate was high in all groups, with a slightly better percentage in the higher fondaparinux group: 96.3% for UFH; 96.5% for fondaparinux 2.5 mg; 98.4% for fondaparinux 5 mg.[74] In patients admitted with ST elevation MI (STEMI), OASIS 6[75] also found reductions in death and recurrent infarction without increased risk of bleeding events when using fondaparinux versus control group.

Further pooled analysis into the OASIS 5 and 6 trials supported the reduction in death rates at 6 months. Despite this positive finding, there was higher rate of catheter-related thrombosis in OASIS 5. The OASIS 6 study showed a significantly higher 30-day rate of death or reinfarction when fondaparinux is used alone during primary PCI as part of therapy for STEMI, compared with the UFH group. This risk of catheter-related thrombus with fondaparinux was minimized when UFH (50–60 IU/kg) was given in the catheterization laboratory immediately before PCI.[76] Based on these findings, current guidelines recommend use of additional agents with activity against factor IIa when using fondaparinux for primary PCI.[12,34]

## Monitoring

Monitoring for fondaparinux is not routinely recommended. A fondaparinux-specific anti-Xa assay can be used when needed, but there is no clearly established therapeutic range, unlike LMWH. Peak steady state when using therapeutic doses of fondaparinux (eg, 7.5 mg) should be 1.20 to 1.26 mg/L 3 hours after dosing.[37] There is no POCT available for use during PCI.[13]

## Reversal

Despite the reductions in major bleeding rates identified in previous trials, there remains a concern for bleeding complications, because of the long half-life of fondaparinux. Fondaparinux does not bind to protamine sulfate, unlike UFH and LMWH.[37] Recombinant factor VIIa is recommended for uncontrolled bleeding attributed to fondaparinux. Recombinant factor VIIa is able to overcome thrombin inhibition by fondaparinux and has been shown to normalize the prolongation of aPTT and prothrombin time (PT).[77]

## Direct Thrombin Inhibitors (Bivalirudin, Argatroban)

Use of direct thrombin inhibitors has shown benefit in preventing ischemic complications from PCI.[78,79] Direct thrombin inhibitors do not require antithrombin as a cofactor, unlike UFH, LMWH, and fondaparinux. Direct thrombin inhibitors are able to directly inhibit both circulating thrombin and clot-bound thrombin.[80] They are also more predictable than heparins, because they do not activate platelets (thus are not neutralized by platelet factor 4 when platelets are activated) and do not bind to plasma proteins.[81] Without platelet activation, there is no interaction with platelet factor 4, thus eliminating the possibility of immune-mediated HIT. This situation makes direct thrombin inhibitors a safe alternative to heparin for PCI in patients with HIT.[82] The direct thrombin inhibitors available for use during PCI are bivalirudin and argatroban.

### Bivalirudin

Bivalirudin is a synthetic analogue of hirudin that is slowly cleaved by thrombin and only transiently inhibits thrombin. It has a quick onset of action, achieving therapeutic ACT within 5 minutes, and a short half-life of approximately 25 minutes.

These characteristics contribute to its safe profile, with lower risk of bleeding; thus making it attractive for use during PCI.[80,83]

Bivalirudin has been extensively studied since its development. Studies have shown reduced incidences of bleeding compared with heparin when used as treatment with a thrombolytic agent for acute MI and unstable angina. After being proved as a safe alternative to heparin in the setting of balloon angioplasty, it was later proved to be more efficacious in addition to having lower risk of bleeding.[78,79,84–86] These initial studies of bivalirudin were performed in the era before use of GP IIb/IIIa inhibitors. The REPLACE-2 (The Randomized Evaluation in PCI Linking Angiomax to Reduced Clinical Events) trial[87] tested the safety and efficacy of using bivalirudin with GP IIb/IIIa inhibitors compared with heparin with planned use of GP IIb/IIIa inhibitors during PCI. The results showed that bivalirudin was noninferior to heparin plus a GP IIb/IIIa antagonist and had significantly less bleeding in the bivalirudin group. The ISAR-REACT 4 (Intracoronary Stenting and Antithrombotic Regimen Rapid Early Action for Coronary Treatment) trial[88] showed similar outcomes rates of death, MI or revascularization between bivalirudin and heparin plus GP IIb/IIIa inhibitor groups when used during PCI in patients with NSTEMI. However, the outcomes of the study did show an increased risk of bleeding in the heparin plus GP IIb/IIIa inhibitor group. ACUITY investigators studied the outcomes of treating moderate-risk to high-risk patients with ACS. Groups were divided as follows: UFH or enoxaparin with GP IIb/IIIa inhibitor; bivalirudin with GP IIb/IIIa inhibitor; or bivalirudin alone. Results showed that bivalirudin had similar rates of ischemia whether or not it was used with GP IIb/IIIa inhibitors but had significantly lower rates of bleeding when used alone when compared with the heparin (or enoxaparin) group.[87] This finding was further expanded on by the HORIZONS-AMI (The Harmonizing Outcomes with RevasculariZatiON and Stents in Acute Myocardial Infarction) trial investigators,[89] who compared outcomes of patients with STEMI treated with either bivalirudin alone or heparin plus GP IIb/IIIa inhibitors. In this trial, there was a higher rate of stent thrombosis within 24 hours (1.3% vs 0.3%, $P<.001$) but significantly reduced 30-day mortality (2.1% vs 3.1%, $P = .047$) in the bivalirudin arm. The reduced 30-day event rate was largely in part caused by the significantly lower rate of major bleeding with bivalirudin compared with heparin plus GP IIb/IIIa inhibitors (4.9 vs 8.3%, $P<.001$). This reduction in mortality persisted at the end of 1-year follow-up also (3.4% vs 4.8%, $P = .029$).

Bivalirudin can typically be given immediately before PCI with 0.75 mg/kg IV bolus then 1.75 mg/kg/h continuous infusion. It is renally excreted; however, no adjustments need to be made until $Cl_{cr}$ is less than 30. If $Cl_{cr}$ is 10–29 mL/min, then infusion rate should be decreased to 1 mg/kg/h and decreased to 0.25 mg/kg/h if the patient is on hemodialysis. This regime can be continued for up to 4 hours after the PCI procedure at the discretion of the physician.[90]

### Argatroban

Argatroban is a small, synthetically derived direct thrombin inhibitor that reversibly binds to the active site of thrombin. It has a half-life of approximately 45 minutes; it is metabolized through the liver and may be an attractive agent in the setting of HIT or renal failure.[83] Argatroban has been approved for use during PCI in the setting of HIT based on the Argatroban-216, Argatroban-310, and Argatroban-311 studies.[82] Use of argatroban in combination with thrombolytic therapy has shown better outcomes in terms of TIMI (Thrombolysis in Myocardial Ischemia) III flow on angiography as well as less bleeding when compared with heparin. Results of the ARGAMI pilot and ARGAMI 2 (Argatroban in Acute Myocardial Infarction-2) studies[81] showed comparable end points (mortality, recurrent MI, cardiac failure, interventions for ischemia or ischemic stroke) and a nonsignificantly lower incidence of bleeding in the argatroban group. The low-dose argatroban group studied in ARGAMI 2 showed no evidence of efficacy, and this arm was closed prematurely.

ARG-E04 (Argatroban for Elective Percutaneous Coronary Intervention Trial) was a prospective trial that tested 3 different doses of argatroban compared with UFH. The results showed that argatroban dose-dependently increased ACT levels. It also rapidly and consistently achieved sufficient ACT prolongation to allow for shortened time to initiate PCI compared with patients receiving UFH (ACT target parameter of 250 seconds used for anticoagulation). There were no significant differences in angiographic success rates, composite end points (death, MI, or revascularization) or incidence of bleeding. This study proved that argatroban dose-dependently achieved ACT prolongation more effectively than UFH in patients undergoing elective PCI with dual antiplatelet therapy (ASA and clopidogrel). This study provides evidence that argatroban has a predictable anticoagulant effect and can be used in patients undergoing PCI with dual antiplatelet therapy (only studied with ASA and clopidogrel). Particular settings in which argatroban may be most attractive is in patients with HIT or with renal dysfunction when undergoing PCI.[91]

### Monitoring of direct thrombin inhibitors

Bivalirudin can cause increases in multiple coagulation assays: aPTT, PT, international normalized ratio, and ACT. Routine monitoring is not required with use of bivalirudin but can be performed with ACT. In REPLACE-2,[87] the median ACT 5 minutes after a bolus infusion (0.75 mg/kg) followed by continuous infusion (1.75 mg/kg/h) was 358. If ACT is less than 225 seconds after first bolus, then an additional bivalirudin bolus of 0.3 mg/kg should be given. If ACT is greater than 225 seconds, then no further monitoring is required, because an infusion dose should maintain appropriate ACT levels. Because of the short half-life of bivalirudin (~25 minutes), an ACT is also not required before sheath removal.[90]

Like bivalirudin, argatroban can cause increases in multiple monitoring assays: aPTT, PT, ACT, and ecarin clotting time, which is sensitive only to direct thrombin inhibitors. There seems to be a consistent dose-effect relationship using argatroban, regardless of the assay used. A study evaluating the pharmacokinetic-pharmacodynamic relationship of argatroban[92] showed that in contrast to UFH, argatroban causes a faster response in all coagulation parameters (a quicker increase after initiation and normalization after stopping medication). This study also concluded that ACT is the most appropriate method for monitoring the effect of argatroban in patients undergoing PCI.

Argatroban is given IV with a bolus dose of 350 µg/kg followed by an initial infusion rate of 25 µg/kg/min. ACT should be checked within 10 minutes and can proceed with PCI if ACT is greater than 300 seconds. If ACT is less than 300 seconds, give an additional 150-µg/kg bolus and increase infusion rate to 30 µg/kg/min. If ACT is greater than 450 seconds, decrease infusion rate to 15 µg/kg/min. An ACT level should be obtained within 10 minutes after any change to the infusion rate of argatroban.

### Reversal of direct thrombin inhibitors

There are no specific reversal agents for direct thrombin inhibitors. In normal healthy individuals with normal kidney function, coagulation times return to normal within 1 hour of discontinuing infusion. Recombinant factor VIIa may reduce some of the bleeding effect from these agents. Hemodialysis can remove approximately 25% of bivalirudin or argatroban.[37]

## ANTIPLATELETS

Platelets are a key player in thrombotic events. Once the integrity of normal endothelium has been compromised, platelet adhesion, activation, and aggregation lead to formation of thrombus. Adhesion of platelets to the site of vessel wall injury occurs via von Willebrand factor and other GP cell receptors (GP Ib/IX/V, GP IV, GP VI, GP Ia/IIa). Once platelets start adhering, they become activated, initiating further activation of surrounding platelets through the secretion of platelet granules from agonists (adenosine diphosphate [ADP], collagen, thrombin), synthesis of thromboxane $A_2$ and increased expression of activated GP IIb/IIIa receptors on the platelet surface. The activation also facilitates binding of factors Va and VIIIa. Platelet aggregation occurs via fibrinogen acting as a bridge between GP IIb/IIIa receptors on neighboring platelets. The aggregation of platelets leads to formation of a platelet plug, which becomes further anchored by fibrin mesh developed from the coagulation cascade.[14,93] This important cascade of events leads to serious complications of MIs and strokes. Steps of the cascade can be interrupted by different classes of antiplatelet agents to minimize the risk of arterial thrombosis (**Table 2**). ASA irreversibly inhibits thromboxane $A_2$ by acetylating cyclooxygenase 1 (COX-1). This situation reduces platelet activation and recruitment to site of injury. Thienopyridines (ticlopidine, clopidogrel, prasugrel) and other ADP antagonists (ticagrelor, cangrelor) inhibit P2Y12, a key ADP receptor on the platelet surface. Ticlopidine, clopidogrel, and prasugrel irreversibly inhibit P2Y12, whereas ticagrelor and cangrelor are reversible inhibitors of P2Y12. GP IIb/IIIa inhibitors (abciximab, eptifibatide, tirofiban) inhibit platelet aggregation by preventing fibrinogen and von Willebrand factor from binding to activated GP IIb/IIIa.[35] Antiplatelet therapy is the standard of care not only in patients undergoing PCI but also in the acute and long-term management of ACS.[93-95]

### ASA

ASA has long been recognized for its protective effect of thrombotic occlusive events and its importance in reducing incidence of MIs and strokes. The large meta-analysis performed by the Antithrombotic Trialists' Collaboration showed that ASA reduced the occurrence of death, MI, and stroke.[96] ASA has also been shown to significantly decrease mortalities in the setting of acute STEMI and severe cardiovascular complications in patients undergoing PCI. Since the benefit of ASA was widely established, it is now the standard of

**Table 2**
**Antiplatelets**

| | Mechanism of Action | Time of Onset (Half-Life) | Recommended PCOT | Reversal for Bleeding |
|---|---|---|---|---|
| ASA | Irreversibly inhibits COX-1,2 and thromboxane-$A_2$ | 1–2 h (~3 h for doses ≤325 mg) | None | Platelets, desmopressin |
| Clopidogrel | Thienopyridine; irreversibly blocks P2Y12 receptor | 20%–30% platelet inhibition at 6 h, 300–600 mg (6 h); 50%–60% platelet inhibition at 5–7 d, 50–100 mg | None | Platelets, desmopressin |
| Prasugrel | | <30 min, 60 mg (7 h) | None | Platelets, desmopressin |
| Ticagrelor | Nonthienopyridine; reversibly inhibiting | 41% platelet inhibition <30 min, 180 mg (6–12 h) | None | Platelets, desmopressin |
| Cangrelor | P2Y12 receptors | Rapid onset (3–6 min) | None | Platelets, desmopressin |
| Abciximab | Near irreversible, GP IIb/IIIa inhibition | <10 min (15–30 min) | None | Platelets, desmopressin |
| Eptifibatide | Reversible GP IIb/IIIa inhibition | <60 min (2–3 h) | None | Hemodialysis, platelets, desmopressin |
| Tirofiban | Reversible GP IIb/IIIa inhibition | <30 min (1.5–2 h) | None | Hemodialysis, platelets, desmopressin |

*Abbreviation:* COX, cyclooxygenase.

therapy in clinical practice and routine background therapy when studying possible additive benefits of other agents used in treatment of ACS or during PCI.[14]

Several studies have attempted to define the optimal dose of ASA. An ASA dose of 75 mg achieves complete inactivation of COX-1.[35] When comparing ASA 75 mg/d with high doses up to 1500 mg/d, there has been no proven benefit, but rather there is increased risk of bleeding (particularly gastrointestinal). There is less conclusive evidence on the benefit of doses less than 75 mg.[97–99] In situations in which an immediate antithrombotic event is needed (ie, ACS, ischemic stroke), a higher dose of ASA (160–325 mg) should be given. Current PCI guidelines recommend giving ASA 325 mg at least 2 hours and preferably 24 hours before PCI.[34,96] Low doses of ASA (75–150 mg/d) are recommended for long-term prevention of vascular events in high-risk patients with less risk of bleeding events.[100]

## Monitoring

Although not routinely used in the clinical setting, multiple methods of monitoring platelet function have been developed over time (**Table 3**). These monitoring methods have been developed and studied in the setting of ASA therapy and in the evaluation of bleeding diatheses without antiplatelet therapy. Ideally, platelet monitoring assays would be able to identify whether a patient who suffered an occlusive event (MI or ischemic stroke) while on ASA therapy was caused by treatment failure or treatment resistance, or prospectively identify the risk of a patient suffering severe bleeding, especially in the setting of surgery.

The bleeding time was the initial and still only in vivo test of platelet function. Initially, it was developed as a measure of bleeding diatheses and the influence of platelet count; after decades of broad clinical use, it was subsequently found to not be predictive of clinical bleeding in the setting of surgery or antiplatelet therapy.[101] Several point-of-care antiplatelet assays have been developed and studied in research settings; however, similar to bleeding time, there has been no clinical evidence that shows the clinical benefit of these monitoring methods. Light transmittance aggregometry (LTA) is the historical gold standard of platelet function testing, which has shown a significantly higher risk of thrombotic events in patients with increased aggregation in the setting of ASA therapy. However, this test is labor intensive and technically demanding, preventing its routine application in clinical practice. Simpler, point-of-care devices such as the Verify-Now (Accumetrics, San Diego, CA) ASA assay

**Table 3**
**Overview of the available platelet function assays**

| | Easy to Use | Total Processing Time | Accurate Detection of ASA Effects | Accurate Detection of Clopidogrel Effects | Accurate Detection of GP IIb/IIIa Inhibitor Effects | ASA Results Correlated with Clinical Outcome | Clopidogrel Results Correlated with Clinical Outcome | GP IIb/IIIa Results Correlated with Clinical Outcome |
|---|---|---|---|---|---|---|---|---|
| Light transmission aggregometry | No | 1–2 h | + | + | + | + | + | + |
| Plateletworks (Helena Laboratories, Beaumont, TX) | Yes | 5 min | + | + | + | – | UNK | – |
| PFA-100 (DiaMed, Switzerland) | Yes | 5 min | + | – | + | – | – | ± |
| VerifyNow (Accumetrics, San Diego, CA) | Yes | 2 min | + | + | + | + | UNK | + |
| Impact-R (Siemens Corporation, Germany) | No | 1 h | UNK | + | + | UNK | + | UNK |
| Thrombo-elastography (TEG) | No | Up to 1 h | UNK | + | + | UNK | + | UNK |

*Abbreviations:* –, no; +, yes; UNK, unknown.
*Data from* van Werkum JW, Hackeng CM, Smit JJ, et al. Monitoring antiplatelet therapy with point-of-care platelet function assays: a review of the evidence. Future Cardiol 2008;4:33–55.

have been developed and shown to correlate well with LTA. Studies using the VerifyNow ASA assay found that patients with increased platelet agglutination while receiving ASA had higher increases of cardiac biomarkers (CK-MB, troponin I) when undergoing elective PCI. Unlike the LTA, the VerifyNow ASA assay has less processing time and is easier to use. Despite these findings, there have been no studies to suggest that change of therapy based on point-of-care ASA assays would have a benefit on clinical outcomes or cost efficiency.[93,102,103]

### Reversal

The antiplatelet effect of ASA can last from 5 to 10 days. Rarely does the antiplatelet effect of ASA need to be reversed with the exceptions of intracranial bleeding. However, if bleeding from ASA needs to be reversed immediately, platelet concentrate can be administered, although banked platelets are also functionally diminished. Desmopressin, or DDAVP, can also be used to correct the antiplatelet effect of ASA. Dosing is similar when used for hemophilia or von Willebrand disease: 0.3 μg/kg in 100 mL infused over 30 minutes.[69]

### P2Y12 Inhibitors (Clopidogrel, Prasugrel, Ticagrelor, Cangrelor)

Thienopyridines provide additional antiplatelet therapy to ASA by inhibiting the P2Y12 receptor for ADP on the platelet surface. This additive, and some studies suggest even synergistic, platelet inhibition provides enhanced protection from thrombotic complications during PCI. The role of dual antiplatelet therapy beyond the setting of PCI is less clear and may be agent specific.[98]

### Clopidogrel

Clopidogrel received approval from the US Food and Drug Administration in 1998 after the results of the CAPRIE (Clopidogrel vs Aspirin in Patients at Risk of Ischaemic Events) trial, which compared ASA only versus clopidogrel alone. The clopidogrel group of patients had a statistically significant ($P = .043$) lower risk of MI, ischemic stroke, or vascular death (9.8%) compared with the ASA group (10.7%). This study showed that clopidogrel is a safe and effective alternative to ASA.[104] The first large-scale prospective trial of dual antiplatelet therapy versus ASA alone was the CURE (Clopidogrel in Unstable Angina to Prevent Recurrent Events) trial, which found that when used for patients with unstable angina or NSTEMI, clopidogrel plus ASA reduces ischemic events relative to ASA regardless of the invasive or noninvasive therapy. There was a higher incidence of major bleeding events, with an increased risk of bleeding related to coronary artery bypass graft (CABG) limited to those who went to surgery sooner than 5 days after discontinuing clopidogrel. The subanalysis of the PCI cohort, PCI-CURE, showed that ASA with clopidogrel pretreatment (median 6 days) followed by long-term therapy after PCI had a 31% reduction in cardiovascular death or MI at 30 days and 9 months ($P = .002$) when compared with no pretreatment and short-term dual therapy (4 weeks after PCI). There was no significant difference in major bleeding between the groups.[105] The CREDO (Clopidogrel for the Reduction of Events During Observation) trial[94] studied the benefits of pretreatment and long-term treatment (1 year) with clopidogrel and ASA in the setting of nonurgent PCI. The results showed a 26.9% relative risk reduction for combined incidence of death, MI, or stroke ($P = .02$) at 1 year, although only a trend toward benefit at 30 days as a result of pretreatment. A post hoc analysis of the results suggested that a longer interval between the loading dose of clopidogrel and PCI may further reduce periprocedural thrombotic events. Patients receiving 300 mg clopidogrel at least 10 to 12 hours before PCI experienced a significant reduction in the combined 30-day end point.[106] The current American College of Cardiology/American Heart Association guidelines recommend dual antiplatelet therapy for at least 1 month after bare metal stent placement and at least 1 year after drug-eluting stent placement.[34]

Use of clopidogrel in the setting of acute STEMI treated with a primary noninvasive strategy gained acceptance after the results of the CLARITY-TIMI 28 (Clopidogrel as Adjunctive Reperfusion Therapy - Thrombolysis in Myocardial Infarction 28) and COMMIT (ClOpidogrel and Metoprolol in Myocardial InfarcTion) trials. CLARITY-TIMI 28[107] found the benefit of adding clopidogrel to ASA and fibrinolytic therapy in the treatment of patients with STEMI younger than 75 years. This study used a loading dose of clopidogrel 300 mg followed by 75 mg daily versus placebo, with all patients receiving ASA. The clopidogrel group improved all angiographic outcome measurements and reduced the 30-day odds of composite end point of death, recurrent MI, or recurrent ischemia needing urgent revascularization (14.1%–11.6%, $P = .03$). The COMMIT trial[108] similarly showed a significant ($P = .002$) reduction in death, reinfarction, or stroke in the clopidogrel group (9.2%) compared with placebo (10.1%) when added to ASA for treatment of acute MI. The COMMIT trial did not show an increased risk of bleeding but did not use a loading dose of clopidogrel.

## Prasugrel

Prasugrel is a new thienopyridine that has been proved to be beneficial in the treatment of patients with ACS undergoing PCI. Similar to clopidogrel, prasugrel irreversibly binds to the P2Y12 receptor. Prasugrel is rapidly absorbed and nearly completely activated. In contrast, clopidogrel is more slowly absorbed and only ~15% undergoes metabolic activation.[35] The quick onset of action for prasugrel makes it attractive to use at the time of PCI, especially in the setting of ACS. Prasugrel 60 mg achieves high levels of platelet inhibition by 30 minutes as opposed to clopidogrel, which requires 4 to 6 hours. The duration of platelet inhibition for both clopidogrel and prasugrel lasts for at least 5 to 7 days, because of its irreversible binding of P2Y12 receptors.[109] In patients with ACS scheduled to undergo PCI, TRITON-TIMI 38 (Trial to Assess Improvement in Therapeutic Outcomes by Optimizing Platelet Inhibition with Prasugrel–Thrombolysis in Myocardial Infarction 38)[110] proved prasugrel to be significantly superior to clopidogrel when initiated at 300 mg at the time of PCI in preventing death, MI, ischemic stroke, urgent revascularization, and stent thrombosis (9.9% vs 12.1%, hazard ratio 0.81, $P<.001$). Most benefit seen with prasugrel was seen early and diminished over time. There was a significantly higher risk of major bleeding, including fatal bleeding.

## Ticagrelor

Ticagrelor is a novel nonthienopyridine, reversible P2Y12 inhibitor that has a rapid onset of action within 30 minutes and a peak platelet inhibition within 2 hours. Because of its reversible receptor-binding properties, ticagrelor has a short half-life of 6 to 12 hours and requires twice-daily dosing.[109] The PLATO (PLATelet inhibition and patient Outcomes) investigators[111] showed superiority of ticagrelor compared with clopidogrel in patients with ACS with or without STEMI, all on a background of ASA. Patients in the ticagrelor group had significantly lower rates of death from vascular causes, MI, or stroke without an increase in the rate of major bleeding. The benefits were evident at 30 days and persisted at follow-up after 1 year.

## Cangrelor

Cangrelor is an IV-administered nonthienopyridine that reversibly inhibits the P2Y12 receptor, achieving high levels of platelet inhibition in vitro and ex vivo. It is notable for its rapid onset of action and short half-life (3–6 minutes).[112] Normalization of platelet function occurs within 60 minutes after discontinuing cangrelor. Despite these advantages over the oral P2Y12 inhibitors, cangrelor has not been shown to be superior to placebo or clopidogrel 600 mg when used in patients with ACS or stable angina when given before PCI in terms of reducing composite end points (death, MI, or revascularization).[113,114]

## Monitoring P2Y12 antagonists

Tailored antiplatelet therapy based on platelet reactivity and responsiveness has been theorized to potentially improve outcomes. One theory regarding the concern of antiplatelet resistance is that there is platelet hyperreactivity in the setting of the acute thrombotic event.[115] The GRAVITAS (Gauging Responsiveness with A VerifyNow assay—Impact on Thrombosis And Safety) trial[116] aimed to evaluate whether tailoring clopidogrel after PCI would improve outcomes based on point-of-care platelet function assays. Despite efforts made to identify an accurate and reliable point-of-care assay for P2Y12 inhibitors at time of PCI and for tailored antiplatelet therapy, there is insufficient evidence that point-of-care platelet function testing for P2Y12 inhibitors would be beneficial.[117]

## Reversing P2Y12 antagonists

Bleeding while on dual antiplatelet therapy remains a difficult situation to manage. Patients who have undergone recent stent implantation are still at high risk of stent thrombosis until complete endothelialization occurs. Besides cangrelor, all P2Y12 antagonists require days off therapy before platelet function is normalized. If a decision is made to reverse bleeding induced by P2Y12 inhibitors, it is recommended to administer platelet concentrate. Desmopressin (DDAVP) can also be used to correct the effect on platelet aggregation.[69]

## GP IIb/IIIa Inhibitors (Abciximab, Eptifibatide, Tirofiban)

Vessel trauma by PCI may lead to adhesion, followed by activation and aggregation of platelets. GP IIb/IIIa inhibitors offer additional protection from thrombus formation by preventing platelet aggregation and reducing risk of intracoronary thrombosis.[118] Three GP IIb/IIIa inhibitors are available for use during PCI: abciximab, eptifibatide, and tirofiban. These agents block fibrinogen from binding to GP IIb/IIIa receptors. Meta-analysis of GP IIb/IIIa inhibitors during PCI has shown a 30-day mortality benefit in addition to fewer incidences of nonfatal MI and urgent repeat revascularizations. The strongest data supporting the use of GP IIb/IIIa inhibitors come from trials studying abciximab.[119] The EPILOG (Evaluation in PTCA to improve Long-Term Outcome with

Abciximab GP IIb/IIIa Blockade) and EPISTENT (Evaluation of Platelet IIb/IIIa Inhibitor for Stenting) trials showed sustained benefits in these end points up to 1 year, whereas EPIC (Evaluation of 7E3 for the Prevention of Ischemic Complication) reported benefit at 3 years.[10,120–122] Select populations may especially experience a protective effect during PCI with GP IIb/IIIa inhibitors including high-risk ACS, diabetics, and patients with chronic kidney disease.[123]

### Abciximab
The first developed GP IIb/IIIa inhibitor, abciximab, is a human-murine chimeric monoclonal antibody with high affinity for GP IIb/IIIa receptors, leading to near-irreversible inhibition, although its plasma half-life is short. Approximately 50% platelet inhibition remains 24 hours after discontinuing abciximab. The EPIC trial was the first study to show its clinical benefit during PCI, with a 35% reduction in rate of primary end points (death from any cause, nonfatal MI, CABG, or repeat PCI for acute ischemia; placement of intra-aortic balloon pump to relieve refractory ischemia); a 10% reduction was observed after abciximab bolus alone.[120,124] The breakthrough trials EPIC, EPILOG, and EPISTENT showed that treatment with abciximab and UFH (abciximab continued after procedure) was superior to UFH alone in reducing major adverse cardiac events after PCI without significant differences in bleeding complications between the treatment groups.[120–122]

Abciximab administration as part of treatment in patients undergoing PCI for STEMI can improve outcomes. The ADMIRAL (Abciximab before Direct angioplasty and stenting in Myocardial Infarction Regarding Acute and Long-term follow-up) trial randomized patients to receive abciximab plus stenting or placebo plus stenting for treatment of STEMI. The abciximab group had improved coronary patency and left ventricular function with fewer incidences of reinfarction and recurrent ischemia. Although not statistically significant, there remained a mortality benefit from 30 days to 3 years after PCI treatment of STEMI in patients who received abciximab. In this 3-year follow-up period, there was a 30% relative risk reduction of the composite end point of death and MI.[125] The CADILLAC (The Controlled Abciximab and Device Investigation to Lower Late Angioplasty COmplications) trial randomized 2082 patients presenting with STEMI to treatment groups of balloon angioplasty alone, balloon angioplasty plus abciximab, stenting alone, and stenting plus abciximab. Use of abciximab showed significant improvements (P<.001) in the primary end point: a composite of death, reinfarction, stroke, and ischemia-driven target vessel

revascularization. The end point occurrences were balloon angioplasty alone 20%, balloon angioplasty plus abciximab 16.5%, bare metal stent alone 11.5%, and bare metal stent plus abciximab 10.2%. These end points were mainly driven by revascularization, because there were no significant differences between the groups treated with stents in terms of rates of death, stroke, or reinfarction.[126] Antoniucci and colleagues[127] evaluated whether treatment of STEMI with bare metal stenting with or without abciximab would have a difference of outcomes. Composite of death, reinfarction, target vessel revascularization, and stroke at 1 month was the primary end point. The event rate was significantly reduced in the group treated with bare metal stent plus abciximab compared with the group treated with bare metal stent (4.5% vs 10.5% respectively, P = .023). There was also smaller infarct size on technetium-99m sestamibi scintigraphy at 1 month. Beyond treatment of STEMI, abciximab is recommended for treatment in high-risk patients undergoing PCI. Abciximab is not recommended for low-risk patients or patients receiving noninvasive treatment of ACS.[128,129]

### Eptifibatide and tirofiban
There has been less convincing evidence for eptifibatide and tirofiban. Both are smaller molecules than abciximab. Eptifibatide is a synthetic heptapeptide (<1000 Da) that reversibly binds to a β subunit of GP IIb/IIIa receptor, causing platelet inhibition correlating to the plasma level of the drug. It is metabolized by the kidneys, with half-life of ~2 to 3 hours. Tirofiban is a tyrosine derivative nonpeptide that is metabolized by the biliary system (30%–40%) and primarily excreted by the kidneys (60%–70%). Tirofiban half-life is ~1.5 to 2 hours.[130]

The IMPACT-II (Integrilin to Minimize Platelet Aggregation and Coronary Thrombosis-II) trial randomized patients undergoing elective, urgent, or emergency PCI to 1 of 3 treatment arms: placebo, eptifibatide 135 μg/kg bolus followed by 0.5 μg/kg/min infusion, or eptifibatide 135 μg/kg bolus followed by 0.75 μg/kg/min infusion. The composite end point was death, MI, unplanned surgical or repeat percutaneous revascularization, or coronary stent implantation for abrupt closure. The primary safety end point was major bleeding. There were nonstatistically significant reduced rates of composite end point in the eptifibatide groups compared with placebo without significant differences between the eptifibatide groups. There was no significant increase in bleeding with eptifibatide.[131] It has been hypothesized that the doses used in this trial may have been insufficient to provide adequate platelet inhibition.[14] The PURSUIT (Platelet Glycoprotein IIb/IIIa in Unstable Angina: Receptor Suppression Using Integrilin Therapy) trial investigators[132] used higher doses of eptifibatide in patients with ACS, but without STEMI. Those patients undergoing early PCI (<72 hours) treated with eptifibatide 180 μg/kg bolus followed by 2.0 μg/kg/min infusion had a significantly lower 30-day composite end point of death or nonfatal MI compared with the placebo group (11.6% vs 16.7, $P$ = .01). The ESPRIT (Enhanced Suppression of Platelet IIb/IIIa Receptor with Integrilin Therapy) trial[133] randomized 2064 patients undergoing PCI to receive a high-dose regimen of eptifibatide or placebo. The eptifibatide group received 2 boluses of 180 μg/kg administered 10 minutes apart followed by 2.0 μg/kg/min infusion for 18 to 24 hours. Both groups also received ASA, heparin, and a thienopyridine as part of standard therapy. The primary end point was composite of death, MI, urgent target vessel revascularization, and thrombotic bailout GP IIb/IIIa inhibitor therapy within 48 hours after randomization. The trial was terminated early because of significant efficacy findings: primary end point reduced from 10.5% in placebo group to 6.6% in eptifibatide group ($P$ = .0015). Although not frequent, major bleeding was more often with eptifibatide (1.3% vs 0.4%, $P$ = .027). This trial proved that pretreatment with eptifibatide as a GP IIb/IIIa inhibitor significantly reduces ischemic complications during PCI. This trial has provided the recommended eptifibatide dosing in current guidelines for patients with STEMI undergoing PCI treated with UFH.[34]

Tirofiban showed a nonsignificant trend toward reduced end points of death, MI, or revascularization in the balloon angioplasty-based RESTORE (Randomized Efficacy Study of Tirofiban for Outcomes and REstenosis) trial[134]; however, there was also higher rates of major bleeding compared with placebo. Later, the PRISM-PLUS (Platelet Receptor Inhibition in Ischemic Syndrome Management in Patients Limited by Unstable Signs and Symptoms) investigators[135] showed greater efficacy in patients with ACS treated with UFH plus tirofiban over UFH alone. The end point of death, MI, or refractory ischemia was reduced from 17.9% in the UFH alone group to 12.9% in the UFH plus tirofiban at 30 days ($P$ = .004). Subgroup analysis of patients who underwent PCI provided further evidence that the combination of tirofiban with UFH compared with UFH alone reduced the end point incidence from 15.3% to 8.8% (risk ratio, 0.55; confidence interval [CI] 95%, 0.32–0.94). In the TARGET (Do Tirofiban and ReoPro Give Similar Efficacy Trial?) trial,[136] tirofiban was compared

head-to-head against abciximab in a noninferiority trial in ~5000 patients undergoing PCI. Tirofiban was found to be inferior to abciximab. Subsequent studies suggested that the dose of tirofiban studied in TARGET was too low. Smaller trials have studied higher doses, with encouraging results.[137] Current PCI guidelines recommend administration of GP IIb/IIIa inhibitors with UFH in high-risk ACS when not treated with bivalirudin and not adequately pretreated with a thienopyridine.[34]

### Monitoring

Although the GP IIb/IIIa inhibitors are beneficial during PCI, there is a narrow therapeutic window. As shown by earlier studies, the GP IIb/IIIa inhibitors have been associated with higher risk of bleeding and thrombocytopenia (especially abciximab). Because of pharmacologic property differences between the GP IIb/IIIa inhibitors, there will be variability. For example, plasma level of eptifibatide correlates closely with platelet inhibition, whereas abciximab does not provide good correlation because it has high affinity to the receptors and is cleared rapidly from the plasma.[138] This finding again brings up the important topic of how to best tailor GP IIb/IIIa therapy not only during PCI but also the value in determining return of normal platelet function. The theoretic benefit of tailored therapy based on monitoring is met with real-life limitations, such as technical experience, expensive equipment and transferring what is found in vitro to the present clinical situation. It remains to be proved whether an assay can provide the most reliable results that can be translated into clinical practice.[139]

Light transmission aggregometry has historically been the gold standard of platelet function testing. Although it is based on the fibrinogen-GP IIb/IIIa aggregation, its poor reproducibility between laboratories, long sampling time, and labor-intensive requirements make it less appealing during PCI.

The best study correlating the efficiency of platelet inhibition through GP IIb/IIIa inhibitors with clinical outcomes was the GOLD multicenter study (AU-Assessing Ultegra multicenter study).[140] This study used the point-of-care Ultegra rapid platelet function assay (RPFA). The Ultegra RPFA, now known as the VerifyNow assay, is able to provide a simple and rapid functional means of monitoring of GP IIb/IIIa inhibitors with results that correlate well with aggregometry and receptor-binding assays. The primary end point was major adverse cardiac events: death, MI, or urgent target vessel revascularization in hospital or within 7 days of PCI. A total of 485 patients were evaluated for the primary end point. Most patients in this study received abciximab (84%); the others received tirofiban (9%) and eptifibatide (7%). The dosing regimens for each medication were based on previously described trials showing potential benefit of their use in PCI. Platelet inhibition was achieved at high percentages in the initial 10 minutes (96% ± 9%), 1 hour (95% ± 8%) and 8 hours (91% ± 11%) after initiating therapy. However, at 24 hours, the mean inhibition decreased to 73% ± 20%, with wide variability. The patients in the lowest quartile of platelet inhibition (<95%) at 10 minutes after GP IIb/IIIa bolus had a substantially higher incidence (14.4%) of major adverse cardiac events compared with those with more than 95% platelet inhibition (6.4%, $P = .006$). This study confirmed that higher incidences of major adverse cardiac events are correlated with lower levels of platelet inhibition. The study did not find a correlation between level of platelet inhibition and major bleeding complications when using the RPFA. However, an increased procedural ACT correlated with major bleeding.[141,142]

### Reversing GP IIb/IIIa inhibitors

Platelet monitoring for return to normal function may be helpful in nonemergent situations; however, immediate reversal is warranted when major bleeding occurs or emergency CABG is needed. The pharmacodynamic properties of each GP IIb/IIIa inhibitor affect how they can be reversed in emergent situations. No direct antidote is available for any of the 3 available GP IIb/IIIa receptor antagonists.

Despite the long dissociation half-life from GP IIb/IIIa receptors of abciximab (up to 6–12 hours), it has a short plasma half-life (15–30 minutes), meaning little of the medication remains in the plasma once discontinued. Platelet transfusion after discontinuing abciximab decreases the platelet receptor occupancy, which is related to platelet function inhibition. Platelet transfusion leads to redistribution of abciximab from platelets saturated with the medication to transfused cells. This situation causes a dilution of bound GP IIb/IIIa receptors by abciximab, with little hemostatic defect.[143,144] In addition to platelet transfusion, administration of desmopressin (DDAVP) may also have an additive effect in normalizing platelet function after GP IIb/IIIa inhibition.[97]

Platelet transfusion is ineffective for the smaller molecule GP IIb/IIIa inhibitors eptifibatide and tirofiban, because of their high plasma levels. The pharmacokinetic effect is dose dependent. The biological half-life is ~2.5 hours for these agents based on the adjusted dosing for $Cl_{cr}$.[124] Reversal of the antiplatelet effect from eptifibatide and tirofiban occurs within 2 to 4 hours after discontinuation. It is typically considered safe to proceed with surgical procedure after the allotted time.[144] In patients with advanced renal insufficiency in whom the time to reversal may be longer, hemodialysis can hasten the reversal of platelet inhibition induced by these agents.[145,146]

## SUMMARY

Anticoagulation and antiplatelet therapy have been heavily studied since their inception. Although certain agents have advantages and disadvantages relative to others, there will likely never be a 1 size fits all medication. The art of practicing medicine requires tailoring therapy based on the unique patient being treated. This statement holds true during PCI as well, in which certain presentations or preexisting comorbidities make 1 anticoagulant or antiplatelet agent better than another. It is important to understand not only which therapies are available but also what other tools are needed to achieve optimal use of the medication. Understanding how to monitor (if possible) the therapy being delivered and, if needed, how to manage the emergency situations (major bleeding) is as crucial as the technical skills required during PCI.

## REFERENCES

1. Kolandaivelu K, Swaminathan R, Gibson WJ, et al. Stent thrombogenicity early in high-risk interventional settings is driven by stent design and deployment and protected by polymer-drug coatings/clinical perspective. Circulation 2011;123: 1400–9.

2. Van Belle E, Tio FO, Couffinhal T, et al. Stent endothelialization. Circulation 1997;95:438–48.

3. Xie Y, Takano M, Murakami D, et al. Comparison of neointimal coverage by optical coherence tomography of a sirolimus-eluting stent versus a bare-metal stent three months after implantation. Am J Cardiol 2008;102:27–31.

4. Levine GN, Bates ER, Blankenship JC, et al. ACCF/AHA/SCAI Guideline for Percutaneous Coronary Intervention: a report of the American College of Cardiology Foundation/American Heart Association Task Force on Practice Guidelines and the Society for Cardiovascular Angiography and Interventions. Circulation 2011;124:e574–651.

5. Popma JJ, Weitz J, Bittl JA, et al. Antithrombotic therapy in patients undergoing coronary angioplasty. Chest 1998;114:728S–41S.

6. Gruntzig A. Transluminal dilatation of coronary-artery stenosis. Lancet 1978;1:263.

7. Gruntzig A, Hirzel H, Goebel N, et al. Percutaneous transluminal dilatation of chronic coronary

stenoses. First experiences. Schweiz Med Wochenschr 1978;108:1721–3 [in German].

8. Fischman DL, Leon MB, Baim DS, et al. A randomized comparison of coronary-stent placement and balloon angioplasty in the treatment of coronary artery disease. N Engl J Med 1994;331:496–501.

9. Serruys PW, Jaegere P, Kiemeneij F, et al. A comparison of balloon-expandable-stent implantation with balloon angioplasty in patients with coronary artery disease. N Engl J Med 1994;331:489–95.

10. Harding SA, Walters DL, Palacios IF, et al. Adjunctive pharmacotherapy for coronary stenting. Curr Opin Cardiol 2001;16:293–9.

11. Hochholzer W, Wiviott SD, Antman EM, et al. Predictors of bleeding and time dependence of association of bleeding with mortality/clinical perspective. Circulation 2011;123:2681–9.

12. Rao SV, Ohman EM. Anticoagulant therapy for percutaneous coronary intervention. Circ Cardiovasc Interv 2010;3:80–8.

13. O'Neill BP, Shaw ES, Cohen MG. Anticoagulation in percutaneous coronary intervention. Intervent Cardiol 2010;2:559–77.

14. Garg R, Uretsky BF, Lev EI. Anti-platelet and antithrombotic approaches in patients undergoing percutaneous coronary intervention. Catheter Cardiovasc Interv 2007;70:388–406.

15. Hirsh JA, Sonia S, Halperin JL, et al. Guide to anticoagulant therapy: heparin: a statement for healthcare professionals from the American Heart Association. Circulation 2001;103:2994–3018.

16. Cohen M, Adams PC, Parry G, et al. Combination antithrombotic therapy in unstable rest angina and non-Q-wave infarction in nonprior aspirin users: primary end points analysis from the ATACS Trial. Antithrombotic Therapy in Acute Coronary Syndromes Research Group. Circulation 1994;89:81–8.

17. Oler AW, Mary A, Oler JG, et al. Adding heparin to aspirin reduces the incidence of myocardial infarction and death in patients with unstable angina: a meta-analysis. JAMA 1996;276:811–5.

18. Neri Serneri GG, Rovelli F, Gensini GF, et al. Effectiveness of low-dose heparin in prevention of myocardial reinfarction. Lancet 1987;1:937–42.

19. Li Y, Rha SW, Chen K, et al. Low-molecular-weight heparin versus unfractionated heparin in acute ST-segment elevation myocardial infarction patients undergoing primary percutaneous coronary intervention with drug-eluting stents. Am Heart J 2010;159:684–690.e1.

20. Montalescot G, Collet JP, Lison L, et al. Effects of various anticoagulant treatments on von Willebrand factor release in unstable angina. J Am Coll Cardiol 2000;36:110–4.

21. de Feyter PJ, van den Brand M, Laarman GJ, et al. Acute coronary artery occlusion during and after percutaneous transluminal coronary angioplasty: frequency, prediction, clinical course, management, and follow-up. Circulation 1991;83:927–36.

22. Young E, Prins M, Levine MN, et al. Heparin binding to plasma proteins, an important mechanism for heparin resistance. Thromb Haemost 1992;67:639–43.

23. Marciniak E. Factor-Xa inactivation by antithrombin. 3. Evidence for biological stabilization of factor Xa by factor V-phospholipid complex. Br J Haematol 1973;24:391–400.

24. Hirsh J, Warkentin TE, Raschke R, et al. Heparin and low-molecular-weight heparin: mechanisms of action, pharmacokinetics, dosing considerations, monitoring, efficacy, and safety. Chest 1998;114:489S–510S.

25. Xiao Z, Theroux P. Platelet activation with unfractionated heparin at therapeutic concentrations and comparisons with a low-molecular-weight heparin and with a direct thrombin inhibitor. Circulation 1998;97:251–6.

26. D'Angelo A, Seveso MP, D'Angelo SV, et al. Effect of clot-detection methods and reagents on activated partial thromboplastin time (APTT). Implications in heparin monitoring by APTT. Am J Clin Pathol 1990;94:297–306.

27. McGarry TF Jr, Gottlieb RS, Morganroth J, et al. The relationship of anticoagulation level and complications after successful percutaneous transluminal coronary angioplasty. Am Heart J 1992;123:1445–51.

28. Ferguson JJ, Dougherty KG, Gaos CM, et al. Relation between procedural activated coagulation time and outcome after percutaneous transluminal coronary angioplasty. J Am Coll Cardiol 1994;23:1061–5.

29. Narins CR, Hillegass WB Jr, Nelson CL, et al. Relation between activated clotting time during angioplasty and abrupt closure. Circulation 1996;93:667–71.

30. Chew DP, Bhatt DL, Lincoff AM, et al. Defining the optimal activated clotting time during percutaneous coronary intervention: aggregate results from 6 randomized, controlled trials. Circulation 2001;103:961–6.

31. Brener SJ, Moliterno DJ, Lincoff AM, et al. Relationship between activated clotting time and ischemic or hemorrhagic complications: analysis of 4 recent randomized clinical trials of percutaneous coronary intervention. Circulation 2004;110:994–8.

32. Montalescot G, Cohen M, Salette G, et al. Impact of anticoagulation levels on outcomes in patients undergoing elective percutaneous coronary intervention: insights from the STEEPLE trial. Eur Heart J 2008;29:462–71.

33. Doherty TM, Shavelle RM, French WJ. Reproducibility and variability of activated clotting time measurements in the cardiac catheterization laboratory. Catheter Cardiovasc Interv 2005;65:330–7.

34. Levine GN, Bates ER, Blankenship JC, et al. 2011 ACCF/AHA/SCAI Guideline for Percutaneous Coronary Intervention. A report of the American College of Cardiology Foundation/American Heart Association Task Force on Practice Guidelines and the Society for Cardiovascular Angiography and Interventions. J Am Coll Cardiol 2011;58: e44–122.

35. Weitz JI. Blood coagulation and anticoagulant, fibrinolytic, and antiplatelet drugs. In: Brunton LL, Chabner BA, Knollmann BC, editors. Goodman & Gilman's the pharmacological basis of therapeutics. 12th edition. New York: McGraw-Hill; 2011. Available at: http://www.accessmedicine.com/content.aspx?aID=16668944. Accessed January 10, 2013.

36. Wakefield TW, Hantler CB, Wrobleski SK, et al. Effects of differing rates of protamine reversal of heparin anticoagulation. Surgery 1996;119:123–8.

37. Garcia DA, Baglin TP, Weitz JI, et al. Parenteral anticoagulants: antithrombotic therapy and prevention of thrombosis, 9th ed: American College of Chest Physicians evidence-based clinical practice guidelines. Chest 2012;141:e24S–43S.

38. Harenberg J. Pharmacology of low molecular weight heparins. Semin Thromb Hemost 1990;16: 12–8.

39. Kadakia RA, Baimeedi SR, Ferguson JJ. Low-molecular-weight heparins in the cardiac catheterization laboratory. Tex Heart Inst J 2004;31:72–83.

40. Kleinschmidt K, Charles R. Pharmacology of low molecular weight heparins. Emerg Med Clin North Am 2001;19:1025–49.

41. Antman EM. The search for replacements for unfractionated heparin. Circulation 2001;103:2310–4.

42. Weitz JI. Low-molecular-weight heparins. N Engl J Med 1997;337:688–99.

43. Ferguson JJ, Antman EM, Bates ER, et al. Combining enoxaparin and glycoprotein IIb/IIIa antagonists for the treatment of acute coronary syndromes: final results of the National Investigators Collaborating on Enoxaparin-3 (NICE-3) study. Am Heart J 2003;146:628–34.

44. Gurfinkel EP, Manos EJ, Mejaíl RI, et al. Low molecular weight heparin versus regular heparin or aspirin in the treatment of unstable angina and silent ischemia. J Am Coll Cardiol 1995;26:313–8.

45. Klein W, Buchwald A, Hillis SE, et al. Comparison of low-molecular-weight heparin with unfractionated heparin acutely and with placebo for 6 weeks in the management of unstable coronary artery disease: Fragmin in Unstable Coronary Artery Disease Study (FRIC). Circulation 1997;96:61–8.

46. Cohen M, Demers C, Gurfinkel EP, et al. A comparison of low-molecular-weight heparin with unfractionated heparin for unstable coronary artery disease. N Engl J Med 1997;337:447–52.

47. Antman EM. The Thrombolysis in Myocardial Infarction B Trial Investigators. TIMI 11B. Enoxaparin versus unfractionated heparin for unstable angina or non-Q-wave myocardial infarction: a double-blind, placebo-controlled, parallel-group, multicenter trial. Rationale, study design, and methods. Am Heart J 1998;135:S353–60.

48. Antman EM, Cohen M, Radley D, et al. Assessment of the treatment effect of enoxaparin for unstable angina/non-Q-wave myocardial infarction: TIMI 11B-ESSENCE meta-analysis. Circulation 1999; 100:1602–8.

49. SYNERGY Trial Investigators. Enoxaparin vs unfractionated heparin in high-risk patients with non-ST-segment elevation acute coronary syndromes managed with an intended early invasive strategy: primary results of the SYNERGY randomized trial. JAMA 2004;292:45–54.

50. Drouet L, Bal dit Sollier C, Martin J. Adding intravenous unfractionated heparin to standard enoxaparin causes excessive anticoagulation not detected by activated clotting time: results of the STACK-on to ENOXaparin (STACKENOX) study. Am Heart J 2009;158:177–84.

51. Montalescot G, White HD, Gallo R, et al. Enoxaparin versus unfractionated heparin in elective percutaneous coronary intervention. N Engl J Med 2006;355:1006–17.

52. Kereiakes DJ, Grines C, Fry E, et al. Enoxaparin and abciximab adjunctive pharmacotherapy during percutaneous coronary intervention. J Invasive Cardiol 2001;13:272–8.

53. Bhatt DL, Lee BI, Casterella PJ, et al. Safety of concomitant therapy with eptifibatide and enoxaparin in patients undergoing percutaneous coronary intervention: results of the coronary revascularization using integrilin and single bolus enoxaparin study. J Am Coll Cardiol 2003;41:20–5.

54. Dumaine R, Borentain M, Bertel O, et al. Intravenous low-molecular-weight heparins compared with unfractionated heparin in percutaneous coronary intervention: quantitative review of randomized trials. Arch Intern Med 2007;167:2423–30.

55. Gallo R, Steinhubl SR, White HD, et al, for the STEEPLE Investigators. Impact of anticoagulation regimens on sheath management and bleeding in patients undergoing elective percutaneous coronary intervention in the STEEPLE trial. Catheter Cardiovasc Interv 2009;73:319–25.

56. Henry TD, Satran D, Knox LL, et al. Are activated clotting times helpful in the management of anticoagulation with subcutaneous low-molecular-weight heparin? Am Heart J 2001;142:590–3.

57. Linkins L, Julian JA, Rischke J, et al. In vitro comparison of the effect of heparin, enoxaparin and fondaparinux on tests of coagulation. Thromb Res 2002;107:241–4.

58. Abbate R, Gori AM, Farsi A, et al. Monitoring of low-molecular-weight heparins in cardiovascular disease. Am J Cardiol 1998;82:33L–6L.

59. Choussat R, Montalescot G, Collet JP, et al. A unique, low dose of intravenous enoxaparin in elective percutaneous coronary intervention. J Am Coll Cardiol 2002;40:1943–50.

60. Collet JP, Montalescot G, Lison L, et al. Percutaneous coronary intervention after subcutaneous enoxaparin pretreatment in patients with unstable angina pectoris. Circulation 2001;103:658–63.

61. Montalescot G, Collet JP, Tanguy ML, et al. Anti-Xa activity relates to survival and efficacy in unselected acute coronary syndrome patients treated with enoxaparin. Circulation 2004;110:392–8.

62. Martin JL, Fry ET, Sanderink GC, et al. Reliable anticoagulation with enoxaparin in patients undergoing percutaneous coronary intervention: the pharmacokinetics of enoxaparin in PCI (PEPCI) study. Catheter Cardiovasc Interv 2004;61:163–70.

63. Rouby SE, Cohen M, Gonzales A, et al. Point-of-care monitoring of enoxaparin in the presence of GpIIb/IIIa combined therapy during percutaneous coronary interventions. Point Care 2005;4:30–5.

64. Moliterno DJ, Mukherjee D. Applications of monitoring platelet glycoprotein IIb/IIIa antagonism and low molecular weight heparins in cardiovascular medicine. Am Heart J 2000;140:S136–42.

65. Moliterno DJ, Hermiller JB, Kereiakes DJ, et al. A novel point-of-care enoxaparin monitor for use during percutaneous coronary intervention. Results of the Evaluating Enoxaparin Clotting Times (ELECT) Study. J Am Coll Cardiol 2003;42:1132–9.

66. Lim W, Dentali F, Eikelboom JW, et al. Meta-analysis: low-molecular-weight heparin and bleeding in patients with severe renal insufficiency. Ann Intern Med 2006;144:673–84.

67. Popma JJ, Berger P, Ohman EM, et al. Antithrombotic therapy during percutaneous coronary intervention: the Seventh ACCP Conference on Antithrombotic and Thrombolytic Therapy. Chest 2004;126:576S–99S.

68. Lindblad B, Borgstrom A, Wakefield TW, et al. Protamine reversal of anticoagulation achieved with a low molecular weight heparin. The effects on eicosanoids, clotting and complement factors. Thromb Res 1987;48:31–40.

69. Levi M, Eerenberg E, Kamphuisen PW. Bleeding risk and reversal strategies for old and new anticoagulants and antiplatelet agents. J Thromb Haemost 2011;9:1705–12.

70. Vuillemenot A, Schiele F, Meneveau N, et al. Efficacy of a synthetic pentasaccharide, a pure factor Xa inhibitor, as an antithrombotic agent–a pilot study in the setting of coronary angioplasty. Thromb Haemost 1999;81:214–20.

71. Coussement PK, Bassand JP, Convens C, et al. A synthetic factor-Xa inhibitor (ORG31540/SR9017A) as an adjunct to fibrinolysis in acute myocardial infarction. The PENTALYSE study. Eur Heart J 2001;22:1716–24.

72. Simoons ML, Bobbink IW, Boland J, et al. A dose-finding study of fondaparinux in patients with non-ST-segment elevation acute coronary syndromes: the Pentasaccharide in Unstable Angina (PENTUA) Study. J Am Coll Cardiol 2004;43:2183–90.

73. Fifth Organization to Assess Strategies in Acute Ischemic Syndromes Investigators, Yusuf S, Mehta SR, et al. Comparison of fondaparinux and enoxaparin in acute coronary syndromes. N Engl J Med 2006;354:1464–76.

74. Mehta SR, Steg PG, Granger CB, et al. Randomized, blinded trial comparing fondaparinux with unfractionated heparin in patients undergoing contemporary percutaneous coronary intervention: Arixtra Study in Percutaneous Coronary Intervention: a Randomized Evaluation (ASPIRE) Pilot Trial. Circulation 2005;111:1390–7.

75. Yusuf S, Mehta SR, Chrolavicius S, et al. Effects of fondaparinux on mortality and reinfarction in patients with acute ST-segment elevation myocardial infarction: the OASIS-6 randomized trial. JAMA 2006;295:1519–30.

76. Mehta SR, Boden WE, Eikelboom JW, et al. Antithrombotic therapy with fondaparinux in relation to interventional management strategy in patients with ST- and non-ST-segment elevation acute coronary syndromes: an individual patient-level combined analysis of the Fifth and Sixth Organization to Assess Strategies in Ischemic Syndromes (OASIS 5 and 6) randomized trials. Circulation 2008;118:2038–46.

77. Bijsterveld NR, Moons AH, Boekholdt SM, et al. Ability of recombinant factor VIIa to reverse the anticoagulant effect of the pentasaccharide fondaparinux in healthy volunteers. Circulation 2002;106:2550–4.

78. Topol EJ, Bonan R, Jewitt D, et al. Use of a direct antithrombin, hirulog, in place of heparin during coronary angioplasty. Circulation 1993;87:1622–9.

79. Bittl JA, Strony J, Brinker JA, et al. Treatment with bivalirudin (hirulog) as compared with heparin during coronary angioplasty for unstable or postinfarction angina. N Engl J Med 1995;333:764–9.

80. Bates SM, Weitz JI. The mechanism of action of thrombin inhibitors. J Invasive Cardiol 2000;12:27F–32F.

81. Wong C, White HD. Direct antithrombins: mechanisms, trials, and role in contemporary interventional medicine. Am J Cardiovasc Drugs 2007; 7:249–57.

82. Lewis BE, Hursting MJ. Direct thrombin inhibition during percutaneous coronary intervention in patients with heparin-induced thrombocytopenia. Expert Rev Cardiovasc Ther 2007;5:57–68.

83. Lee CJ, Ansell JE. Direct thrombin inhibitors. Br J Clin Pharmacol 2011;72:581–92.

84. White HD, Aylward PE, Frey MJ, et al. Randomized, double-blind comparison of hirulog versus heparin in patients receiving streptokinase and aspirin for acute myocardial infarction (HERO). Circulation 1997;96:2155–61.

85. Kong DF, Topol EJ, Bittl JA, et al. Clinical outcomes of bivalirudin for ischemic heart disease. Circulation 1999;100:2049–53.

86. Bittl JA, Chaitman BR, Feit F, et al. Bivalirudin versus heparin during coronary angioplasty for unstable or postinfarction angina: final report reanalysis of the Bivalirudin Angioplasty Study. Am Heart J 2001;142:952–9.

87. Lincoff A, Michael Bittl JA, Harrington RA, et al. Bivalirudin and provisional glycoprotein IIb/IIIa blockade compared with heparin and planned glycoprotein IIb/IIIa blockade during percutaneous coronary intervention: REPLACE-2 Randomized Trial. JAMA 2003;289:853–63.

88. Kastrati A, Neumann F, Schulz S, et al. Abciximab and heparin versus bivalirudin for non–ST-elevation myocardial infarction. N Engl J Med 2011;365: 1980–9.

89. Stone GW, Witzenbichler B, Guagliumi G, et al. Bivalirudin during primary PCI in acute myocardial infarction. N Engl J Med 2008;358:2218–30.

90. Moen MD, Keating GM, Wellington K. Bivalirudin: a review of its use in patients undergoing percutaneous coronary intervention. Drugs 2005;65: 1869–91.

91. Rossig L, Genth-Zotz S, Rau M, et al. Argatroban for elective percutaneous coronary intervention: the ARG-E04 multi-center study. Int J Cardiol 2011;148:214–9.

92. Akimoto K, Klinkhardt U, Zeiher A, et al. Anticoagulation with argatroban for elective percutaneous coronary intervention: population pharmacokinetics and pharmacokinetic-pharmacodynamic relationship of coagulation parameters. J Clin Pharmacol 2011;51:805–18.

93. van Werkum JW, Hackeng CM, Smit JJ, et al. Monitoring antiplatelet therapy with point-of-care platelet function assays: a review of the evidence. Future Cardiol 2008;4:33–55.

94. Steinhubl SR, Berger PB, Mann JT 3rd, et al, CREDO Investigators, Clopidogrel for the Reduction of Events During Observation. Early and sustained dual oral antiplatelet therapy following percutaneous coronary intervention: a randomized controlled trial. JAMA 2002;288:2411–20.

95. Becker R, Meade T, Berger P, et al. The primary and secondary prevention of coronary artery disease: American College of Chest Physicians evidence-based clinical practice guidelines (8th edition). Chest 2008;133:776S–814S.

96. Antithrombotic Trialists' Collaboration. Collaborative meta-analysis of randomised trials of antiplatelet therapy for prevention of death, myocardial infarction, and stroke in high risk patients. BMJ 2002;324:71–86.

97. Reiter RA, Jilma B. Platelets and new antiplatelet drugs. Therapy 2005;2:465–502.

98. Holmes DR Jr, Kereiakes DJ, Kleiman NS, et al. Combining antiplatelet and anticoagulant therapies. J Am Coll Cardiol 2009;54:95–109.

99. Campbell CL, Smyth S, Montalescot G, et al. Aspirin dose for the prevention of cardiovascular disease: a systematic review. JAMA 2007;297: 2018–24.

100. Peters RJ, Mehta SR, Fox KA, et al. Effects of aspirin dose when used alone or in combination with clopidogrel in patients with acute coronary syndromes: observations from the Clopidogrel in Unstable angina to prevent Recurrent Events (CURE) study. Circulation 2003;108:1682–7.

101. Steinhubl SR. Historical observations on the discovery of platelets, platelet function testing and the first antiplatelet agent. Curr Drug Targets 2011;12:1792–804.

102. Polena S, Zazzali KM, Shaikh HD, et al. Comparison of a point-of-care platelet function testing to light transmission aggregometry in patients undergoing percutaneous coronary intervention pretreated with aspirin and clopidogrel. Point Care 2011;10:35–9.

103. Hezard N, TessierMarteau A, Macchi L. New insight in antiplatelet therapy monitoring in cardiovascular patients: from aspirin to thienopyridine. Cardiovasc Hematol Disord Drug Targets 2010; 10:224–33.

104. CAPRIE Steering Committee. A randomised, blinded, trial of clopidogrel versus aspirin in patients at risk of ischaemic events (CAPRIE). Lancet 1996;348:1329–39.

105. Mehta SR, Yusuf S, Peters RJ, et al. Effects of pretreatment with clopidogrel and aspirin followed by long-term therapy in patients undergoing percutaneous coronary intervention: the PCI-CURE study. Lancet 2002;359:527–33.

106. Steinhubl SR, Berger PB, Brennan DM, et al, CREDO Investigators. Optimal timing for the initiation of pre-treatment with 300 mg clopidogrel

before percutaneous coronary intervention. J Am Coll Cardiol 2006;47:939–43.

107. Sabatine MS, Cannon CP, Gibson CM, et al. Addition of clopidogrel to aspirin and fibrinolytic therapy for myocardial infarction with ST-segment elevation. N Engl J Med 2005;352:1179–89.

108. Chen ZM, Jiang LX, Chen YP, et al. Addition of clopidogrel to aspirin in 45,852 patients with acute myocardial infarction: randomised placebo-controlled trial. Lancet 2005;366:1607–21.

109. Wong YW, Prakash R, Chew DP. Antiplatelet therapy in percutaneous coronary intervention: recent advances in oral antiplatelet agents. Curr Opin Cardiol 2010;25:305–11.

110. Antman EM, Wiviott SD, Murphy SA, et al. Early and late benefits of prasugrel in patients with acute coronary syndromes undergoing percutaneous coronary intervention: a TRITON-TIMI 38 (TRial to Assess Improvement in Therapeutic Outcomes by Optimizing Platelet InhibitioN with Prasugrel-Thrombolysis In Myocardial Infarction) analysis. J Am Coll Cardiol 2008;51:2028–33.

111. Wallentin L, Becker RC, Budaj A, et al. Ticagrelor versus clopidogrel in patients with acute coronary syndromes. N Engl J Med 2009;361:1045–57.

112. Akers WS, Oh JJ, Oestreich JH, et al. Pharmacokinetics and pharmacodynamics of a bolus and infusion of cangrelor: a direct, parenteral P2Y12 receptor antagonist. J Clin Pharmacol 2010;50: 27–35.

113. Bhatt DL, Lincoff AM, Gibson CM, et al. Intravenous platelet blockade with cangrelor during PCI. N Engl J Med 2009;361:2330–41.

114. Harrington RA, Stone GW, McNulty S, et al. Platelet inhibition with cangrelor in patients undergoing PCI. N Engl J Med 2009;361:2318–29.

115. Linden MD, Tran H, Woods R, et al. High platelet reactivity and antiplatelet therapy resistance. Semin Thromb Hemost 2012;38:200–12.

116. Price MJ, Berger PB, Angiolillo DJ, et al. Evaluation of individualized clopidogrel therapy after drug-eluting stent implantation in patients with high residual platelet reactivity: Design and rationale of the GRAVITAS trial. Am Heart J 2009;157: 818–824.e1.

117. Steinhubl SR. The illusion of "optimal" platelet inhibition. JACC Cardiovasc Interv 2012;5:278–80.

118. Dangas G, Colombo A. Platelet glycoprotein IIb/IIIa antagonists in percutaneous coronary revascularization. Am Heart J 1999;138:S16–23.

119. Kong DF, Hasselblad V, Harrington RA, et al. Meta-analysis of survival with platelet glycoprotein IIb/IIIa antagonists for percutaneous coronary interventions. Am J Cardiol 2003;92:651–5.

120. The EPIC Investigators. Use of a monoclonal antibody directed against the platelet glycoprotein IIb/IIIa receptor in high-risk coronary angioplasty. The EPIC Investigation. N Engl J Med 1994;330: 956–61.

121. The EPILOG Investigators. Platelet glycoprotein IIb/IIIa receptor blockade and low-dose heparin during percutaneous coronary revascularization. The EPILOG Investigators. N Engl J Med 1997; 336:1689–96.

122. The EPISTENT Investigators. Randomised placebo-controlled and balloon-angioplasty-controlled trial to assess safety of coronary stenting with use of platelet glycoprotein-IIb/IIIa blockade. The EPISTENT Investigators. Evaluation of Platelet IIb/IIIa Inhibitor for Stenting. Lancet 1998;352:87–92.

123. Zimarino M, De Caterina R. Glycoprotein IIb-IIIa antagonists in non-ST elevation acute coronary syndromes and percutaneous interventions: from pharmacology to individual patient's therapy: part 1: the evidence of benefit. J Cardiovasc Pharmacol 2004;43:325–32.

124. Nguyen CM, Harrington RA. Glycoprotein IIb/IIIa receptor antagonists: a comparative review of their use in percutaneous coronary intervention. Am J Cardiovasc Drugs 2003;3:423–36.

125. The ADMIRAL Investigators. Three-year duration of benefit from abciximab in patients receiving stents for acute myocardial infarction in the randomized double-blind ADMIRAL study. Eur Heart J 2005; 26:2520–3.

126. Stone GW, Grines CL, Cox DA, et al. Comparison of angioplasty with stenting, with or without abciximab, in acute myocardial infarction. N Engl J Med 2002;346:957–66.

127. Antoniucci D, Rodriguez A, Hempel A, et al. A randomized trial comparing primary infarct artery stenting with or without abciximab in acute myocardial infarction. J Am Coll Cardiol 2003;42: 1879–85.

128. The GUSTO IV-ACS Investigators. Effect of glycoprotein IIb/IIIa receptor blocker abciximab on outcome in patients with acute coronary syndromes without early coronary revascularisation: the GUSTO IV-ACS randomised trial. Lancet 2001;357:1915–24.

129. Kastrati A, Mehilli J, Neumann F, et al. Abciximab in patients with acute coronary syndromes undergoing percutaneous coronary intervention after clopidogrel pretreatment: the ISAR-REACT 2 Randomized Trial. JAMA 2006;295:1531–8.

130. Koutouzis M, Grip L. Glycoprotein IIb/IIIa inhibitors during percutaneous coronary interventions. Intervent Cardiol 2010;2:301–18.

131. The IMPACT-II Investigators. Randomised placebo-controlled trial of effect of eptifibatide on complications of percutaneous coronary intervention: IMPACT-II. Integrilin to Minimise Platelet Aggregation and Coronary Thrombosis-II. Lancet 1997; 349:1422–8.

132. The PURSUIT Trial Investigators. Inhibition of platelet glycoprotein IIb/IIIa with eptifibatide in patients with acute coronary syndromes. N Engl J Med 1998;339:436–43.

133. The ESPRIT Investigators. Novel dosing regimen of eptifibatide in planned coronary stent implantation (ESPRIT): a randomised, placebo-controlled trial. Lancet 2000;356:2037–44.

134. The RESTORE Investigators. Effects of platelet glycoprotein IIb/IIIa blockade with tirofiban on adverse cardiac events in patients with unstable angina or acute myocardial infarction undergoing coronary angioplasty. Circulation 1997;96: 1445–53.

135. The Platelet Receptor Inhibition in Ischemic Syndrome Management in Patients Limited by Unstable Signs and SYmptoms (PRISM-PLUS) Study Investigators. Inhibition of the Platelet Glycoprotein IIb/IIIa Receptor with Tirofiban in Unstable Angina and Non-Q-Qave Myocardial Infarction. N Engl J Med 1998;338:1488–97.

136. Topol EJ, Moliterno DJ, Herrmann HC, et al. Comparison of two platelet glycoprotein IIb/IIIa inhibitors, tirofiban and abciximab, for the prevention of ischemic events with percutaneous coronary revascularization. N Engl J Med 2001;344:1888–94.

137. Moliterno DJ, TENACITY Steering Committee and Investigators. A randomized two-by-two comparison of high-dose bolus tirofiban versus abciximab and unfractionated heparin versus bivalirudin during percutaneous coronary revascularization and stent placement: the tirofiban evaluation of novel dosing versus abciximab with clopidogrel and inhibition of thrombin (TENACITY) study trial. Catheter Cardiovasc Interv 2011;77:1001–9.

138. Warltier DC, Kam PC, Egan MK. Platelet glycoprotein IIb/IIIa antagonists: pharmacology and clinical developments. Anesthesiology 2002;96:1237–49.

139. Coller BS. Monitoring platelet GP IIb/IIIa antagonist therapy. Circulation 1998;97:5–9.

140. Wheeler GL, Braden GA, Steinhubl SR, et al. The Ultegra rapid platelet-function assay: comparison to standard platelet function assays in patients undergoing percutaneous coronary intervention with abciximab therapy. Am Heart J 2002;143: 602–11.

141. Steinhubl SR, Talley J, David Braden GA, et al. Point-of-care measured platelet inhibition correlates with a reduced risk of an adverse cardiac event after percutaneous coronary intervention: results of the GOLD (AU-Assessing Ultegra) multicenter study. Circulation 2001;103:2572–8.

142. Tamberella M, Bhatt D, Chew D, et al. Relation of platelet inactivation with intravenous glycoprotein IIb/IIIa antagonists to major bleeding (from the GOLD study). Am J Cardiol 2002;89:1429–31.

143. Mascelli M, Lance E, Damaraju L, et al. Pharmacodynamic profile of short-term abciximab treatment demonstrates prolonged platelet inhibition with gradual recovery from GP IIb/IIIa receptor blockade. Circulation 1998;97:1680–8.

144. Tcheng J. Clinical challenges of platelet glycoprotein IIb/IIIa receptor inhibitor therapy: bleeding, reversal, thrombocytopenia, and retreatment. Am Heart J 2000;139:s38–45.

145. Schroeder WS, Gandhi PJ. Emergency management of hemorrhagic complications in the era of glycoprotein IIb/IIIa receptor antagonists, clopidogrel, low molecular weight heparin, and third-generation fibrinolytic agents. Curr Cardiol Rep 2003;5:310–7.

146. Sperling RT, Pinto DS, Ho KK, et al. Platelet glycoprotein IIb/IIIa inhibition with eptifibatide: prolongation of inhibition of aggregation in acute renal failure and reversal with hemodialysis. Catheter Cardiovasc Interv 2003;59:459–62.

# Vasoactive and Antiarrhythmic Drugs During Percutaneous Coronary Intervention

Bimmer E. Claessen, MD, PhD*, José P.S. Henriques, MD, PhD

## KEYWORDS

- Percutaneous coronary intervention • Adjunct pharmacology • Drug discontinuation
- Periprocedural myocardial infarction • Vasodilators • Antiarrhythmics

## KEY POINTS

- Procedural sedation is used to create a state of depressed consciousness with the ability to respond purposefully to verbal commands.
- Vasoactive drugs, such as nitric oxide donors, adenosine, and calcium-channel blockers (either alone or as a "cocktail"), are used to facilitate standardized vessel measurements, achieve maximal hyperemia, or to treat no-reflow.
- Several drugs, such as nonsteroidal anti-inflammatory drugs, diuretics, angiotensin-converting enzyme inhibitors, aminoglycoside antibiotics, and metformin, should be discontinued 24 to 48 hours before percutaneous coronary intervention and restarted 48 hours after percutaneous coronary intervention after assessment of renal function.

## INTRODUCTION

Patients undergoing percutaneous coronary intervention (PCI) are administered a large variety of pharmacologic agents during this procedure. In addition to antithrombotic drugs to minimize the risk of thrombotic complications of the mechanical intervention performed during PCI, patients are often administered sedatives, analgesics, vasodilators, and antiarrhythmic agents. Sedative and analgesic drugs are used to increase patient well-being during the procedure. Vasodilators can be administered for a variety of indications (eg, to facilitate standardized and accurate vessel size measurements, treatment of the no-reflow phenomenon after PCI, treatment of arterial spasm during PCI, or inducing maximal hyperemia to facilitate measurement of fractional flow reserve [FFR]). Antiarrhythmic drugs are indicated for recurrent ventricular fibrillation or ventricular tachycardia or to prevent ventricular extrasystoles during ventriculography. Moreover, several drugs should be interrupted before coronary angiography or PCI, such as metformin and angiotensin-converting enzyme inhibitors. These various drugs are discussed in further detail in this review article.

## VASODILATORS: MOST COMMONLY USED VASODILATING AGENTS

Several medications, such as nitroglycerine, verapamil, and adenosine, are frequently used during PCI to achieve vasodilation. Nitroglycerin was discovered by Asciano Sobrero in 1847, who first noted a violent headache after administering a small quantity of nitroglycerine on his tongue.[1] He also discovered its explosive properties and was badly scarred on the face after a nitroglycerine

Department of Cardiology, Academic Medical Center, University of Amsterdam, Meibergdreef 9, 1105 AZ, Amsterdam, The Netherlands
* Corresponding author. Department of Cardiology, Academic Medical Center, University of Amsterdam, Room B2-213, Meibergdreef 9, 1105 AZ, Amsterdam, The Netherlands.
*E-mail address:* BimmerClaessen@gmail.com

Intervent Cardiol Clin 2 (2013) 665–670
http://dx.doi.org/10.1016/j.iccl.2013.06.002
2211-7458/13/$ – see front matter © 2013 Elsevier Inc. All rights reserved.

explosion. Nitroglycerine (glycerine trinitrate) is an organic nitrate that releases nitric oxide (NO) through an enzymatic reaction.[2] Nitroglycerine causes vasodilation without a reduction in blood pressure in doses up to 200 μg. However, when doses exceeding 250 μg are administered, hypotension may result without a further increase in coronary vasodilation.[3] Direct NO donors, such as nitroprusside and molsidomine, release NO directly without the need for activation by molecular metabolism.[4,5]

Verapamil, a calcium channel blocker, is considered a class IV antiarrhythmic agent. Verapamil has negative chronotropic effects by decreasing the electrical impulse conduction in the atrioventricular (AV) node, where there is a high concentration of calcium channels.[6] By blocking calcium channels in the smooth muscle of coronary arteries, verapamil also induces vasodilation.[7] Because of the different mechanisms by which verapamil and nitroglycerin cause coronary artery vasodilation, they are often combined and administered together as an intracoronary "cocktail." Because of its negative chronotropic properties, verapamil is contraindicated in patients with severe bradycardia. Furthermore, verapamil is contraindicated in patients with left ventricular dysfunction due to its negative inotropic properties. Diltiazem, another calcium channel blocker, has stronger vasodilating and weaker negative chronotropic effects compared with verapamil.[8]

Adenosine is a purine nucleoside that can bind to purinergic receptors in different cell types. Vasodilation results by binding to adenosine type 2A ($A_{2a}$) receptors in vascular smooth muscle cells. Moreover, adenosine inhibits calcium entry into the cell through L-type calcium channels, which are present in vascular smooth muscle cells and also in the sinoatrial node and the atrioventricular node, resulting in negative chronotropic and dromotropic effects.[9] Adenosine is used to induce hyperemia to assess accurately the severity of intermediate coronary artery stenoses by FFR.[10] Adenosine can be administered by both intracoronary or intravenous infusion. Intravenous adenosine is usually administered as a continuous infusion of 140 μg/kg/min, achieving a peak effect in approximately 1 minute, and the effect will wear off 1 minute after stopping the infusion. In the case of an intermediate FFR measurement, the dose can be increased to 180 μg/kg/min. Important side effects of adenosine include bradycardia, hypotension, and bronchospasm. Intracoronary adenosine requires lower doses (bolus infusion of 15–50 μg) and has fewer side effects. However, intracoronary adenosine may induce suboptimal hyperemia in a small

proportion of patients (8%).[11] A recent study by Leone and colleagues[12] compared intracoronary infusion of incremental boluses of adenosine (ranging from 60 to 600 μg) and intravenous infusion of adenosine (140 μg/kg/min) in 45 patients with 50 intermediate stenoses. This study suggested that only a high dose of intracoronary adenosine (600 μg) yielded similar FFR values compared with intravenous adenosine. In this study, the use of high-dose intracoronary adenosine was not associated with a higher rate of unwanted side effects.

## VASODILATORS IN THE TREATMENT OF NO-REFLOW

The no-reflow phenomenon may describe vasospasm and downstream embolization of debris during PCI or suboptimal reperfusion of an infarct artery attributed to endothelial injury in addition to embolization and vasospasm.[13] Most studies investigating the utility of vasoactive drugs to treat or prevent no-reflow have been conducted in the setting of PCI for acute coronary syndromes. Typically, greater effectiveness is realized if these agents are administered in the culprit distal vascular bed through an infusion microcatheter rather than when they are given intravenously or via the guiding catheter that is sitting at the ostium of the coronary artery. A recent meta-analysis of 3821 patients from 10 randomized controlled trials undergoing PCI for acute coronary syndromes investigated whether adjunct therapy with adenosine was associated with a reduction in no-reflow and subsequently clinical outcomes.[14] Compared with placebo, adenosine was significantly associated with a reduction of postprocedural no-reflow with an odds ratio of 0.25 (95% confidence interval 0.08–0.73, $P = .01$). However, adenosine failed to reduce mortality, reinfarction, symptoms of heart failure, and ST-segment resolution. Nicorandil and nitroprusside have also been associated with improved coronary flow,[15,16] again without a benefit in terms of hard clinical endpoints. Therefore, these agents are not commonly used in everyday clinical practice. The administration of an intracoronary vasodilator to treat PCI-related no reflow carries a class IIa recommendation with a level of evidence B in the current interventional guidelines.[13]

## VASODILATORS IN THE TREATMENT OF ARTERIAL SPASM—RADIAL ARTERY SPASM

Transradial vascular access is rapidly becoming the standard of care for coronary angiography and percutaneous PCI. Compared with the transfemoral approach, transradial access is associated with reduced bleeding complications, early ambulation, reduced procedural cost, and potentially a reduction in mortality in patients undergoing PCI for ST-segment elevation myocardial infarction.[17] However, radial artery spasm (RAS) causes reduced success rates and patient discomfort during cardiac catheterization via the radial approach in approximately 10% of patients.[18] Risk factors for the development of RAS include smaller diameter radial arteries, female gender, larger sheath size, and operator inexperience.[19] RAS can be prevented and treated by using intra-arterial nitroglycerin or a cocktail of vasodilating agents (ie, 100 μg nitroglycerine with 1.25 mg of verapamil).[20]

## ANTIARRHYTHMIC DRUGS IN PCI

Ischemia or pain during PCI results in an increased sympathoadrenal tone, which may induce an increase in heart rate, blood pressure, and myocardial contractility, resulting in increased oxygen demand. β-Blockers decrease myocardial oxygen demand by lowering heart rate and blood pressure.[21] Several animal studies have shown that the administration of β-blockers can reduce myocardial injury in animal models of myocardial infarction.[22,23] Moreover, clinical studies established that the administration of intracoronary β-blockers during PCI may reduce adverse clinical events and myocardial injury after PCI.[24–26] However, intracoronary β-blockers during PCI are currently not routinely administered.

Other anti-arrhythmic drugs are sporadically used during PCI. Lidocaine, a class Ib antiarrhythmic drug, acts by blocking the rapid influx of sodium ions during the depolarization of cardiac myocytes. Class Ib antiarrhythmics primarily affect the His-Purkinje system and are used to treat ventricular tachycardias. Ventricular extrasystoles occur frequently during left ventriculography. Sporadically, sustained ventricular tachycardia may ensue. A bolus of intravenous lidocaine can be injected to stop the ventricular tachycardia.

## PERIPROCEDURAL SEDATION

Periprocedural sedation is applied to achieve a minimally depressed state of consciousness in which the patient is able to respond to verbal comments while minimizing the risk of a compromised airway.[27] Usually, benzodiazepines are used to achieve conscious sedation. Benzodiazepines, such as midazolam, diazepam, and oxazepam, have sedative, hypnotic, muscle relaxant, and anxiolytic effects by selectively enhancing the inhibitory activity of γ-aminobutyric acid (GABA) by binding to the benzodiazepine site of the $GABA_a$ receptor in the central nervous system.[28] Anterograde amnesia can sometimes be a welcome side effect of benzodiazepines, causing patients to forget any unpleasantness during the procedure.

When using procedural sedation, one should always be prepared to react to the probability that a level of sedation deeper than desired is induced. For this reason, current guidelines recommend that level of consciousness, respiratory rate, blood pressure, and oxygen saturation should be monitored.[13] In addition, catheterization laboratories should be outfitted with oxygen and suction ports and a resuscitation cart. Other, less frequently used drugs used for periprocedural sedation include the opioid, fentanyl, and the hypnotic, propofol.[13] **Table 1** shows an overview of commonly used short-acting drugs used in periprocedural sedation.

## WHICH DRUGS SHOULD BE DISCONTINUED

Drugs that should be stopped before PCI are summarized in **Table 2**.

The use of contrast agents in PCI can lead to contrast-induced acute kidney injury (CI-AKI), which is associated with prolonged hospital stay. CI-AKI is an infrequent complication in nondiabetic patients with normal renal function (~2%).[29] However, CI-AKI has been reported to occur in up to 50% of patients with diabetic nephropathy and a mean serum creatinine of 5.9 mg/dl.[30] Several studies have reported an association between CI-AKI and an increased incidence of myocardial

**Table 1**
**Overview of short-acting drugs used in periprocedural sedation**

| Class | Drugs | Effects | Onset | Duration | Reversal Agents |
|---|---|---|---|---|---|
| Benzodiazepines | Midazolam | Sedative, anxiolytic | 2–3 min | 45–60 min | Flumazenil |
| Opioids | Fentanyl | Analgesic | 3–5 min | 30–60 min | Anexate |
| Other | Propofol | Sedative, anxiolytic | <1 min | 5–15 min | None |

**Table 2**
**Drugs that should be stopped before PCI**

| Class | Drugs | Reason to Discontinue |
|-------|-------|----------------------|
| Diuretics | Furosemide, bumetanide, hydrochlorothiazide, chlorthalidone, etc | May cause prerenal kidney injury |
| Angiotensin-converting enzyme inhibitors | Captopril, enalapril, ramipril, lisinopril, etc | May cause prerenal kidney injury |
| Nonsteroidal anti-inflammatory drugs | Ibuprofen, Diclofenac, naproxen, etc | May cause prerenal kidney injury |
| Aminoglycoside antibiotics | Gentamicin, amikacin, tobramycin, etc | Nephrotoxicity by inhibiting protein synthesis in renal cells |
| Biguanides | Metformin | Increased risk of lactate acidosis |

infarction, target vessel revascularization, and death after PCI.[31,32] Currently, the mechanism causing CI-AKI is incompletely understood, but direct cytotoxicity of iodinated contrast agents and disturbances in renal hemodynamics have been identified to be contributing factors.[33]

Patients undergoing PCI will often use medication that is associated with an increased risk of CI-AKI, such as diuretics, nonsteroidal anti-inflammatory drugs, and angiotensin-converting enzyme inhibitors (ACEI). These drugs are associated with prerenal kidney insufficiency and are routinely discontinued 24 to 48 hours before PCI and restarted after 24 to 48 hours after PCI. However, no clinical trials have ever investigated whether discontinuation of angiotensin-converting enzyme inhibitors or diuretics is associated with reduction in CI-AKI and subsequently a reduction in clinical outcome. Interestingly, it was once thought that prophylactic treatment with diuretics during PCI could prevent CI-AKI by inducing and maintaining diuresis and blocking of the oxygen-demanding active ionic transport processes in the loop of Henle. Solomon and colleagues[34] randomized 78 patients with chronic renal insufficiency who underwent cardiac angiography to receive saline alone, saline plus mannitol, or saline plus furosemide during a period of 12 hours before and 12 hours after angiography. The incidence of CI-AKI, defined as a rise in serum creatinine of 0.5 mg/dl within 48 hours after angiography, was 11%, 28%, and 40% in the saline, mannitol, and furosemide groups, respectively ($P = .05$). Prehydration with saline became the standard of care after the publication of this landmark trial.

Metformin, an anti-diabetic agent from the class of biguanides, is associated with the incidence of potentially lethal lactate acidosis.[35] The risk of lactate acidosis is increased in patients with acute renal insufficiency; therefore, metformin is usually discontinued 24 to 38 hours after PCI and restarted 48 hours after the procedure after renal function has been assessed.

## HIGH-DOSE STATIN TREATMENT TO REDUCE THE RISK OF PERIPROCEDURAL MYOCARDIAL INFARCTION

Periprocedural myocardial injury, assessed by a rise in cardiac biomarkers after PCI, remains a common complication. Pretreatment with high doses of hydroxymethyl-glutaryl-CoA reductase inhibitors, commonly known as statins, has been shown to reduce the incidence of periprocedural myocardial injury in several trials. A study by Pasceri and colleagues[36] randomized 153 patients with chronic stable angina undergoing elective PCI to pretreatment with atorvastatin 40 mg once daily versus placebo. In this study, the detection of cardiac biomarkers above the upper limit of normal was significantly reduced with statin pretreatment compared with placebo (20% vs 48% for troponin I, $P = .0004$). A single loading dose of 80 mg atorvastatin or 40 mg rosuvastatin has also been found to reduce periprocedural myocardial injury.[37,38] A small number of other studies and meta-analyses have confirmed the protective effects of statin pretreatment before PCI.[39,40] The exact mechanism by which statins reduce peri-procedural myocardial injury is not well understood. These effects of statins occur before significant lipid lowering has occurred; therefore, it is hypothesized that pleitropic effects of statins, such as anti-inflammatory effects, a reduction in oxidative stress, or improvement of endothelial function, are involved. Additional data have been emerging, suggesting a possible benefit of statins in the prevention of post-PCI AKI; these data are not detailed here as they are still not widely accepted as a practice standard.

## SUMMARY

A large number of adjunct drugs are used during PCI for a variety of indications. This review focused on the use of sedative, vasoactive, antiarrhythmic, and risk-factor-modifying drugs during PCI. Moreover, an overview was provided detailing which drugs should be interrupted before PCI.

## REFERENCES

1. Marsh N, Marsh A. A short history of nitroglycerine and nitric oxide in pharmacology and physiology. Clin Exp Pharmacol Physiol 2000;27:313–9.
2. Mayer B, Beretta M. The enigma of nitroglycerin bioactivation and nitrate tolerance: news, views and troubles. Br J Pharmacol 2008;155:170–84.
3. Jost S, Nolte CW, Sturm M, et al. How to standardize vasomotor tone in serial studies based on quantitation of coronary dimensions? Int J Cardiovasc Imaging 1998;14:357–72.
4. Ignarro LJ, Lippton H, Edwards JC, et al. Mechanism of vascular smooth muscle relaxation by organic nitrates, nitrites, nitroprusside and nitric oxide: evidence for the involvement of s-nitrosothiols as active intermediates. J Pharmacol Exp Ther 1981; 218:739–49.
5. Rosenkranz B, Winkelmann BR, Parnham MJ. Clinical pharmacokinetics of molsidomine. Clin Pharm 1996;30:372–84.
6. Katz AM. Calcium channel diversity in the cardiovascular system. J Am Coll Cardiol 1996;28:522–9.
7. Braun LT. Calcium channel blockers for the treatment of coronary artery spasm: rationale, effects, and nursing responsibilities. Heart Lung 1983;12: 226–32.
8. Fugit MD, Rubal BJ, Donovan DJ. Effects of intracoronary nicardipine, diltiazem and verapamil on coronary blood flow. J Invasive Cardiol 2000;12:80–5.
9. Martynyuk AE, Kane KA, Cobbe SM, et al. Role of nitric oxide, cyclic GMP and superoxide in inhibition by adenosine of calcium current in rabbit atrioventricular nodal cells. Cardiovasc Res 1997;34:360–7.
10. Park SJ, Ahn JM, Kang SJ. Paradigm shift to functional angioplasty: new insights for fractional flow reserve- and intravascular ultrasound-guided percutaneous coronary intervention. Circulation 2011;124: 951–7.
11. Jeremias A, Whitbourn RJ, Filardo SD, et al. Adequacy of intracoronary versus intravenous adenosine-induced maximal coronary hyperemia for fractional flow reserve measurements. Am Heart J 2000;140:651–7.
12. Leone AM, Porto I, De Caterina AR, et al. Maximal hyperemia in the assessment of fractional flow reserve: intracoronary adenosine versus intracoronary sodium nitroprusside versus intravenous adenosine: the NASCI (Nitroprussiato versus Adenosina nelle Stenosi Coronariche Intermedie) study. JACC Cardiovasc Interv 2012;5:402–8.
13. Levine GN, Bates ER, Blankenship JC, et al. 2011 ACCF/AHA/SCAI Guideline for Percutaneous Coronary Intervention. A report of the American College of Cardiology Foundation/American Heart Association Task Force on Practice Guidelines and the Society for Cardiovascular Angiography and Interventions. J Am Coll Cardiol 2011;58:e44–122.
14. Navarese EP, Buffon A, Andreotti F, et al. Adenosine improves post-procedural coronary flow but not clinical outcomes in patients with acute coronary syndrome: a meta-analysis of randomized trials. Atherosclerosis 2012;222:1–7.
15. Ito H, Taniyama Y, Iwakura K, et al. Intravenous nicorandil can preserve microvascular integrity and myocardial viability in patients with reperfused anterior wall myocardial infarction. J Am Coll Cardiol 1999;33:654–60.
16. Amit G, Cafri C, Yaroslavtsev S, et al. Intracoronary nitroprusside for the prevention of the no-reflow phenomenon after primary percutaneous coronary intervention in acute myocardial infarction. A randomized, double-blind, placebo-controlled clinical trial. Am Heart J 2006;152:887.e1–14.
17. Romagnoli E, Biondi-Zoccai G, Sciahbasi A, et al. Radial versus femoral randomized investigation in st-segment elevation acute coronary syndrome: the rifle-steacs (radial versus femoral randomized investigation in ST-elevation acute coronary syndrome) study. J Am Coll Cardiol 2012;60:2481–9.
18. Gorgulu S, Norgaz T, Karaahmet T, et al. Incidence and predictors of radial artery spasm at the beginning of a transradial coronary procedure. J Interv Cardiol 2013;26:208–13.
19. Kiemeneij F. Prevention and management of radial artery spasm. J Invasive Cardiol 2006;18:159–60.
20. Ho HH, Jafary FH, Ong PJ. Radial artery spasm during transradial cardiac catheterization and percutaneous coronary intervention: incidence, predisposing factors, prevention, and management. Cardiovasc Revasc Med 2012;13:193–5.
21. Viskin S, Kitzis I, Lev E, et al. Treatment with beta-adrenergic blocking agents after myocardial infarction: from randomized trials to clinical practice. J Am Coll Cardiol 1995;25:1327–32.
22. Miura M, Thomas R, Ganz W, et al. The effect of delay in propranolol administration on reduction of myocardial infarct size after experimental coronary artery occlusion in dogs. Circulation 1979;59:1148–57.
23. Reimer KA, Rasmussen MM, Jennings RB. Reduction by propranolol of myocardial necrosis following

temporary coronary artery occlusion in dogs. Circ Res 1973;33:353–63.

24. Zalewski A, Goldberg S, Dervan JP, et al. Myocardial protection during transient coronary artery occlusion in man: beneficial effects of regional beta-adrenergic blockade. Circulation 1986;73:734–9.

25. Sharma SK, Kini A, Marmur JD, et al. Cardioprotective effect of prior beta-blocker therapy in reducing creatine kinase-mb elevation after coronary intervention: benefit is extended to improvement in intermediate-term survival. Circulation 2000;102:166–72.

26. Park H, Otani H, Noda T, et al. Intracoronary followed by intravenous administration of the short-acting beta-blocker landiolol prevents myocardial injury in the face of elective percutaneous coronary intervention. Int J Cardiol 2012. [Epub ahead of print].

27. Venneman I, Lamy M. Sedation, analgesia and anesthesia for interventional radiological procedures in adults. Part II. Recommendations for interventional radiologists. JBR-BTR 2000;83:116–20.

28. Barnard EA, Skolnick P, Olsen RW, et al. International union of pharmacology. Xv. Subtypes of gamma-aminobutyric acida receptors: classification on the basis of subunit structure and receptor function. Pharmacol Rev 1998;50:291–313.

29. Rihal CS, Textor SC, Grill DE, et al. Incidence and prognostic importance of acute renal failure after percutaneous coronary intervention. Circulation 2002;105:2259–64.

30. Manske CL, Sprafka JM, Strony JT, et al. Contrast nephropathy in azotemic diabetic patients undergoing coronary angiography. Am J Med 1990;89:615–20.

31. Lindsay J, Apple S, Pinnow EE, et al. Percutaneous coronary intervention-associated nephropathy foreshadows increased risk of late adverse events in patients with normal baseline serum creatinine. Catheter Cardiovasc Interv 2003;59:338–43.

32. Lindsay J, Canos DA, Apple S, et al. Causes of acute renal dysfunction after percutaneous coronary intervention and comparison of late mortality rates with postprocedure rise of creatine kinase-mb versus rise of serum creatinine. Am J Cardiol 2004; 94:786–9.

33. Heyman SN, Rosen S, Brezis M. Radiocontrast nephropathy: a paradigm for the synergism between toxic and hypoxic insults in the kidney. Exp Nephrol 1994;2:153–7.

34. Solomon R, Werner C, Mann D, et al. Effects of saline, mannitol, and furosemide to prevent acute decreases in renal function induced by radiocontrast agents. N Engl J Med 1994;331:1416–20.

35. Kajbaf F, Lalau JD. The criteria for metformin-associated lactic acidosis: the quality of reporting in a large pharmacovigilance database. Diabet Med 2013;30:345–8.

36. Pasceri V, Patti G, Nusca A, et al. Randomized trial of atorvastatin for reduction of myocardial damage during coronary intervention: results from the ARMYDA (atorvastatin for reduction of myocardial damage during angioplasty) study. Circulation 2004;110:674–8.

37. Briguori C, Visconti G, Focaccio A, et al. Novel approaches for preventing or limiting events (NAPLES) II trial: impact of a single high loading dose of atorvastatin on periprocedural myocardial infarction. J Am Coll Cardiol 2009;54:2157–63.

38. Yun KH, Jeong MH, Oh SK, et al. The beneficial effect of high loading dose of rosuvastatin before percutaneous coronary intervention in patients with acute coronary syndrome. Int J Cardiol 2009;137: 246–51.

39. Zhang F, Dong L, Ge J. Effect of statins pretreatment on periprocedural myocardial infarction in patients undergoing percutaneous coronary intervention: a meta-analysis. Annu Mediaev 2010;42:171–7.

40. Winchester DE, Wen X, Xie L, et al. Evidence of preprocedural statin therapy a meta-analysis of randomized trials. J Am Coll Cardiol 2010;56:1099–109.

# Index

*Note:* Page numbers of article titles are in **boldface** type.

## A

Abciximab
  for acute coronary syndromes, 565–567
  for complication prevention, 522
  for endovascular interventions, 630
  for STEMI, 576–577
  mechanism of action of, 504
  parenteral, 538, 540–541, 543
  properties of, 652
ACE trial, 538
ACUITY trial, 518, 520, 544, 558, 565, 649
Acute coronary syndromes, non-ST segment
  elevation, antithrombotic therapy for, **553–571**
ACUTE-II trial, 542
ADAPT-DES trial, 592, 609
Adenosine, 665–667
Adenosine diphosphate
  in thrombus formation, 501
  platelet function testing and, 608–609
ADMIRAL trial, 540, 543, 655
ADVANCE trial, 541, 543
Aggregometry, 608–609
AIDA trial, 577
Alteplase, 648
Antiarrhythmic drugs, 667
Anticoagulants
  for acute coronary syndromes, 554–559
  for STEMI, 577–578, 580
  for stent placement, 597–604
  mechanism of action of, 506–509
  monitoring of, 644–650
  properties of, 644–650
  reversal of, 644–650
Antihistamines, for anticoagulant reversal, 645
Antiplatelet agents. *See also specific agents.*
  for acute coronary syndromes, 559, 562–565
  for complication prevention, 519, 521–522
  for STEMI, 579–580
  for stent placement, **585–594**
  in triple therapy, **585–594**
  mechanism of action of, 500–506
  monitoring of, **607–614**
  parenteral, 538–545
  pharmacology of, 527–535
  properties of, 650–657
  strategies for, 608
Antithrombotic therapy. *See also specific agents.*
  basic principles of, **499–513**
  combination

after stent placement, **595–606**
  duration of, **585–594**
  for acute coronary syndromes, **533–571**
  for STEMI, **573–583**
complications of, **515–525**
for endovascular interventions, **627–633**
for valvular and structural disease interventions,
  **635–642**
monitoring of, **643–663**
oral antiplatelets, **527–535**
parenteral, **537–551**
pharmacogenomics of, **615–625**
platelet function testing in, **607–614**
Aortic valve, transcatheter implantation of,
  635–640
Apixaban
  for stent placement, 597–598, 601
  mechanism of action of, 508
APPRAISE trials, 508, 597–598, 601
ARCTIC trial, 609, 611
ARGAMI trials, 649
Argatroban
  mechanism of action of, 507
  monitoring of, 650
  parenteral, 540, 544, 548
  properties of, 649–650
  reversal of, 650
ARG-E04 trial, 649
ARISTOTLE trial, 600
ARMYDA-PROVE study, 533
ASPIRE trial, 547, 648
Aspirin
  for acute coronary syndromes, 559, 568–569
  for endovascular interventions, 628
  for STEMI, 574, 579–580
  for stent placement, 587, 592, 596–597, 600–602
  for valvular and structural interventions, 638
  mechanism of action of, 502
  monitoring of, 651–653
  pharmacology of, 527–528
  properties of, 650–652
  reversal of, 653
Atherosclerosis, antithrombotic therapy action on,
  **499–513**
ATLAS ACS TIMI trials, 508, 522, 598
Atopaxar, mechanism of action of, 505
Atorvastatin, periprocedural, 668–669
Atrial fibrillation, 602–603
Atrial septal defect closure, 636–639

interventional.theclinics.com

**B**

Benzodiazepines, for sedation, 667
Beta blockers, for arrhythmias, 667
Bivalrudin
    for acute coronary syndromes, 558–559
    for complication prevention, 518, 520
    for endovascular interventions, 631
    for STEMI, 577–578
    mechanism of action of, 507
    monitoring of, 650
    parenteral, 539, 544, 547–548
    properties of, 648–649
    reversal of, 650
Bleeding Academic Research Consortium, 589
Bleeding complications. *See* Complications,
    ischemic or bleeding.
BRAVE trials, 576, 639–640
BRIDGE trial, 504, 592

**C**

CADILLAC trial, 538, 543, 655
Calcium channel blockers, 665–667
Candidate gene studies, for pharmacogenomics,
    616–617
Cangrelor
    for acute coronary syndromes, 564–565
    for STEMI, 576
    for stent placement, 592
    mechanism of action of, 503–504
    pharmacology of, 531–532
    properties of, 652
CAPRIE trial, 652
CAPTURE trial, 538, 540, 543
CHADS2 score, 702
CHAMPION trials, 503–504, 565, 576
Cilostazol
    for endovascular interventions, 631
    for stent placement, 596–597, 603–604
    mechanism of action of, 505
CLARITY-TIMI trial, 652
Clopidogrel
    for acute coronary syndromes, 561–564, 569
    for complication prevention, 521–522
    for endovascular interventions, 628–629
    for STEMI, 574–576, 579–580
    for stent placement, 587–589, 592–593, 596, 600,
        602
    for valvular and structural interventions, 638–639
    mechanism of action of, 502
    metabolism of, 618
    pharmacogenomics of, 617–620
    pharmacology of, 529–530
    platelet function testing and, 611–612
    properties of, 652
CLOSURE-1 trial, 639

COMMIT trial, 652
Complications, ischemic or bleeding, **515–525**
    definitions of, 515–516
    outcomes of, 516–517
    preventive strategies for, 518–522
    risk assessment for, 517–518
Contrast agents, discontinuation of, 667–668
Corticosteroids, for anticoagulant reversal, 645
CPY450 polymorphisms, in pharmacogenomics,
    617–621
CREDO trial, 652
CRUISE trial, 546
CRUSADE trial, 601
CURE trial, 562, 619, 652

**D**

Dabigatran
    for stent placement, 598–604
    mechanism of action of, 507
Dalteparin, parenteral, 546
DATE trial, 590
DECREASE trial, 596
Desmopressin
    for aspirin reversal, 653
    for cangrelor reversal, 654
    for glycoprotein IIb/IIIa inhibitor reversal, 657
Diltiazem, 666
Dipyridamole
    for endovascular interventions, 629
    mechanism of action of, 505
Direct antithrombin agents, parenteral, 547–548
Direct factor-Xa inhibitors, mechanism of action of,
    508
Direct thrombin inhibitors, mechanism of action of,
    507
Diuretics, discontinuation of, 668
Dual antiplatelet therapy
    for stent implantation, **585–594**
        addition to for triple therapy, 595–606
        cessation of, 591–592
        long-term outcomes of, 588–590
        perioperative management in, 591–592
        practice guidelines for, 587–588
        short-term outcomes of, 590–591
        ultrasound guidance for, 591
    for valvular and structural interventions, 638
    platelet function testing in, 607–614
Dual therapy, for acute coronary syndromes, non-ST
    segment elevation, **553–571**
DX9065a, mechanism of action of, 508

**E**

ELECT trial, 647
ELEVATE-TIMI trial, 609, 620
Elinogrel

mechanism of action of, 504
pharmacology of, 532
ENDOMAX trial, 631
Endovascular interventions, antithrombotic agents for, **627–633**
pathophysiology of, 627–628
types of, 628–631
ENGAGE-AF trial, 600
Enoxaparin
for acute coronary syndromes, 555–557, 568
for complication prevention, 518
for STEMI, 580
monitoring of, 646–647
parenteral, 539, 542, 546
properties of, 645–646
reversal of, 647
EPIC trial, 538, 540, 543, 655
Epifibtide, parenteral, 538, 541
EPILOG trial, 538, 540, 543, 654–655
EPISTENT trial, 538, 540–541, 543, 655
Eptifibatide
for acute coronary syndromes, 565–568
for complication prevention, 522
for STEMI, 577
mechanism of action of, 504
parenteral, 543
properties of, 652
ESPRIT trial, 538, 541, 543, 656
ESPS trial, 505
ESSENCE/TIMI-11B trial, 542, 646
EUCLID trial, 629
EVEREST trial, 636, 639
Everolimus-coated stents, 590–591
EXCELLENT trial, 590–591
Exome sequencing, in pharmacogenomics, 617
ExTRACT-TIMI trial, 542, 546, 580

**F**

Factor VIIa, recombinant, for anticoagulant reversal, 648, 650
Factor-XA inhibitors, mechanism of action of, 507–508
Fentanyl, for sedation, 667
Fibrin, in thrombus formation, 501
Fibrinolysis, PCI after, 578–580
FINESSE trial, 576–577
Fondaparinux
for acute coronary syndromes, 559–560, 568
for complication prevention, 518
for STEMI, 580
mechanism of action of, 507–508
monitoring of, 648
parenteral, 540, 544, 547
properties of, 647–648
reversal of, 648
FRANCE-2 trial, 638

**G**

Genome-wide association studies, in pharmacogenomics, 616–617
Genomics, for pharmacology. See Pharmacogenomics.
GIFT study, 620
Glycoprotein IIb/IIIa inhibitors
for acute coronary syndromes, 565–567
for endovascular interventions, 630
for STEMI, 576–577
for stent placement, 597, 604
mechanism of action of, 504
monitoring of, 656–657
parenteral, 538–545
properties of, 654–656
reversal of, 657
GOLD multicenter study, 656
GRACE trial, 516, 518
GRACIA trial, 578–579
GRAVITAS trial, 609, 611, 620, 654
GUSTO trial, 516
GUSTO trials, 546
Guthrie PCI Registry, 590

**H**

HAS-BLED risk score, 518, 520, 601
HEMONOX assay, 647
Heparins
for acute coronary syndromes, 554–555
for complication prevention, 520
for endovascular interventions, 630
for STEMI, 577–578, 580
for valvular and structural interventions, 639
mechanism of action of, 506–507
monitoring of, 645
parenteral, 539, 542, 545–547
properties of, 644–645
reversal of, 645
Hirudin, mechanism of action of, 507
HMO Research Network Stent registry, 589
HORIZONS-AMI trials, 516, 518–519, 544, 548, 576–578, 590, 648
Hybridization oligonucleotide capture, in pharmacogenomics, 617

**I**

Idrabiotaparinux, mechanism of action of, 507–508
Idraparinux, mechanism of action of, 507–508
IMPACT trials, 538, 541, 655
Impact-F assay, 652
INFUSE-AMI trial, 576–577
INTERACT A to Z trial, 542
Intravascular ultrasonography, for stent implantation, 591
ISAR trials, 538, 543

ISAR-REACT trials, 538, 541, 543–544, 548, 649
Ischemic complications. *See* Complications,
    ischemic or bleeding.
ISR-SAFE trial, 591

**K**

Kidney, drugs toxic to, 667–668

**L**

LANCELOT trials, 505
Lepirudin
    mechanism of action of, 507
    parenteral, 548
Lidocaine, for arrhythmias, 667
Light remittance aggregometry, 651–652, 656

**M**

MATRIX trial, 592
Mean platelet volume, in antiplatelet therapy, 533
Metformin, discontinuation of, 668
Midazolam, for sedation, 667
MitraClip, 636–639
Mitral valve repair, 636–639
Mortality, in antithrombotic therapy complications,
    516–517
MULTISTRATEGY trial, 576
Myocardial infarction
    definition of, 516
    ST segment elevation (STEMI), **573–583**
        primary percutaneous coronary intervention
            for, 574–578
        rescue percutaneous coronary intervention for,
            578–580

**N**

NICE-1 registry, 546
NICE trials, 646
Nitroglycerin, 665–667
Nonsteroidal anti-inflammatory drugs,
    discontinuation of, 668
No-reflow phenomenon, vasodilators for, 666

**O**

OASIS trials, 519, 544, 547, 559–560, 580, 648
Opioids, for sedation, 667
Oral anticoagulants, for stent placement, 597–604
Otamixaban, mechanism of action of, 508

**P**

Paclitaxel-coated stents, 590–591
PAR-1 inhibitors, mechanism of action of, 505
PARIS trial, 592
PARTNER trial, 636

Patent foramen ovale closure, 636–639
PCI. *See* Percutaneous intervention.
PENTUA trial, 544, 648
Percutaneous intervention
    primary, antithrombotic therapy for, 574–578
    rescue, antithrombotic therapy for, 578–580
Personalized therapy
    pharmacogenomics for, **615–625**
    platelet function testing for, 609–610
PFA-100 assay, 652
Pharmacogenomics, **615–625**
    basic principles of, 616–617
    of clopidogrel, 617–620
    of ticagrelor, 621
Phosphodiesterase inhibitors, mechanism of action
    of, 505
Platelet(s), in thrombus formation, 500–502
Platelet concentrate
    for aspirin reversal, 653
    for cangrelor reversal, 654
    for glycoprotein IIb/IIIa inhibitor reversal, 657
Platelet function testing, **607–614**. *See also individual
    drugs,* monitoring of.
    bleeding during surgery and, 611–612
    cutoff values in, 609
    importance of, 608–609
    in personalized therapy, 609–610
    methods for, 652
    therapeutic window concept in, 610–611
PLATFORM trial, 503
PLATO trial, 503, 521–522, 575–576, 654
POPULAR trial, 611
Prasugrel
    for acute coronary syndromes, 561–563
    for complication prevention, 521–522
    for endovascular interventions, 629
    for STEMI, 574–576, 580
    for stent placement, 587, 596
    mechanism of action of, 502–503
    pharmacogenomics of, 620–621
    pharmacology of, 530–531
    properties of, 652
PREMIER registry, 516
PRISM trials, 541, 656
PRODIGY trials, 589–590
PRoFESS trial, 505
Propofol, for sedation, 667
Protamine sulfate, for anticoagulant reversal, 645,
    647
PURSUIT trial, 656
P2Y12 inhibitors. *See also specific agents, eg,*
    Clopidogrel.
    for acute coronary syndromes, 561–564
    for STEMI, 574–576
    monitoring of, 654
    properties of, 653–654
    reversal of, 654

**R**

RADAR trial, 509
Radial arterial spasm, vasodilators for, 666–667
RAPPORT trial, 540, 543
REAL-LATE trial, 589–590
Receiver operating characteristic curve, in platelet function testing, 609
RE-DEEM trial, 507, 598–599
REG1 system, mechanism of action of, 509
RE-LY trials, 600–601
REPLACE trials, 518, 520, 544, 547–548, 649–650
RESET trial, 590
RESORT trial, 538
RESPECT trial, 636–637
RESTORE trial, 541, 656
Rivaroxaban
    for stent placement, 598
    mechanism of action of, 508
RNA aptamer technology, 509
ROCKET-AE trial, 600
Rosuvastatin, periprocedural, 668–669

**S**

SCAAR registry, 576
Sedation, periprocedural, 667
Sirolimus-coated stents, 589–590
Spasm, radial artery, vasodilators for, 666–667
SR 123781, mechanism of action of, 507–508
STACKENOX trial, 646
Statins, periprocedural, 668–669
STEEPLE trial, 545–546, 645–646
Stents
    antithrombotic therapy for, 565, 569
    dual combination antiplatelet therapy for, duration of, **585–594**
    thrombosis of, 516–517
    triple therapy for, **585–594**
STREAM trial, 578
Stroke
    definition of, 516
    in valvular and structural interventions, prevention of, 636–642
Structural heart disorders, interventions for, **636–642**
SYNERGY trial, 542, 546, 555, 646

**T**

TARGET trial, 541, 611–612, 656
TAVI (transcatheter aortic valve implantation), 635–640
TENACITY trial, 541, 545
Tenecteplase, for STEMI, 578–579
Terutroban, mechanism of action of, 506
Therapeutic window, in platelet function testing, 610–611
Thienopyridines, pharmacology of, 528–531

Thrombin, in thrombus formation, 502
Thrombin inhibitors, mechanism of action of, 506–507
Thromboelastography, 652
Thrombosis
    in valvular and structural interventions, prevention of, 636–642
    pathophysiology of, 596, 627–628
    stent, 516–517
Thromboxane, in thrombus formation, 501
Thromboxane inhibitors, mechanism of action of, 505–506
Thrombus, formation of, 500–502
Ticagrelor
    for acute coronary syndromes, 561–564, 568
    for complication prevention, 521–522
    for endovascular interventions, 629
    for STEMI, 574–576
    for stent placement, 502, 587–588
    mechanism of action of, 503
    pharmacogenomics of, 621
    pharmacology of, 531
    properties of, 652
Ticlopidine, pharmacology of, 528–529
TIMI risk score, 518
TIMI trial, 591
Tirofiban
    for acute coronary syndromes, 566–567
    for complication prevention, 522
    for STEMI, 577
    mechanism of action of, 504
    parenteral, 538, 543
    properties of, 652
Tissue factor, in thrombus formation, 501
TOPSTAR trial, 541
TRA 2P-TIMI trial, 505
TRACER trial, 505
Transcatheter aortic valve implantation (TAVI), 635–640
TRANSFER-AMI trial, 578–579
TRIGGER-PCI trial, 609, 611
TRILOGY-ACS trial, 503
Triple therapy
    for acute coronary syndrome, 569
    for stent placement, **585–594**
TRITON-TIMI trial, 502–503, 521, 561, 575, 580, 654

**U**

Ultrasonography, intravascular, for stent implantation, 591
Urokinase, for endovascular interventions, 630

**V**

Valvular diseases, interventions for, **636–642**
Varoxaban, for complication prevention, 522
Vasodilators, 665–667

Vasodilators-stimulated phosphoprotein
phosphorylation analysis, 621
Vasospasm, vasodilators for, 666–667
Verapamil, 665–667
VerifyNow Assay, 532–533, 651–652, 656–657
Vorapaxar, mechanism of action of, 505

**W**

Warfarin
for acute coronary syndromes, 569

for endovascular interventions, 630–631
for stent placement, 597, 599–603
WEST trial, 578–579
Whole exome sequencing, in pharmacogenomics,
617
WOEST trial, 569, 601

**Z**

ZEST-LATE trial, 589–590
Zotarolimus-coated stents, 589–590

Printed and bound by CPI Group (UK) Ltd, Croydon, CR0 4YY

03/10/2024

01040370-0005